2012
YEAR BOOK OF
PULMONARY DISEASE®

The 2012 Year Book Series

Year Book of Anesthesiology and Pain Management™: Drs Chestnut, Abram, Black, Gravlee, Lien, Mathru, and Roizen

Year Book of Cardiology®: Drs Gersh, Cheitlin, Elliott, Gold, Graham, and Thourani

Year Book of Critical Care Medicine®: Drs Dries, Zanotti-Cavazzoni, Latenser, Martinez, Rincon, and Zwank

Year Book of Dermatology and Dermatologic Surgery™: Dr Del Rosso

Year Book of Diagnostic Radiology®: Drs Elster, Abbara, Oestreich, Offiah, Rosado de Christenson, Stephens, and Strickland

Year Book of Emergency Medicine®: Drs Hamilton, Bruno, Handly, Minczak, Mullin, Quintana, and Ramoska

Year Book of Endocrinology®: Drs Schott, Apovian, Clarke, Eugster, Ludlam, Meikle, Oetjen, Schteingart, and Toth

Year Book of Gastroenterology™: Drs Talley, DeVault, Harnois, Murray, Pearson, Philcox, Picco, and Smith

Year Book of Hand and Upper Limb Surgery®: Drs Yao and Steinmann

Year Book of Medicine®: Drs Barker, Garrick, Gersh, Khardori, LeRoith, Panush, Talley, and Thigpen

Year Book of Neonatal and Perinatal Medicine®: Drs Fanaroff, Benitz, Donn, Neu, Papile, Polin, and Van Marter

Year Book of Neurology and Neurosurgery®: Drs Klimo, Minagar, Breningstall, Gandhi, House, Kevill, Liu, Mazia, Panagariya, Ragel, Riesenburger, Shafazand, Uhm, and Yang

Year Book of Obstetrics, Gynecology, and Women's Health®: Drs Dungan and Shulman

Year Book of Oncology®: Drs Arceci, Bauer, Chiorean, Gordon, Lawton, Murphy, Thigpen, and Tsao

Year Book of Ophthalmology®: Drs Rapuano, Cohen, Flanders, Hammersmith, Milman, Myers, Nagra, Nelson, Penne, Pyfer, Sergott, Shields, Talekar, and Vander

Year Book of Orthopedics®: Drs Morrey, Huddleston, Swiontkowski, and Trigg

Year Book of Otolaryngology-Head and Neck Surgery®: Drs Sindwani, Balough, Franco, Gapany, and Mitchell

Year Book of Pathology and Laboratory Medicine®: Drs Raab and Bissell

Year Book of Pediatrics®: Dr Stockman

Year Book of Plastic and Aesthetic Surgery™: Drs Miller, Gosman, Gurtner, Gutowski, Ruberg, Salisbury, and Smith

Year Book of Psychiatry and Applied Mental Health®: Drs Talbott, Ballenger, Buckley, Frances, Krupnick, and Mack

Year Book of Pulmonary Disease®: Drs Barker, Jones, Maurer, Spradley, Tanoue, and Willsie

Year Book of Sports Medicine®: Drs Shephard, Cantu, Feldman, Galea, Jankowski, Janssen, Lebrun, and Nieman

Year Book of Surgery®: Drs Copeland, Behrns, Daly, Eberlein, Fahey, Huber, Klodell, Mozingo, and Pruett

Year Book of Urology®: Drs Andriole and Coplen

Year Book of Vascular Surgery®: Drs Moneta, Gillespie, Starnes, and Watkins

2012

The Year Book of PULMONARY DISEASE®

Editor-in-Chief
James A. Barker, MD, FACP, FCCP
Chief, Pulmonary, Critical Care Medicine, and Sleep Internal Medicine, Scott & White Health System; Professor of Medicine, Texas A&M Health Science Center, Temple, Texas

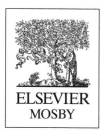

ELSEVIER
MOSBY

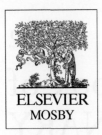

ELSEVIER
MOSBY

Vice President, Continuity: Kimberly Murphy
Developmental Editor: Patrick Manley
Production Supervisor, Electronic Year Books: Donna M. Skelton
Electronic Article Manager: Emily Ogle
Illustrations and Permissions Coordinator: Dawn A. Vohsen

2012 EDITION

Printed and bound by CPI Group (UK) Ltd, Croydon, CR0 4YY

Composition by TNQ Books and Journals Pvt Ltd, India

Transferred to Digital Print 2012

Editorial Office:
Elsevier, Inc.
Suite 1800
1600 John F. Kennedy Blvd
Philadelphia, PA 19103-2899

International Standard Serial Number: 8756-3452
International Standard Book Number: 978-0-323-08893-0

Associate Editors

Shirley F. Jones, MD, FCCP, DABSM
Assistant Professor of Internal Medicine, Division of Pulmonary, Critical Care, and Sleep Medicine, Scott & White Memorial Hospital/Texas A&M Health Science Center, Temple, Texas

Janet R. Maurer, MD, MBA
Vice President, Medical Director, Health Dialog Services Corp, Scottsdale, Arizona

Christopher D. Spradley, MD, FCCP
Director, Medical Intensive Care Unit, Pulmonary Hypertension Clinic, Sleep Medicine, Scott & White Memorial Hospital, Temple, Texas

Lynn T. Tanoue, MD
Professor of Medicine, Section of Pulmonary and Critical Care Medicine, Yale School of Medicine, Yale University, New Haven, Connecticut

Sandra K. Willsie, DO
Professor of Medicine; Executive Dean, Heartland Health Sciences University, Inc; Dean, College of Osteopathic Medicine, Overland Park, Kansas

Table of Contents

JOURNALS REPRESENTED   xi

1. Asthma, Allergy, and Cystic Fibrosis   1
   Introduction   1
   Asthma   2
   Cystic Fibrosis   23
2. Chronic Obstructive Pulmonary Disease   29
   Introduction   29
3. Lung Cancer   59
   Introduction   59
   Epidemiology of Lung Cancer   62
   Tobacco-Related Issues   72
   Lung Cancer Screening   78
   Diagnostic Evaluation   85
   Lung Cancer Treatment   99
   Molecular Approach to Lung Cancer   108
4. Pleural, Interstitial Lung, and Pulmonary Vascular Disease . . .   115
   Introduction   115
   Pulmonary Vascular Disease   116
   Interstitial Lung Disease   129
   Pleural Disease   135
5. Community-Acquired Pneumonia   137
   Introduction   137
6. Lung Transplantation   161
7. Sleep Disorders   181
   Introduction   181
   Diagnosis of Sleep-Disordered Breathing   182
   Epidemiology of Sleep-Disordered Breathing   185
   Consequences of Sleep-Disordered Breathing   186
   CPAP Treatment and Benefits   191
   Non-CPAP Treatment of Sleep-Disordered Breathing   195

Pediatric Sleep-Disordered Breathing 197
Non-Pulmonary Sleep 198
8. Critical Care Medicine 211
Introduction 211
Ventilator Weaning 213
Ventilator-Associated Pneumonia 215
Acute Respiratory Disorder Syndrome 216
Acute Respiratory Failure 219
Airway Management 220
Imaging and Monitoring in the ICU 223
Cardiopulmonary Interactions 224
Pulmonary Hypertension in the ICU 227
Trauma Issues 228
Miscellaneous 233

ARTICLE INDEX 245
AUTHOR INDEX 253

Journals Represented

Journals represented in this YEAR BOOK are listed below.

Academic Emergency Medicine
Acta Anaesthesiologica Scandinavica
Allergy
American Journal of Cardiology
American Journal of Medicine
American Journal of Respiratory and Critical Care Medicine
American Journal of Transplantation
Anaesthesia
Anesthesiology
Annals of Allergy, Asthma & Immunology
Annals of Emergency Medicine
Annals of Internal Medicine
Annals of Thoracic Surgery
Archives of Internal Medicine
Archives of Pediatrics & Adolescent Medicine
Archives of Surgery
British Journal of Ophthalmology
British Medical Journal
CA: A Cancer Journal for Clinicians
Cancer Prevention Research
Chest
Circulation
Clinical Cancer Research
Clinical Infectious Diseases
Clinical Lung Cancer
Critical Care Medicine
European Heart Journal
European Journal of Internal Medicine
European Respiratory Journal
Intensive Care Medicine
Journal of Allergy and Clinical Immunology
Journal of Clinical Oncology
Journal of Heart and Lung Transplantation
Journal of Neurological Sciences
Journal of Pain and Symptom Management
Journal of Rheumatology
Journal of the American Geriatrics Society
Journal of the American Medical Association
Journal of the National Cancer Institute
Journal of Thoracic Oncology
JPEN Journal of Parenteral and Enteral Nutrition
Lancet
Lancet Oncology
Medicine
MMWR Morbidity and Mortality Weekly Report
Nephrology Dialysis Transplantation
New England Journal of Medicine

Pediatrics
Pharmacotherapy
Proceedings of the National Academy of Sciences of the United States of America
Respiratory Medicine
Sleep
Surgery
Thorax
Transfusion
Transplantation

STANDARD ABBREVIATIONS

The following terms are abbreviated in this edition: acquired immunodeficiency syndrome (AIDS), cardiopulmonary resuscitation (CPR), central nervous system (CNS), cerebrospinal fluid (CSF), computed tomography (CT), deoxyribonucleic acid (DNA), electrocardiography (ECG), health maintenance organization (HMO), human immunodeficiency virus (HIV), intensive care unit (ICU), intramuscular (IM), intravenous (IV), magnetic resonance (MR) imaging (MRI), ribonucleic acid (RNA), and ultrasound (US).

NOTE

The YEAR BOOK OF PULMONARY DISEASE is a literature survey service providing abstracts of articles published in the professional literature. Every effort is made to assure the accuracy of the information presented in these pages. Neither the editors nor the publisher of the YEAR BOOK OF PULMONARY DISEASE can be responsible for errors in the original materials. The editors' comments are their own opinions. Mention of specific products within this publication does not constitute endorsement.

To facilitate the use of the YEAR BOOK OF PULMONARY DISEASE as a reference tool, all illustrations and tables included in this publication are now identified as they appear in the original article. This change is meant to help the reader recognize that any illustration or table appearing in the YEAR BOOK OF PULMONARY DISEASE may be only one of many in the original article. For this reason, figure and table numbers will often appear to be out of sequence within the YEAR BOOK OF PULMONARY DISEASE.

1 Asthma, Allergy, and Cystic Fibrosis

Introduction

During the latter quarter of the 20th century, major advances in understanding asthma as an inflammatory disease and development of antiinflammatory therapies served as the primary foci for clinical research in this field. More recently, the discovery of relationships between asthma and a variety of systemic diseases/conditions has taken on a more prominent role with the interplay between genetics and asthma recently coming to the forefront. How else, besides genetic influences, might we explain why 8 patients respond well to a particular pharmacologic treatment while 2 other patients have no response whatsoever?

This amalgamation of new approaches to therapy, definition of patient factors, the role of genetics, and associated diseases and conditions has effectively functioned to expand the role of healthcare providers caring for patients with asthma. Added responsibilities include appropriately screening for associated diseases/conditions and management of asthma in the electronic world. Failure by healthcare providers to effectively address the multivariate aspects of asthma will adversely affect the morbidity and mortality of patients with asthma.

As healthcare providers caring for patients with asthma, we are obligated to keep up with recent advances and evidence-based guidelines for asthma. Asthma-related publications selected for highlighting in this year's YEAR BOOK OF PULMONARY DISEASE range from discussing and reviewing the role and efficacy of bronchoscopic intervention[1] to the use of internet-based tapering of steroids.[2] In between the technology-driven intervention for the most difficult-to-control asthma and the technology-supported algorithms for steroid tapering, you'll find a variety of important articles and investigations, including the American Thoracic Society's clinical practice guideline for interpretation of exhaled nitric oxide levels (FE_{NO}).[3] This technique, which can be used to monitor the status of airway inflammation, has effectively come out of the research labs and is now ready for prime time in healthcare providers' offices (providing that adequate instrument quality control is performed and educated practitioners are interpreting the data). I hope you will enjoy the opportunity to review the updates in asthma.

Survival with cystic fibrosis (CF) has continued to improve over the past 20 years. In the mid-1980s, the mean predicted survival for a patient diagnosed with CF was 25 years, whereas now the mean predicted survival approaches the fifth decade of life.[4] Many advancements in the care of CF are responsible for prolonged survival and, in particular, improved quality of life in patients with CF. Robust investigations continue in this field. The highlighted publications in this year's edition of YEAR BOOK OF PULMONARY DISEASE are small in number but represent important and continued advancements in therapy. Two investigations highlighted are promising and relate to agents formulated to increase the activity of the CF transmembrane conductance regulator (CRTR) proteins.[5,6]

Sandra K. Willsie, DO, MA

References

1. Shifren A, Chen A, Castro M. Point: efficacy of bronchial thermoplasty for patients with severe asthma. Is there sufficient evidence? Yes. *Chest.* 2011;140: 573-575.
2. Hashimoto S, Brinke AT, Roldaan AC, et al. Internet-based tapering of oral corticosteroids in severe asthma: a pragmatic randomised controlled trial. *Thorax.* 2011;66:514-520.
3. Dweik RA, Boggs PB, Erzurum SC, et al; American Thoracic Society Committee on Interpretation of Exhaled Nitric Oxide Levels (FENO) for Clinical Applications. An official ATS clinical practice guideline: interpretation of exhaled nitric oxide levels (FENO) for clinical applications. *Am J Respir Crit Care Med.* 2011; 184:602-615.
4. Strausbaugh SD, Davis PB. Cystic fibrosis: a review of epidemiology and pathobiology. *Clin Chest Med.* 2007;28:279-288.
5. Ramsey BW, Davies J, McElvaney NG, et al; VX08-770-102 Study Group. A CFTR potentiator in patients with cystic fibrosis and the G551D mutation. *N Engl J Med.* 2011;365:1663-1672.
6. Clancy JP, Rowe SM, Accurso FJ, et al. Results of a phase IIa study of VX-809, an investigational CFTR corrector compound, in subjects with cystic fibrosis homozygous for the F508del-CFTR mutation. *Thorax.* 2012;67:12-18.

Asthma

Two Days of Dexamethasone Versus 5 Days of Prednisone in the Treatment of Acute Asthma: A Randomized Controlled Trial

Kravitz J, Dominici P, Ufberg J, et al (St Barnabas Health System, Toms River, NJ; Albert Einstein Med Ctr, Philadelphia, PA; Temple Univ, Philadelphia, PA; et al)
Ann Emerg Med 58:200-204, 2011

Study Objective.—Dexamethasone has a longer half-life than prednisone and is well tolerated orally. We compare the time needed to return to normal activity and the frequency of relapse after acute exacerbation in adults receiving either 5 days of prednisone or 2 days of dexamethasone.

Methods.—We randomized adult emergency department patients (aged 18 to 45 years) with acute exacerbations of asthma (peak expiratory flow

TABLE 2.—Outcome Measures

Outcome Measure	Prednisone (%), N=96	Dexamethasone (%), N=104	Difference (%)	95% CI*
Days to return to normal, 0–3 days[†]	72 (80)	91 (90)	10	(0 to 20)
Any hospital admissions	1 (1)	3 (3)	2	(−6 to 2)
Any ED visits since discharge	6 (6)	5 (5)	1	(−5 to 8)
Any primary care provider visits since discharge	5 (5)	3 (3)	2	(−3 to 8)

*P=.049.
[†]Return to normal daily activity information missing for 6 prednisone and 3 dexamethasone patients.

rate less than 80% of ideal) to receive either 50 mg of daily oral prednisone for 5 days or 16 mg of daily oral dexamethasone for 2 days. Outcomes were assessed by telephone follow-up.

Results.—Ninety-six prednisone and 104 dexamethasone subjects completed the study regimen and follow-up. More patients in the dexamethasone group reported a return to normal activities within 3 days compared with the prednisone group (90% versus 80%; difference 10%; 95% confidence interval 0% to 20%; P=.049). Relapse was similar between groups (13% versus 11%; difference 2%; 95% confidence interval −7% to 11%, P=.67).

Conclusion.—In acute exacerbations of asthma in adults, 2 days of oral dexamethasone is at least as effective as 5 days of oral prednisone in returning patients to their normal level of activity and preventing relapse (Table 2).

▶ Based on previous pediatric studies, this randomized controlled trial compared 2 days of 16 mg oral dexamethasone (D) to 5 days of 50 mg oral prednisone (P). Table 2 demonstrates that a statistically significant increase in numbers of D subjects returned to baseline activity levels at 3 days versus the group assigned to P. There was no significant difference between relapse rates, exacerbations, or visits to primary care practitioners. Weaknesses identified in the study design include telephone follow-up only and lack of objective scoring systems/pulmonary function outcomes. Several studies have demonstrated that as many as 28% of patients leaving an emergency department (ED) following treatment for an acute exacerbation of asthma fail to fill prescriptions.[1,2] This study bears repeating with collection of objective data pre- and postdosing of steroids, assessment of safety parameters including a follow-up visit after the ED visit and an in-clinic evaluation following treatment. Other useful data would be an objective evaluation of practitioner visits, prescription usage, ED visits, and use of reliever medications post ED visit. Based on this investigation, use of a long-acting, higher-potency, compressed steroid dosing regimen appears to offer potential advantages, particularly if the first dose of D is administered in the ED and the following day's dose is dispensed to the patient on discharge from the ED. In addition, long-term administration of inhaled corticosteroids should be addressed at the time of ED admission for those patients not receiving controller medications on a regular basis.

S. K. Willsie, DO, MA

References

1. Thomas EJ, Burstin HR, O'Neil AC, Orav EJ, Brennan TA. Patient noncompliance with medical advice after the emergency department visit. *Ann Emerg Med.* 1996; 27:49-55.
2. Saunders CE. Patient compliance in filling prescriptions after discharge from the emergency department. *Am J Emerg Med.* 1987;5:283-286.

Nebulized Budesonide Added to Standard Pediatric Emergency Department Treatment of Acute Asthma: A Randomized, Double-blind Trial
Upham BD, Mollen CJ, Scarfone RJ, et al (Univ of New Mexico, Albuquerque; Children's Hosp of Philadelphia, PA)
Acad Emerg Med 18:665-673, 2011

Objectives.—The goal was to determine if adding inhaled budesonide to standard asthma therapy improves outcomes of pediatric patients presenting to the emergency department (ED) with acute asthma.

Methods.—The authors conducted a randomized, double-blind, placebo-controlled trial in a tertiary care, urban pediatric ED. Patients 2 to 18 years of age with moderate to severe acute asthma were randomized to receive either a single 2-mg dose of budesonide inhalation suspension (BUD) or normal sterile saline (NSS) placebo, added to albuterol, ipratropium bromide (IB), and systemic corticosteroids (SCS). The primary outcome was the difference in median asthma scores between treatment groups at 2 hours. Secondary outcomes included differences in vital signs and hospitalization rates.

Results.—A total of 180 patients were enrolled. Treatment groups had similar baseline demographics, asthma scores, and vital signs. A total of 169 patients (88 BUD, 81 NSS) were assessed for the primary outcome. No significant difference was found between groups in the change in median asthma score at 2 hours (BUD −3, NSS −3, p = 0.64). Vital signs at 2 hours were also similar between groups. Fifty-six children (62%) were admitted to the hospital in the BUD group and 55 (62%) in the NSS group (difference 0%, 95% confidence interval [CI] = −14% to 14%). Neither multivariate adjustment nor planned subgroup analysis by inhaled corticosteroids (ICS) use prior to the ED significantly altered the results.

Conclusions.—For children 2 to 18 years of age treated in the ED for acute asthma, a single 2-mg dose of budesonide added to standard therapy did not improve asthma severity scores or other short-term ED-based outcomes (Tables 3 and 4).

▶ This is a well-designed emergency department study randomizing pediatric asthmatic patients (ages 2−18 years) to receive either a single 2-mg dose of budesonide (B) inhalation or placebo added to usual care: nebulized albuterol,

TABLE 3.—Change in Asthma Score and Vital Signs from Baseline to 2 Hours After Intervention, Initial Hospital Admissions

Mean Changes	Budesonide Group ($n = 91$)	Placebo Group ($n = 88$)	Difference Between Groups (95% CI)	p-value
Asthma score (IQR) n	−3 (−4 to −2) 89	−3 (−4 to −2) 81	0	0.64
Respiratory rate, breaths/min (95% CI) n	−6 (−8 to −4) 83	−6 (−8 to −3) 71	0 (−3 to 3)	
Heart rate, beats/min (95% CI) n	12 (7 to 17) 82	13 (9 to 17) 72	−1 (−7 to 6)	
Median change in O_2 saturation, % (IQR) n	1 (−1 to 3) 72	1 (−1 to 3) 64	0	0.91
Hospital admission, % (95% CI) n	62 (51 to 72) 56	62 (52 to 73) 55	0 (−14 to 14)	

IQR = interquartile range.

TABLE 4.—Change in Asthma Score and Vital Signs from Baseline to 2 Hours After Intervention and Initial Hospital Admissions by Prior ICS Status

	Budesonide Group	Placebo Group	Difference Between Groups (95% CI)	p-value
Patients on ICS	$n = 45$	$n = 44$		
Median change in asthma score (IQR) n	−3 (−4 to −1.5) 44	−3 (−4 to −1) 41	0	0.44
Mean change in respiratory rate, breaths/min (95% CI) n	−5 (−8 to −2) 41	−6 (−8 to −2) 36	1 (−4 to 5)	
Mean change in heart rate, beats/min (95% CI) n	11 (4 to 18) 41	12 (7 to 17) 37	−1 (−9 to 8)	
Median change in O_2 saturation, % (IQR) n	1 (−1 to 3) 35	1 (0 to 4) 31	0	0.15
Hospital admission, % (95% CI) n	58 (42 to 72) 26	61 (45 to 76) 27	−3 (−24 to 17)	
Patients not on ICS	$n = 46$	$n = 44$		
Median change in asthma score (IQR) n	−3 (−5 to −2) 45	−3.5 (−4.5 to −2) 40	0.5	0.84
Mean change in respiratory rate, breaths/min (95% CI) n	−6 (−9 to −4) 42	−6 (−10 to −2) 35	0 (−4 to 5)	
Mean change in heart rate, beats/min (95% CI) n	14 (7 to 21) 41	14 (8 to 20) 35	0 (−9 to 9)	
Median change in O_2 saturation % (IQR) n	1.5 (0 to 3) 37	0 (−2 to 2) 33	1.5	0.13
Hospital admission, % (95% CI) n	65 (50 to 79) 30	64 (48 to 78) 28	1 (−18 to 21)	

ICS = inhaled corticosteroids; IQR = interquartile range.

ipratropium bromide, and systemic corticosteroids. Outcome assessed was median asthma scores at 2 hours after treatment, vital signs, and hospitalization rates. Tables 3 and 4 show asthma scores in the B and placebo groups. Use of B resulted in no significant change, including no reduction in hospital admission, no improvement in asthma scores, and no significant change in vital signs. Currently, there is no evidence to warrant addition of inhaled B to the usual treatment of childhood acute asthma in the emergency department.

S. K. Willsie, DO, MA

Tiotropium improves lung function in patients with severe uncontrolled asthma: A randomized controlled trial
Kerstjens HAM, Disse B, Schröder-Babo W, et al (Univ of Groningen, The Netherlands; Boehringer Ingelheim Pharma GmbH & Co. KG, Biberach, Germany; Krankenhaus Gelnhausen, Germany; et al)
J Allergy Clin Immunol 128:308-314, 2011

Background.—Some patients with severe asthma remain symptomatic and obstructed despite maximal recommended treatment. Tiotropium, a long-acting inhaled anticholinergic agent, might be an effective bronchodilator in such patients.

Objective.—We sought to compare the efficacy and safety of 2 doses of tiotropium (5 and 10 µg daily) administered through the Respimat inhaler with placebo as add-on therapy in patients with uncontrolled severe asthma (Asthma Control Questionnaire score, ≥1.5; postbronchodilator FEV_1, ≤80% of predicted value) despite maintenance treatment with at least a high-dose inhaled corticosteroid plus a long-acting β_2-agonist.

Methods.—This was a randomized, double-blind, crossover study with three 8—week treatment periods. The primary end point was peak FEV_1 at the end of each treatment period.

Results.—Of 107 randomized patients (54% female patients; mean, 55 years of age; postbronchodilator FEV_1, 65% of predicted value), 100 completed all periods. Peak FEV_1 was significantly higher with 5 µg (difference, 139 mL; 95% CI, 96—181 mL) and 10 µg (difference, 170 mL; 95% CI, 128—213 mL) of tiotropium than with placebo (both $P < .0001$). There was no significant difference between the active doses. Trough FEV_1 at the end of the dosing interval was higher with tiotropium (5 µg: 86 mL [95% CI, 41—132 mL]; 10 µg: 113 mL [95% CI, 67—159 mL]; both $P < .0004$). Daily home peak expiratory flow measurements were higher with both tiotropium doses. There were no significant differences in asthma-related health status or symptoms. Adverse events were balanced across groups except for dry mouth, which was more common on 10 µg of tiotropium.

Conclusion.—The addition of once-daily tiotropium to asthma treatment, including a high-dose inhaled corticosteroid plus a long-acting β_2-agonist, significantly improves lung function over 24 hours in patients with inadequately controlled, severe, persistent asthma (Figs 2 and 3).

▶ Symptomatic severe asthmatics already being treated with maximized therapy, including inhaled corticosteroids and long-acting β-agonists, were randomly assigned to receive placebo, tiotropium 5 µg (T5) or 10 µg (T10) inhaled daily. Figs 2 and 3 show improvement in FEV_1, FVC, and peak expiratory flow over

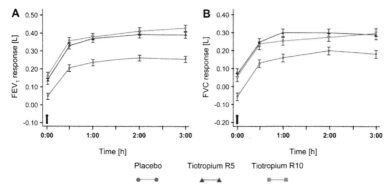

FIGURE 2.—FEV$_1$ (**A**) and FVC (**B**) responses relative to baseline values within 3 hours after dosing after 8 weeks of treatment. The difference in level at *0:00* h is the trough effect of tiotropium administered 24 hours earlier. The measurement obtained at baseline (visit 2 before any maintenance or study medication) is defined as the baseline value. At the on-treatment visits, this was immediately followed by the usual medication (including ICS plus LABA), and this in turn was followed by the study medication. *Error bars* represent SEMs. *Arrows* indicate the timing of the maintenance medication: ICS plus LABA. *Tiotropium R5*, 5 µg of tiotropium; *Tiotropium R10*, 10 µg of tiotropium. (Reprinted from The Journal of Allergy and Clinical Immunology, Kerstjens HAM, Disse B, Schröder-Babo W, et al. Tiotropium improves lung function in patients with severe uncontrolled asthma: a randomized controlled trial. *J Allergy Clin Immunol.* 2011;128:308-314. Copyright 2011, with permission from Elsevier.)

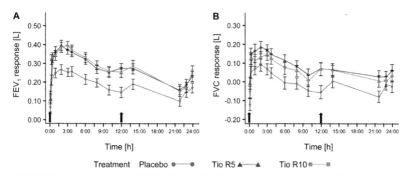

FIGURE 3.—Twenty-four-hour FEV$_1$ (**A**) and FVC (**B**) responses as shown in Fig 2 in the subgroup of patients with 24-hour assessments (n = 67). The baseline value was defined on visit 2 before any maintenance or study medication. At the on-treatment visits, this was immediately followed by the usual medication (including ICS plus LABA), which was followed in turn by the study medication. The afternoon dosing of ICS plus LABA treatment was also taken. *Error bars* represent SEMs. *Arrows* indicate the timing of the maintenance medication: ICS plus LABA. *Tio R5*, 5 µg of tiotropium; *Tio R10*, 10 µg of tiotropium. (Reprinted from The Journal of Allergy and Clinical Immunology, Kerstjens HAM, Disse B, Schröder-Babo W, et al. Tiotropium improves lung function in patients with severe uncontrolled asthma: a randomized controlled trial. *J Allergy Clin Immunol.* 2011;128:308-314. Copyright 2011, with permission from Elsevier.)

time. The only adverse event that was more prominent in the treated group versus placebo was dry mouth, which was most prominent in the T10 group. Improvement in pulmonary function was not statistically different between the T5 and T10 groups. Health care providers should consider adding T5 to their armamentarium for severe asthmatics not responding appropriately to guideline-directed care.

S. K. Willsie, DO, MA

Point: Efficacy of Bronchial Thermoplasty for Patients With Severe Asthma. Is There Sufficient Evidence? Yes

Shifren A, Chen A, Castro M, et al (Washington Univ School of Medicine, St. Louis, MO)
Chest 140:573-579, 2011

Background.—Currently patients with severe asthma have no effective therapy for controlling their symptoms and minimizing their impaired health status. Generally add-on therapy with long-acting beta agonists, leukotriene modifiers, theophylline, and omalizumab is used for patients whose asthma is uncontrolled with inhaled corticosteroids. However, studies are showing that this approach tends to be ineffective in many patients, does not improve quality of life, is expensive, carries substantial side effects, and requires strict adherence to daily medications or monthly or biweekly injections. An alternative, more efficacious approach is desirable for these patients.

Alternative Treatment.—The controlled heating of the airway will diminish the amount of airway smooth muscle and reduce the airway's ability to bronchoconstrict in response to agonists such as methacholine. Bronchial thermoplasty is performed with the Alair Bronchial Thermoplasty System, which delivers a specific amount of radiofrequency (thermal) energy through a dedicated catheter. Treatments are delivered in three sessions and include careful preprocedure and postprocedure monitoring of the patient to manage any respiratory complications that may occur. This treatment can be delivered safely and effectively by pulmonologists.

Evidentiary Support.—Three controlled clinical trials of bronchial thermoplasty covering more than 275 patients have been conducted. In the first, patients demonstrated improved asthma symptoms and an encouraging reduction in mild exacerbations after 1 year of bronchial thermoplasty. The second revealed major improvements in various asthma measures, including forced expiratory volume at 1 second, quality of life, asthma control, and use of rescue medications, compared to a control group. A trend toward a greater reduction in the use of oral corticosteroids was noted in the treated group compared with controls after 1 year. The third study showed a significant improvement in asthma quality of life from baseline to 1 year when bronchial thermoplasty was compared with sham bronchoscopy. Treated patients showed a significant decline in severe exacerbations, emergency department visits, and days lost from work or school. The effects extended for over 2 years in patients receiving bronchial thermoplasty.

The most common adverse reactions to bronchial thermoplasty are breathlessness, wheeze, cough, chest discomfort, night awakenings, and productive cough. These generally occur within a day of the procedure and resolve in an average of 7 days with bronchodilators and corticosteroids. Computed tomography scans of the chest have shown no evidence of airway or parenchymal injury related to the procedure after 5 years.

Conclusions.—Patients with resistant asthma should be evaluated systematically to confirm the diagnosis, exclude any alternative diagnosis, identify comorbid conditions, evaluate treatment compliance, and assess treatment-induced side effects. With appropriate patient selection, management, and follow-up, bronchial thermoplasty may be an effective alternative treatment for severe asthma.

▶ This is a point—counterpoint discussing bronchial thermoplasty as an alternative for patients with severe, uncontrolled asthma and nowhere to turn. Summarized are the clinical trials that led to initial Food and Drug Administration approval of this technique in the United States. More than 55 centers worldwide now have clinicians who are reportedly applying this technique. Health care providers considering this technique for specific patients are encouraged to contact referral centers with experience in applying the technology.

S. K. Willsie, DO, MA

Internet-based tapering of oral corticosteroids in severe asthma: a pragmatic randomised controlled trial
Hashimoto S, Ten Brinke A, Roldaan AC, et al (Univ of Amsterdam, The Netherlands; Med Centre Leeuwarden, The Netherlands; Haga Ziekenhuis, Den Haag, The Netherlands; et al)
Thorax 66:514-520, 2011

Background.—In patients with prednisone-dependent asthma the dose of oral corticosteroids should be adjusted to the lowest possible level to reduce long-term adverse effects. However, the optimal strategy for tapering oral corticosteroids is unknown.

Objective.—To investigate whether an internet-based management tool including home monitoring of symptoms, lung function and fraction of exhaled nitric oxide (FE_{NO}) facilitates tapering of oral corticosteroids and leads to reduction of corticosteroid consumption without worsening asthma control or asthma-related quality of life.

Methods.—In a 6-month pragmatic randomised prospective multicentre study, 95 adults with prednisone-dependent asthma from six pulmonary outpatient clinics were allocated to two tapering strategies: according to conventional treatment (n=43) or guided by a novel internet-based monitoring system (internet strategy) (n=52). Primary outcomes were cumulative sparing of prednisone, asthma control and asthma-related quality of life. Secondary outcomes were forced expiratory volume in 1 s (FEV_1), exacerbations, hospitalisations and patient's satisfaction with the tapering strategy.

Results.—Median cumulative sparing of prednisone was 205 (25—75th percentile −221 to 777) mg in the Internet strategy group compared with 0 (−497 to 282) mg in the conventional treatment group (p=0.02). Changes in prednisone dose (mixed effect regression model) from baseline were −4.79 mg/day and +1.59 mg/day, respectively (p<0.001). Asthma control, asthma-related quality of life, FEV_1, exacerbations, hospitalisations and satisfaction with the strategy were not different between groups.

Conclusions.—An internet-based management tool including home monitoring of symptoms, lung function and FE_{NO} in severe asthma is superior to conventional treatment in reducing total corticosteroid consumption without compromising asthma control or asthma-related quality of life.

Clinical Trial Registration Number.—Clinical trial registered with http://www.trialregister.nl (Netherlands Trial Register number 1146).

▶ This is a novel and sophisticated instrument- and technology-laden approach compared with usual care (UC) in tapering prednisone dose in severe uncontrolled steroid-dependent asthmatics over 6 months. There have been successful efforts with reduction in prednisone (−4.79 mg/d vs +1.59 mg/d—usual care; *P* < .001). Drawbacks to this program appear to be individual use of sophisticated equipment (spirometry, fractional excretion of nitric oxide), required computers, required computer skills of subjects, and intensive nursing interventions. Despite this, the treatment algorithm appears to have potential merit, and further studies appear warranted with an evaluation of alternate delivery techniques that may be more cost effective.

S. K. Willsie, DO, MA

Management of asthma in pregnancy guided by measurement of fraction of exhaled nitric oxide: a double-blind, randomised controlled trial
Powell H, Murphy VE, Taylor DR, et al (Univ of Newcastle and Hunter Med Res Inst, New South Wales, Australia; Univ of Otago, Dunedin, New Zealand; et al)
Lancet 378:983-990, 2011

Background.—Asthma exacerbations during pregnancy are common and can be associated with substantial maternal and fetal morbidity. Treatment decisions based on sputum eosinophil counts reduce exacerbations in non-pregnant women with asthma, but results with the fraction of exhaled nitric oxide (F_ENO) to guide management are equivocal. We tested the hypothesis that a management algorithm for asthma in pregnancy based on F_ENO and symptoms would reduce asthma exacerbations.

Methods.—We undertook a double-blind, parallel-group, controlled trial in two antenatal clinics in Australia. 220 pregnant, non-smoking women with asthma were randomly assigned, by a computer-generated random number list, before 22 weeks' gestation to treatment adjustment at monthly visits by an algorithm using clinical symptoms (control group) or F_ENO concentrations (active intervention group) used to uptitrate (F_ENO >29 ppb) or downtitrate (F_ENO <16 ppb) inhaled corticosteroid dose. Participants, caregivers, and outcome assessors were masked to group assignment. Longacting β2 agonist and minimum dose inhaled corticosteroid were used to treat symptoms when F_ENO was not increased. The primary outcome was total asthma exacerbations (moderate and severe). Analysis was by intention to treat. This study is registered with the Australian and New Zealand Clinical Trials Registry, number 12607000561482.

Findings.—111 women were randomly assigned to the $F_E NO$ group (100 completed) and 109 to the control group (103 completed). The exacerbation rate was lower in the $F_E NO$ group than in the control group (0·288 *vs* 0·615 exacerbations per pregnancy; incidence rate ratio 0·496, 95% CI 0·325—0·755; p=0·001). The number needed to treat was 6. In the $F_E NO$ group, quality of life was improved (score on short form 12 mental summary was 56·9 [95% CI 50·2—59·3] in $F_E NO$ group vs 54·2 [46·1—57·6] in control group; p=0·037) and neonatal hospitalisations were reduced (eight [8%] vs 18 [17%]; p=0·046).

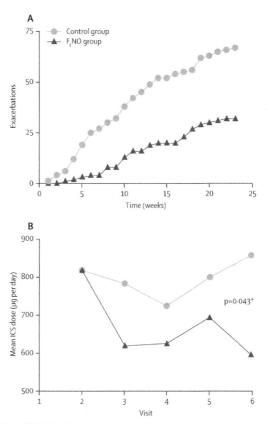

FIGURE 2.—Effect of $F_E NO$-guided asthma management during pregnancy on number of asthma exacerbations (A) and maintenance mean daily ICS dose (B) ICS=inhaled corticosteroids. $F_E NO$=fraction of exhaled nitric oxide. *From generalised linear mixed model model analysis. (Reprinted from The Lancet, Powell H, Murphy VE, Taylor DR, et al. Management of asthma in pregnancy guided by measurement of fraction of exhaled nitric oxide: a double-blind, randomised controlled trial. *Lancet.* 2011;378:983-990. © 2011, with permission from Elsevier.)

TABLE 1.—Dose Changes Based on F_ENO and ACQ Results for the F_ENO Intervention Algorithm

	F_ENO Concentration (ppb)	Symptoms (ACQ Score)	ICS Dose Change	β2-Agonist Dose Change
Level 1	>29	NA	↑ ICS × 1 step	No change
Level 2	16–29	≤1·5	No change	No change
Level 3	16–29	>1·5	No change	↑ LABA × 1 step
Level 4	<16	≤1·5	↓ ICS × 1 step	No change
Level 5	<16	>1·5	↓ ICS × 1 step	↑ LABA × 1 step

F_ENO=fraction of exhaled nitric oxide. ACQ=asthma control questionnaire. ICS=inhaled corticosteroid. NA=not part of the assessment at this F_ENO level. LABA=longacting β2 agonist.

TABLE 2.—F_ENO Algorithm Treatment Steps

	ICS Step	β2 Step
Step 1	0	Salbutamol as required
Step 2	Budesonide 100 μg twice per day	Formoterol 6 μg twice per day
Step 3	Budesonide 200 μg twice per day	Formoterol 12 μg twice per day
Step 4	Budesonide 400 μg twice per day	Formoterol 2 × 12 μg twice per day
Step 5	Budesonide 800 μg twice per day	Formoterol 2 × 12 μg twice per day

F_ENO=fraction of exhaled nitric oxide. ICS=inhaled corticosteroid.

TABLE 3.—Dose Changes Based on Clinical Assessment for the Clinical Algorithm (control)

	ACQ Score	Treatment Adjustment
Level 1	>1·5	↑ 1 step
Level 2	0·75–1·5	No change
Level 3	<0·75	↓ 1 step

ACQ=asthma control questionnaire.

Interpretation.—Asthma exacerbations during pregnancy can be significantly reduced with a validated F_ENO-based treatment algorithm (Fig 2, Tables 1-4).

▶ Uncontrolled asthma during pregnancy can lead to increased maternal-fetal morbidity and mortality.[1-3] This sentinel investigation has found that using fraction of exhaled nitric oxide (F_ENO) and results of the Asthma Control Questionnaire (ACQ) resulted in improved management of asthma during pregnancy. Tables 1-4 detail the decision-making processes used to guide asthma care within a double-blinded protocol. Specifically, F_ENO was used to guide the dosing of budesonide (ICS), and ACQ results were used to guide the dose of formoterol. Fig 2 shows that F_ENO-guided therapy resulted in a reduction of exacerbations during pregnancy ($P = .001$), reduced use of short-acting beta

TABLE 4.—Clinical Algorithm Treatment Steps

	Treatment
Step 1	Salbutamol as required
Step 2	Budesonide 200 μg twice per day
Step 3	Budesonide 400 μg twice per day
Step 4	Budesonide 400 μg and formoterol 12 μg twice per day
Step 5	Budesonide 800 μg and formoterol 24 μg twice per day

agonists, and a longer exacerbation-free period ($P = .018$). This resulted in 6 women being treated according to $F_E NO$ to prevent one woman from experiencing an exacerbation during pregnancy (number needed to treat). In addition, women whose therapy was guided during pregnancy by $F_E NO$ were more likely to be treated with ICS, and, when treated with ICS, received a lower dose. The results of this investigation provide a reasonable basis on which to begin using $F_E NO$ in the management of asthma during pregnancy. Results of larger multicenter trials may provide numbers needed on which to make determinations about whether $F_E NO$-guided care can impact neonatal morbidity/mortality.

S. K. Willsie, DO, MA

References

1. National Heart, Lung, and Blood Institute. NAEPP expert panel report. Managing asthma during pregnancy: recommendations for pharmacologic treatment-2004 update. *J Allergy Clin Immunol.* 2005;115:36-46.
2. Murphy VE, Gibson PG, Giles WB, et al. Maternal asthma is associated with reduced female fetal growth. *Am J Respir Crit Care Med.* 2003;168:1317-1323.
3. Murphy VE, Clifton VL, Gibson PG. Asthma exacerbations during pregnancy: incidence and association with adverse pregnancy outcomes. *Thorax.* 2006;61:169-176.

Daily exhaled nitric oxide measurements and asthma exacerbations in children

van der Valk RJP, Baraldi E, Stern G, et al (Erasmus Univ Med Ctr — Sophia Children's Hosp, Rotterdam, the Netherlands; Univ of Padova, Italy; Univ of Berne, Switzerland; et al)

Allergy 67:265-271, 2012

Background.—Fractional exhaled Nitric Oxide (FeNO) is a biomarker for eosinophilic airway inflammation and can be measured at home on a daily basis. A short-term increase in FeNO may indicate a higher risk of future asthma exacerbations.

Objective.—To assess changes in FeNO before and after asthma exacerbations compared to a stable control period.

Methods.—A *post hoc* analysis was performed on daily FeNO measurements over 30 weeks in children with asthma ($n = 77$). Moderate

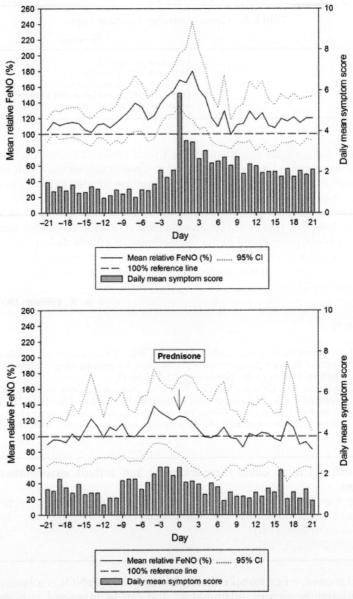

FIGURE 2.—Percentage change in Fractional exhaled Nitric Oxide (FeNO) before and after exacerbations. Mean relative FeNO time series for 3-week periods centered around moderate exacerbations (upper panel) and severe exacerbations (lower panel) (onset exacerbation at day 0). Relative FeNO = FeNO divided by the median of the reference period. Bars show average daily symptom scores (sum of wheezing, shortness of breath, coughing, and sleep disturbances). (Reprinted from van der Valk RJP, Baraldi E, Stern G, et al. Daily exhaled nitric oxide measurements and asthma exacerbations in children. *Allergy.* 2012;67:265-271, with permission from John Wiley & Sons (www.interscience.wiley.com).)

exacerbations were defined by an increase in symptom scores and severe exacerbations by prescription of prednisone. Individual mean and maximum FeNO, the variability of FeNO assessed by the coefficient of variation (CV), and slopes of FeNO in time were all quantified in 3-week blocks. Cross-correlation of FeNO with symptoms and autocorrelation of FeNO were assessed in relation to exacerbations and examined as predictors for exacerbations compared to reference periods using logistic regression.

Results.—Fractional exhaled nitric oxide could be assessed in relation to 25 moderate and 12 severe exacerbations. The CV, slope, cross-correlation, and autocorrelation of daily FeNO increased before moderate exacerbations. Increases in slope were also randomly seen in 19% of 2-week blocks of children without exacerbations. At least 3—5 FeNO measurements in the 3 weeks before an exacerbation were needed to calculate a slope that could predict moderate exacerbations. No specific pattern of FeNO was seen before severe exacerbations.

Conclusion.—Fractional exhaled nitric oxide monitoring revealed changes in FeNO prior to moderate exacerbations. Whether this can be used to prevent loss of asthma control should be further explored (Fig 2).

▶ Headline: Peak flow meters traded in for daily fractional exhaled nitric oxide (FENO) measurements at home! This is 1 of 2 primary publications we have reviewed this year that have focused on the clinical utility of FENO in asthma; the first article[1] dealt with use of FENO, spirometry, and a treatment algorithm to reduce corticosteroid use in uncontrolled asthmatics; this investigation by van der Valk et al focuses on the predictability of moderate exacerbations in children based on changes in FENO. Fig 2 depicts percentage change in FENO detectable prior to development of moderate asthma exacerbation. What is clear is that this marker of airway inflammation is becoming more and more available to the public outside of sophisticated health centers for monitoring asthma and asthmatic treatment. As usually happens with technology, over time it sells at a reduced price. It appears that sooner rather than later, regular home-based assessment of FENO may become standard of care for self-monitoring asthma instead of asking about nighttime awakenings, use of beta agonists, and periodic spirometry measurements in the ambulatory care clinic setting.

S. K. Willsie, DO, MA

Reference

1. Hashimoto S, Brinke AT, Roldaan AC, van Heen IH, Möller GM, Sont JK. Internet-based tapering of oral corticosteroids in severe asthma: a pragmatic randomised controlled trial. *Thorax.* 2007;66:514-520.

An Official ATS Clinical Practice Guideline: Interpretation of Exhaled Nitric Oxide Levels (FE_NO) for Clinical Applications

Dweik RA, Boggs PB, Erzurum SC, et al; American Thoracic Society Committee on Interpretation of Exhaled Nitric Oxide Levels (FE_NO) for Clinical Applications
Am J Respir Crit Care Med 184:602-615, 2011

Background.—Measurement of fractional nitric oxide (NO) concentration in exhaled breath (FE_NO) is a quantitative, noninvasive, simple, and safe method of measuring airway inflammation that provides a complementary tool to other ways of assessing airways disease, including asthma. While FE_NO measurement has been standardized, there is currently no reference guideline for practicing health care providers to guide them in the appropriate use and interpretation of FE_NO in clinical practice.

Purpose.—To develop evidence-based guidelines for the interpretation of FE_NO measurements that incorporate evidence that has accumulated over the past decade.

Methods.—We created a multidisciplinary committee with expertise in the clinical care, clinical science, or basic science of airway disease and/or NO. The committee identified important clinical questions, synthesized the evidence, and formulated recommendations. Recommendations were developed using pragmatic systematic reviews of the literature and the GRADE approach.

Results.—The evidence related to the use of FE_NO measurements is reviewed and clinical practice recommendations are provided.

Conclusions.—In the setting of chronic inflammatory airway disease including asthma, conventional tests such as FEV_1 reversibility or provocation tests are only indirectly associated with airway inflammation. FE_NO offers added advantages for patient care including, but not limited to (1) detecting of eosinophilic airway inflammation, (2) determining the likelihood of corticosteroid responsiveness, (3) monitoring of airway inflammation to determine the potential need for corticosteroid, and (4) unmasking of otherwise unsuspected nonadherence to corticosteroid therapy.

▶ This is a clinical practice guideline from the American Thoracic Society and describes the basis for the use and interpretation of exhaled nitric oxide levels (FE_NO) in clinical medicine. This should become a familiar reference for all health care practitioners in the field of pulmonary medicine and will provide a roadmap for optimized use of this marker of airway inflammation. Never to be used as a test to diagnose asthma, FE_NO is rather an arrow in the armamentarium of a health care provider, allowing for improved differential diagnosis, optimized prescribing, and triaging of care. The FE_NO will best be used only if we understand its physiologic role and apply it appropriately. Read and reread this clinical practice guideline and keep it close at hand as a ready tool, because more and more investigations are showing the use of FE_NO in the everyday management of patients with asthma and other inflammatory airway conditions.

S. K. Willsie, DO, MA

Age and Risks of FDA-Approved Long-Acting β_2-Adrenergic Receptor Agonists
McMahon AW, Levenson MS, McEvoy BW, et al (Food and Drug Administration, Silver Spring, MD; Ctr for Drug Evaluation and Res, MD)
Pediatrics 128:e1147-e1154, 2011

Objective.—To determine the risk, by age group, of serious asthma-related events with long-acting β_2-adrenergic receptor agonists marketed in the United States for asthma.

Methods.—The US Food and Drug Administration performed a meta-analysis of controlled clinical trials comparing the risk of LABA use with no LABA use for patients 4 to 11, 12 to 17, 18 to 64, and older than 64 years old. The effects of age on a composite of asthma-related deaths, intubations, and hospitalizations (asthma composite index) and the effects of concomitant inhaled corticosteroid (ICS) use were analyzed.

Results.—One hundred ten trials with 60 954 patients were included in the meta-analysis. The composite event incidence difference for all ages was 6.3 events per 1000 patient-years (95% confidence interval [CI]: 2.2−10.3) for using LABAs compared with not using LABAs. The largest incidence difference was observed for the 4- to 11-year age group (30.4 events per 1000 patient-years [95% CI: 5.7−55.1]). Differences according to age were statistically significant ($P = .020$). Results for the subgroup of patients with concomitant ICS use ($n = 36\,210$) were similar to the overall results; with assigned ICSs ($n = 15\,192$), the incidence difference was 0.4 events per 1000 patient-years (95% CI: −3.8 to 4.6), and there was no statistically significant difference according to age group.

Conclusions.—The excess of serious asthma-related events attributable to LABAs was greatest among children. Additional data are needed to assess risks of LABA use for children with simultaneous ICS use.

▶ Meta-analysis of controlled clinical trials evaluating the risk of long-acting beta agonist (LABA) use versus no LABA for 4 subgroups by age: 4 to 11 years, 12 to 17 years, 18 to 64 years, and older than 64 years. This meta-analysis, undertaken by the US Food and Drug Administration, included 110 clinical research studies and greater than 60 000 asthmatics. Two trials in particular showed greater risk of LABA use for children.[1,2] Fig 4 in the original article shows a comparison, by age group, of LABA plus inhaled corticosteroids (ICS) versus ICS alone. Neutralization of adverse effects of LABA by concomitant use of ICS cannot be relied on in children. Until these findings can be explained, health care providers should take great care in using LABAs in children with asthma, and for the time being, using them with ICS and only when there is no other viable option for achieving and maintaining asthma control, seems appropriate.

S. K. Willsie, DO, MA

References

1. Salpeter SR, Buckley NS, Ormiston TM, Salpeter EE. Meta-analysis: effect of long-acting β-agonists on severe asthma exacerbations and asthma related deaths. *Ann Intern Med.* 2006;144:904-912.
2. Cates CJ, Cates MJ, Lasserson TJ. Regular treatment with formoterol for chronic asthma: serious adverse events. *Cochrane Database Syst Rev.* 2008;(4). CD006923.

Efficacy of budesonide/formoterol pressurized metered-dose inhaler versus budesonide pressurized metered-dose inhaler alone in Hispanic adults and adolescents with asthma: a randomized, controlled trial
Zangrilli J, Mansfield LE, Uryniak T, et al (AstraZeneca LP, Wilmington, DE; Texas Tech Univ, El Paso)
Ann Allergy Asthma Immunol 107:258-265, 2011

Background.—Few clinical trials in asthma have focused on Hispanic populations.

Objective.—To compare the efficacy and safety of budesonide/formoterol (BUD/FM) with BUD in an ethnically diverse group of Hispanic participants with asthma previously treated with inhaled corticosteroids (ICS).

Methods.—This 12-week, randomized, double-blind, active-controlled study (NCT00419757) was designed to enroll Hispanic participants (self-reported) ($\geq$12 years of age) with moderate to severe asthma requiring medium- to high-dose ICS. After a 2-week run-in period (low-dose BUD pressurized metered-dose inhaler [pMDI] 80 μg $\times$ 2 inhalations [160 μg] twice daily), participants with a symptom score greater than 0 (scale: 0–3) on 3 or more of 7 run-in days and forced expiratory volume in 1 second (FEV$_1$) 45%–85% predicted were randomized to BUD/FM pMDI 160/4.5 μg $\times$ 2 inhalations (320/9 μg) twice daily or BUD pMDI 160 μg $\times$ 2 inhalations (320 μg) twice daily.

Results.—Randomized participants ($n = 127$ BUD/FM; $n = 123$ BUD) were predominately Mexican (51%) or Puerto Rican (21%). During low-dose ICS run-in, the mean symptom score was 1.0; however, mean predose FEV$_1$ improved (2.10–2.21 L). During randomized treatment, small, but not statistically significant, improvements favored BUD/FM vs BUD (AM peak expiratory flow [PEF; primary efficacy variable] 25.4 vs 19.9 L/min; PM PEF 20.6 vs 15.8 L/min; predose FEV$_1$ 0.16 vs 0.11 L; rescue medication use −0.7 vs −0.6 inhalations/d). Most adverse events were mild or moderate in intensity.

Conclusions.—Improvement in clinically relevant control end points occurred in both BUD/FM and BUD groups; both treatments were well tolerated in this Hispanic asthma population but were not significantly differentiated.

▶ This 12 week-long investigation limited to Hispanic subjects evaluated outcomes following treatment with budesonide plus long-acting beta agonist (BLABA) versus budesonide alone (B). Hispanic asthmatics enrolled were of variable ethnicity (51% Mexican; 21% Puerto Rican). After 12 weeks, no statistically significant differences were noted between BLABA and B groups, although small differences were noted that appeared to trend to favor BLABA. Both treatments were well tolerated by all subjects. Consistent with current recommendations from the National Asthma Education and Prevention Program for all comers, efficacy of inhaled corticosteroids (ICS) alone versus ICS plus LABA appears to be comparable in Hispanics receiving dosage for 12 weeks.

S. K. Willsie, DO, MA

Fluticasone furoate demonstrates efficacy in patients with asthma symptomatic on medium doses of inhaled corticosteroid therapy: an 8-week, randomised, placebo-controlled trial
Busse WW, Bleecker ER, Bateman ED, et al (Univ of Wisconsin, Madison; Wake Forest Univ Health Sciences, Winston-Salem, NC; Univ of Cape Town, South Africa; et al)
Thorax 67:35-41, 2012

Background.—Fluticasone furoate (FF) is a novel inhaled corticosteroid with 24 h activity. FF is being developed as a once-daily treatment in combination with the long-acting β_2 agonist vilanterol trifenatate for asthma and chronic obstructive pulmonary disease.

Objectives.—To determine the optimal dose(s) of FF for treating patients with asthma.

Methods.—An 8-week multicentre, randomised, double-blind study. 627 patients with persistent moderate-to-severe asthma, symptomatic on medium-dose inhaled corticosteroid therapy, were randomised to placebo, FF 200, 400, 600 or 800 µg (once daily in the evening using a novel dry powder inhaler), or fluticasone propionate 500 µg twice daily (via Diskus™/Accuhaler™). The primary efficacy measure was mean change from baseline in pre-dose evening forced expiratory volume in one second (FEV_1). Other endpoints included morning and evening peak expiratory flow, and rescue/symptom-free 24 h periods.

Results.—Each dose was significantly superior to placebo for the primary endpoint ($p < 0.001$) with efficacy at least similar to that reported with fluticasone propionate. There was no dose—response relationship across the FF doses studied. Peak expiratory flow improved in all groups ($p<0.001$ vs placebo), and there were significant treatment effects on rescue/symptom-free 24 h periods with all active treatments. FF was generally well tolerated. The incidence of oral candidiasis was higher with FF 800 µg than placebo; pharmacokinetic and 24 h urinary cortisol analyses confirmed a higher systemic exposure of FF at this highest dose level.

Conclusions.—FF doses <800 µg have a favourable therapeutic index. The absence of an efficacy dose response suggests that 200 µg is an appropriate dose in patients with moderate persistent asthma.

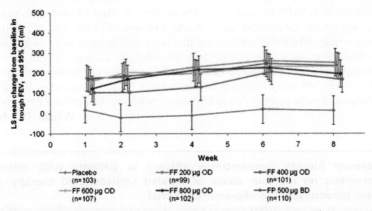

FIGURE 3.—Least squares mean change from baseline in trough FEV₁. Repeated measures analysis (intent-to-treat population). Error bars indicate 95% CI. Data points are offset for clarity. BD, twice daily; FEV_1, forced expiratory volume in 1 s; FF, fluticasone furoate; FP, fluticasone propionate; LS, least squares; OD, once daily; PBO, placebo. (Reproduced from Thorax, Busse WW, Bleecker ER, Bateman ED, et al. Fluticasone furoate demonstrates efficacy in patients with asthma symptomatic on medium doses of inhaled corticosteroid therapy: An 8-week, randomised, placebo-controlled trial. *Thorax.* 2012;67:35-41, with permission from BMJ Publishing Group Ltd.)

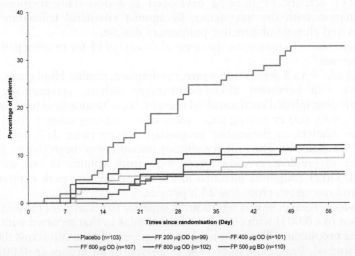

FIGURE 5.—Time to withdrawals due to lack of efficacy (cumulative incidence curve) (intent-to-treat population). BD, twice daily; FF, fluticasone furoate; FP, fluticasone propionate; OD, once daily. (Reproduced from Thorax, Busse WW, Bleecker ER, Bateman ED, et al. Fluticasone furoate demonstrates efficacy in patients with asthma symptomatic on medium doses of inhaled corticosteroid therapy: An 8-week, randomised, placebo-controlled trial. *Thorax.* 2012;67:35-41, with permission from BMJ Publishing Group Ltd.)

ClinicalTrials.gov identifier: NCT00603746 (Figs 3 and 5).

▶ Compliance with long-term medications in uncontrolled asthma remains problematic. This investigation evaluated an inhaled corticosteroid (ICS) with 24-hour activity, fluticasone furoate (FF), with regard to tolerance and efficacy in moderate-to-severe persistent asthmatics symptomatic on medium-dosed ICS therapy. Fig 3 depicts least squares mean change in baseline FEV_1 over time, and Fig 5 demonstrates time to withdrawal from trial due to lack of efficacy. Incidence of oral candidiasis was significantly more common, as was urinary cortisol suppression with the 800 µg FF dose versus 200, 400, 500 and 600 µg daily doses. Given that efficacy was not dose dependent at the 800 µg dose, the recommended starting dose for FF in asthmatics with difficulty with compliance on bid ICS is 200 µg/d. Longer duration studies are indicated.

S. K. Willsie, DO, MA

Reslizumab for Poorly Controlled, Eosinophilic Asthma: A Randomized, Placebo-Controlled Study
Castro M, for the Res-5-0010 Study Group (Washington Univ School of Medicine, St Louis, MO; et al)
Am J Respir Crit Care Med 184:1125-1132, 2011

Rationale.—Eosinophilic asthma is a phenotype of asthma characterized by the persistence of eosinophils in the airways. IL-5 is involved in the activation and survival of eosinophils.

Objectives.—To evaluate the effect of the antibody to IL-5, reslizumab, in patients with eosinophilic asthma that is poorly controlled with high-dose inhaled corticosteroid.

Methods.—Patients were randomly assigned to receive infusions of reslizumab at 3.0 mg/kg (n = 53) or placebo (n = 53) at baseline and at Weeks 4, 8, and 12, with stratification by baseline Asthma Control Questionnaire (ACQ) score less than or equal to 2 or greater than 2. The primary efficacy measure was the difference between the reslizumab- and placebo groups in the change in ACQ score from baseline to end of therapy (Week 15 or early withdrawal).

Measurements and Main Results.—Mean changes from baseline to end of therapy in ACQ score were −0.7 in the reslizumab group and −0.3 in the placebo group (P = 0.054) and in FEV_1 were 0.18 and −0.08 L, respectively (P = 0.002). In those patients with nasal polyps, the changes in ACQ score were −1.0 and −0.1, respectively (P = 0.012). Median percentage reductions from baseline in sputum eosinophils were 95.4 and 38.7%, respectively (P = 0.007). Eight percent of patients in the reslizumab group and 19% of patients in the placebo group had an asthma exacerbation (P = 0.083). The most common adverse events with reslizumab were nasopharyngitis, fatigue, and pharyngolaryngeal pain.

Conclusions.—Patients receiving reslizumab showed significantly greater reductions in sputum eosinophils, improvements in airway function, and a trend toward greater asthma control than those receiving placebo. Reslizumab was generally well tolerated.

▶ This was an investigation evaluating monoclonal antibody targeting interleukin (IL)-5 for patients who met the following inclusion criteria: phenotypic eosinophilic asthma, uncontrolled asthma despite therapy with high-dose inhaled corticosteroids and at least 1 other agent; Asthma Control Questionnaire score greater than 1.5, and induced sputum eosinophilia (>3%) despite baseline therapy. Changes in pulmonary function following treatment ($P = .002$) was statistically significant, whereas clinical improvement overall did not reach statistical significance (Fig 2 in the original article). The greatest improvement (reduction in sputum eosinophils; reduction in asthma exacerbations) was seen in subjects who had nasal polyposis. This monoclonal antibody targeting IL-5 shows promise for uncontrolled asthmatics with nasal polyposis who meet criteria for the eosinophilic phenotype. Therein remains the challenge: appropriate selection of patients for treatment with what no doubt will be costly therapy.

S. K. Willsie, DO, MA

Association between childhood asthma and ADHD symptoms in adolescence — a prospective population-based twin study

Mogensen N, Larsson H, Lundholm C, et al (Karolinska Institutet, Stockholm, Sweden)
Allergy 66:1224-1230, 2011

Background.—Cross-sectional studies report a relationship between childhood asthma and attention-deficit hyperactivity disorder (ADHD) symptoms, but the mechanisms are yet unclear. Our objective was to investigate the longitudinal link between childhood asthma and the two dimensions of ADHD (hyperactivity–impulsivity, HI, and inattention, IN) in adolescence. We also aimed to explore the genetic and environmental contributions and the impact of asthma medication.

Methods.—Data on asthma, HI and IN, birth weight, socioeconomic status, zygosity, and medication were collected from the Swedish Medical Birth Register and through parental questionnaires at ages 8–9 and 13–14 years on 1480 Swedish twin pairs born 1985–1986. The association between asthma at age 8–9 and ADHD symptoms at age 13–14 was assessed with generalized estimating equations, and twin analyses to assess the genetic or environmental determinants were performed.

Results.—Children with asthma at age 8–9 had an almost twofold increased risk of having one or more symptoms of HI (OR 1.88, 95% CI 1.18–3.00) and a more than twofold increased risk to have three symptoms or more of HI (OR 2.73, 95% CI 1.49–5.00) at age 13–14, independent of asthma medication. For IN, no significant relationship was seen. Results from twin modeling indicate that 68% of the phenotypic correlation between asthma and HI ($r = 0.23$, 0.04–0.37) was because of genetic influences.

Conclusions.—Our findings suggest that childhood asthma is associated with subsequent development of HI in early adolescence, which could be partly explained by genetic influences. Early strategies to identify children at risk may reduce burden of the disease in adolescence.

▶ Asthma and attention deficit and hyperactivity disorder (ADHD) have been suggested as important comorbid conditions in children with asthma.[1-4] This investigation entailed utilizing twin registry data from the Swedish Medical Birth Registry, 1985–1986 births. Parental responses were sought at 2 time points: ages 8 and 9 (incidence of asthma) and 13 and 14 (presence of inattention and hyperactivity). The results of this study showed that children with asthma at ages 8 and 9 were almost 2-fold more likely to have hyperactivity and inattention at ages 13 and 14. The study suggested an influence of genetics. Given that ADHD can have a significant negative impact on learning and academic performance, health care providers should screen childhood asthmatics for ADHD if history is suggestive.

S. K. Willsie, DO, MA

References

1. McQuaid EL, Weiss-Laxer N, Kopel SJ, et al. Pediatric asthma and problems in attention, concentration, and impulsivity: disruption of the family management system. *Fam Syst Health*. 2008;26:16-29.
2. Yuksel H, Sogut A, Yilmaz O. Attention deficit and hyperactivity symptoms in children with asthma. *J Asthma*. 2008;45:545-547.
3. McGee R, Stanton WR, Sears MR. Allergic disorders and attention deficit disorder in children. *J Abnorm Child Psychol*. 1993;21:79-88.
4. Biederman J, Milberger S, Faraone SV, Guite J, Warburton R. Associations between childhood asthma and ADHD: issues of psychiatric comorbidity and familiality. *J Am Acad Child Adolesc Psychiatry*. 1994;33:842-848.

Cystic Fibrosis

Results of a phase IIa study of VX-809, an investigational CFTR corrector compound, in subjects with cystic fibrosis homozygous for the *F508del-CFTR* mutation

Clancy JP, Rowe SM, Accurso FJ, et al (Cincinnati Children's Hosp Med Ctr, OH; Univ of Alabama at Birmingham; Univ of Colorado Health Sciences Ctr, Denver; et al)
Thorax 67:12-18, 2012

Background.—VX-809, a cystic fibrosis transmembrane conductance regulator (CFTR) modulator, has been shown to increase the cell surface density of functional *F508del-CFTR* in vitro.

Methods.—A randomised, double-blind, placebo-controlled study evaluated the safety, tolerability and pharmacodynamics of VX-809 in adult patients with cystic fibrosis (n=89) who were homozygous for the *F508del-CFTR* mutation. Subjects were randomised to one of four VX-809 28 day dose groups (25, 50, 100 and 200 mg) or matching placebo.

Results.—The type and incidence of adverse events were similar among VX-809- and placebo-treated subjects. Respiratory events were the most

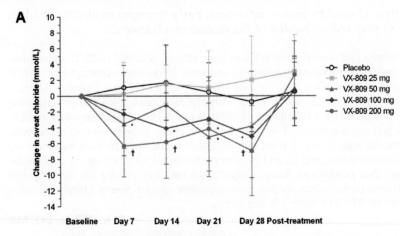

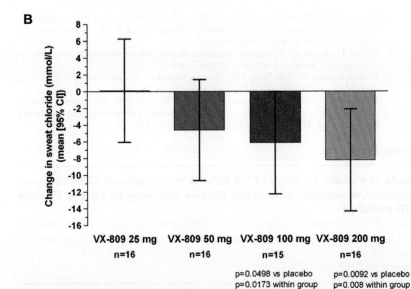

FIGURE 1.—(A) Change in sweat chloride measurements from baseline for placebo- and VX-809-treated subjects. Mean values are shown (± 95% CI, based on analysis of covariance (ANCOVA) analysis) predose, at weekly intervals over the course of treatment, and 1 week following discontinuation of study drug. (B) Sweat chloride change from baseline to day 28 treatment, difference versus placebo (mean (95% CI, based on ANCOVA analysis)). Sweat Cl⁻ changes were seen as early as day 7 of treatment (data not shown), and reached statistical significance for the 100 and 200 mg dose groups (p<0.05 and p<0.01, respectively). (Reproduced from Thorax, Clancy JP, Rowe SM, Accurso FJ, et al. Results of a phase IIa study of VX-809, an investigational CFTR corrector compound, in subjects with cystic fibrosis homozygous for the *F508del-CFTR* mutation. *Thorax.* 2012;67:12-18, with permission from BMJ Publishing Group Ltd.)

commonly reported and led to discontinuation by one subject in each active treatment arm. Pharmacokinetic data supported a once-daily oral dosing regimen. Pharmacodynamic data suggested that VX-809 improved CFTR function in at least one organ (sweat gland). VX-809 reduced elevated sweat chloride values in a dose-dependent manner (p=0.0013) that was statistically significant in the 100 and 200 mg dose groups. There was no statistically significant improvement in CFTR function in the nasal epithelium as measured by nasal potential difference, nor were there statistically significant changes in lung function or patient-reported outcomes. No maturation of immature *F508del-CFTR* was detected in the subgroup that provided rectal biopsy specimens.

Conclusions.—In this study, VX-809 had a similar adverse event profile to placebo for 28 days in *F508del-CFTR* homozygous patients, and demonstrated biological activity with positive impact on CFTR function in the sweat gland. Additional data are needed to determine how improvements detected in CFTR function secondary to VX-809 in the sweat gland relate to those measurable in the respiratory tract and to long-term measures of clinical benefit.

Clinical Trial Number.—NCT00865904 (Fig 1).

▶ This is a potentially promising and interesting therapeutic advance still in the investigational phase: cystic fibrosis (CF) transmembrane conductance regulator (CFTR) impacting sweat chloride. This is a phase IIA study evaluating sweat gland's biologic activity. Fig 1 depicts, by dose of investigational agent, reduction in sweat chloride, reaching statistical significance in adult patients with CF who were homozygotes for *F508del-CFTR* after 28 days of consecutive dose administration. Additional studies are warranted with this and other agents on the horizon for this genetic disease with little but reactive treatment (eg, for infections; pancreatic insufficiency) to currently offer.

S. K. Willsie, DO, MA

A CFTR Potentiator in Patients with Cystic Fibrosis and the *G551D* Mutation

Ramsey BW, for the VX08-770-102 Study Group (Seattle Children's Hosp and Univ of Washington School of Medicine; et al)
N Engl J Med 365:1663-1672, 2011

Background.—Increasing the activity of defective cystic fibrosis transmembrane conductance regulator (CFTR) protein is a potential treatment for cystic fibrosis.

Methods.—We conducted a randomized, double-blind, placebo-controlled trial to evaluate ivacaftor (VX-770), a CFTR potentiator, in subjects 12 years of age or older with cystic fibrosis and at least one *G551D-CFTR* mutation. Subjects were randomly assigned to receive 150 mg of ivacaftor every 12 hours (84 subjects, of whom 83 received at least one dose) or placebo (83, of whom 78 received at least one dose) for 48 weeks. The primary end point was the estimated mean change from baseline through week 24 in the percent of predicted forced expiratory volume in 1 second (FEV_1).

Results.—The change from baseline through week 24 in the percent of predicted FEV_1 was greater by 10.6 percentage points in the ivacaftor group than in the placebo group (P<0.001). Effects on pulmonary function were noted by 2 weeks, and a significant treatment effect was maintained through week 48. Subjects receiving ivacaftor were 55% less likely to have a pulmonary exacerbation than were patients receiving placebo, through week 48 (P<0.001). In addition, through week 48, subjects in the ivacaftor group scored 8.6 points higher than did subjects in the placebo group on the respiratory-symptoms domain of the Cystic Fibrosis Questionnaire–revised instrument (a 100-point scale, with higher numbers indicating a lower effect of symptoms on the patient's quality of life) (P<0.001). By 48 weeks, patients treated with ivacaftor had gained, on average, 2.7 kg more weight than had patients receiving placebo (P<0.001). The change from baseline through week 48 in the concentration of sweat chloride, a measure of CFTR activity, with ivacaftor as compared with placebo was −48.1 mmol per liter (P<0.001). The incidence of adverse events was similar with ivacaftor and placebo, with a lower proportion of serious adverse events with ivacaftor than with placebo (24% vs. 42%).

Conclusions.—Ivacaftor was associated with improvements in lung function at 2 weeks that were sustained through 48 weeks. Substantial improvements were also observed in the risk of pulmonary exacerbations, patient-reported respiratory symptoms, weight, and concentration of sweat chloride. (Funded by Vertex Pharmaceuticals and others; VX08-770-102 ClinicalTrials.gov number, NCT00909532.)

▶ Late Breaking Development in Cystic Fibrosis: January 31, 2012: New drug approved for use in Cystic Fibrosis. Ivacaftor was approved by the US Food and Drug Administration (FDA) on January 31, 2012, for use in cystic fibrosis patients aged 6 and older who have at least 1 copy of the G551D mutation in the cystic fibrosis transmembrane conductance regulator (CFTR) gene. This investigation, published in the New England Journal of Medicine, was part of the research considered by the FDA in making its decision to approve this drug for use in the United States. Fig 1 in the original article depicts changes from baseline in percentage of predicted forced expiratory volume in 1 second, respiratory symptoms, and weight, and time to the first pulmonary exacerbation, according to the study group. The estimated annual cost of twice-daily dosing for ivacaftor is nearly $300 000; however, Vertex has announced plans to provide the drug for free to patients without insurance and who make less than $150 000 annually. FDA approval of this drug represents expedited approval of a genetic-based approach to disease management. The biggest winners in 2012 are the patients who will benefit from this new drug.

S. K. Willsie, DO, MA

Comparative Efficacy and Safety of 4 Randomized Regimens to Treat Early
***Pseudomonas aeruginosa* Infection in Children With Cystic Fibrosis**
Treggiari MM, for the Early Pseudomonas Infection Control (EPIC)
Investigators (Univ of Washington, Seattle, et al)
Arch Pediatr Adolesc Med 165:847-856, 2011

Objective.—To investigate the efficacy and safety of 4 antipseudomonal treatments in children with cystic fibrosis with recently acquired *Pseudomonas aeruginosa* infection.

Design.—Randomized controlled trial.

Setting.—Multicenter trial in the United States.

Participants.—Three hundred four children with cystic fibrosis aged 1 to 12 years within 6 months of *P aeruginosa* detection.

Interventions.—Participants were randomized to 1 of 4 antibiotic regimens for 18 months (six 12-week quarters) between December 2004 and June 2009. Participants randomized to cycled therapy received tobramycin inhalation solution (300 mg twice a day) for 28 days, with oral ciprofloxacin (15-20 mg/kg twice a day) or oral placebo for 14 days every quarter, while participants randomized to culture-based therapy received the same treatments only during quarters with positive *P aeruginosa* cultures.

Main Outcome Measures.—The primary end points were time to pulmonary exacerbation requiring intravenous antibiotics and proportion of *P aeruginosa*—positive cultures.

Results.—The intention-to-treat analysis included 304 participants. There was no interaction between treatments. There were no statistically significant differences in exacerbation rates between cycled and culture-based groups (hazard ratio, 0.95; 95% confidence interval [CI], 0.54-1.66) or ciprofloxacin and placebo (hazard ratio, 1.45; 95% CI, 0.82-2.54). The odds ratios of *P aeruginosa*—positive culture comparing the cycled vs culture-based group were 0.78 (95% CI, 0.49-1.23) and 1.10 (95% CI, 0.71-1.71) comparing ciprofloxacin vs placebo. Adverse events were similar across groups.

Conclusions.—No difference in the rate of exacerbation or prevalence of *P aeruginosa* positivity was detected between cycled and culture-based therapies. Adding ciprofloxacin produced no benefits.

Trial Registration.—ClinicalTrials.gov Identifier: NCT00097773.

▶ This is the largest randomized trial to date of young patients (1 to < 12 years) with cystic fibrosis enrolled within 6 months of sentinel isolation of respiratory tract *Pseudomonas aeruginosa* (PA). Groups (4) were randomly assigned to 1 of 4 antibiotic regimens (every 3 months from 2004 through June 2009), which included tobramycin inhaled solution (TIS) with ciprofloxacin or placebo as cycled therapy versus therapy based on results of respiratory cultures (TIS with or with ciprofloxacin vs placebo). Fig 3 in the original article depicts results of the study. Overall, the addition of ciprofloxacin produced no benefit; a trend was seen toward increased cough in the group receiving ciprofloxacin treatments. Regular use of TIS for new-onset colonization of the lower airways in cystic fibrosis patients is not supported by this study. Based on the results of this investigation, routine surveillance cultures and judicious treatment of emerging infections is the recommended approach in this population.

S. K. Willsie, DO, MA

Improved treatment response to dornase alfa in cystic fibrosis patients using controlled inhalation
Bakker EM, Volpi S, Salonini E, et al (Erasmus MC — Sophia Children's Hosp, Rotterdam, The Netherlands; et al)
Eur Respir J 38:1328-1335, 2011

Better treatment of obstructed small airways is needed in cystic fibrosis. This study investigated whether efficient deposition of dornase alfa in the small airways improves small airway obstruction.

In a multicentre, double-blind, randomised controlled clinical trial, cystic fibrosis patients on maintenance treatment with 2.5 mL dornase alfa once daily were switched to a smart nebuliser and randomised to small airway deposition (n=24) or large airway deposition (n=25) for 4 weeks. The primary outcome parameter was forced expiratory flow at 75% of forced vital capacity ($FEF_{75\%}$).

$FEF_{75\%}$ increased significantly by 0.7 SD (5.2% predicted) in the large airways group and 1.2 SD (8.8% pred) in the small airways group. Intention-to-treat analysis did not show a significant difference in treatment effect between groups. Per-protocol analysis, excluding patients not completing the trial or with adherence <70%, showed a trend (p=0.06) in $FEF_{75\%}$ Z-score and a significant difference (p=0.04) between groups in absolute $FEF_{75\%}$ ($L \cdot s^{-1}$) favouring small airway deposition.

Improved delivery of dornase alfa using a smart nebuliser that aids patients in correct inhalation technique resulted in significant improvement of $FEF_{75\%}$ in children with stable cystic fibrosis. Adherent children showed a larger treatment response for small airway deposition.

▶ Cystic fibrosis (CF) patients receiving stable inhaled dornase alfa were randomly assigned to 4 weeks of dornase alfa delivered via a smart nebulizer to deliver either large or small airway deposition; serial lung function studies were performed to determine whether the new delivery technique led to improved lung function. Fig 3 in the original article depicts the differences between small and large airway deposition of the dornase alfa using the smart nebulizer. Improved small airway delivery via smart nebulizer led to statistically significant improvement of the $FEF_{75\%}$ and $FEF_{25\%-75\%}$ (note both large and small airway delivery led to improvement). Studies over longer terms with efficacy testing to determine whether the improvement in airway function is maintained are needed.

S. K. Willsie, DO, MA

2 Chronic Obstructive Pulmonary Disease

Introduction

This year's chapter on chronic obstructive lung disease is divided into 4 sections. The first section deals with epidemiological studies and other population-related investigations that describe the manifestation of chronic obstructive pulmonary disease (COPD) in various population groups. The ability to look at the bigger picture of COPD has been more possible in the last decade or so with the formation of investigator groups able to perform multicenter studies and collect data on large numbers of patients. Other investigators have used government, government-supported, and other centralized databases to access population-related information. From these efforts, characteristics of manifestations of the disease across different sexes, ethnicities, and geographies have been described. Some of the US-based groups have included the Lung Health Study, the National Emphysema Treatment Trial Investigators, the COPD Clinical Research Network, and the Genetic Epidemiology of COPD Investigators. Similar groups have been active internationally. In this YEAR BOOK, we have included studies from several of these types of sources. Topics include the lifetime risk of developing COPD, risks of COPD mortality related to geography, additional insights into risks of COPD patients for developing lung cancer, racial differences in the way COPD is experienced, factors associated with early-onset COPD, heterogeneity in the progression of COPD, and a description of the bronchitic phenotype of COPD. These studies have been very helpful in giving us a more complete and accurate picture of the prevalence, broad range of presentations, and progression of COPD.

A second group of articles deals with acute exacerbations of COPD. Acute exacerbations continue to be a difficult aspect of treatment and greatly affect not only quality of life, but also disease progression. The first article represents early attempts to characterize exacerbations by using biomarkers; this approach may be able to classify exacerbations in such a way that therapy can be specifically directed. A second study presents an approach to closing a gap in the early assessment of COPD exacerbations. Unlike in community-acquired pneumonia, an outcome risk score by which prognosis can be predicted does not exist for COPD exacerbations. The authors propose such a scoring system which could be helpful in the treatment of these patients.

Other studies address self-management through the use of an action plan and the use of azithromycin for possible prevention of exacerbations.

A number of systemic reviews and meta-analyses addressing various aspects of COPD and COPD management were published in 2011. Two addressing medication management were selected for the YEAR BOOK. The first is a meta-analysis that evaluates the troubling question raised in several studies of increased cardiovascular events with anticholinergic medications. This particular meta-analysis looks at tiotropium and mortality. The second study is also a meta-analysis of medication complications—in this case, fracture risk with inhaled corticosteroids.

The final section is a potpourri of 3 articles. Two address important but often neglected areas of interest in COPD patients: first, the effect of anxiety and depression on rehabilitation outcomes and second, the role of bronchiectasis in COPD. The third article is about the importance of beta blockers in COPD. New data suggest that, unlike the standard dogma about beta blockers, not only are beta blockers generally well tolerated, they may extend life. More to come in this area.

Janet R. Maurer, MD, MBA

Lifetime risk of developing chronic obstructive pulmonary disease: a longitudinal population study

Gershon AS, Warner L, Cascagnette P, et al (Inst for Clinical Evaluative Sciences, Toronto, Ontario, Canada; et al)
Lancet 378:991-996, 2011

Background.—Although chronic obstructive pulmonary disease (COPD) is one of the most deadly, prevalent, and costly chronic diseases, no comprehensive estimates of the risk of developing COPD in the general population have been published. We aimed to quantify the lifetime risk of developing physician-diagnosed COPD in a large, multicultural North American population.

Methods.—We did a retrospective longitudinal cohort study using population-based health administrative data from Ontario, Canada (total population roughly 13 million). All individuals free of COPD in 1996 were monitored for up to 14 years for three possible outcomes; diagnosis of COPD by a physician, reached 80 years of age, or death. COPD was identified with a previously validated case definition based on COPD health services claims. The cumulative incidence of physician-diagnosed COPD over a lifetime adjusted for the competing risk of death was calculated by a modified survival analysis technique. Results were stratified by sex, socioeconomic status, and whether individuals lived in a rural or urban setting.

Findings.—A total of 579 466 individuals were diagnosed with COPD by a physician over the study period. The overall lifetime risk of physician-diagnosed COPD at age 80 years was 27·6%. Lifetime risk was higher in men than in women (29·7% vs 25·6%), individuals of lower socioeconomic status than in those of higher socioeconomic status (32·1% vs 23·0%), and individuals who lived in a rural setting than in those who lived in an urban setting (32·4% vs 26·7%).

Interpretation.—About one in four individuals are likely to be diagnosed and receive medical attention for COPD during their lifetime. Clinical evidence-based approaches, public health action, and more research are needed to identify effective strategies to prevent COPD and ensure that those with the disease have the highest quality of life possible (Fig 1).

▶ Despite increased attention to chronic obstructive pulmonary disease (COPD) in recent years, it remains both an underfunded and underrecognized disease.[1] Gershon et al note that although it is currently the fourth most common cause of death worldwide and expected by the World Health Organization to be the third most common cause by 2030, there is a general paucity of public knowledge about the disease. That, they speculate, is because the average person believes that this is a disease people "bring on themselves" through unhealthy behaviors such as smoking. Although smoking-related disease is a common cause of the disease, biofuel use is increasingly recognized as a causative factor, and it is increasingly recognized that among the general public, there is a significant rate of COPD that does not (at present) have a specific known cause. The authors believe that increased public awareness through articles such as this showing a general population risk of disease will help to funnel more funding to better understand the causes and impact of chronic pulmonary disease. The strength of this study is that covers the lifetime risk of physician-diagnosed COPD (Fig 1) in a complete population of a specific region (Ontario, Canada); however, that the study uses physician diagnoses and not confirmatory spirometry is also its greatest limitation. Physicians frequently assign a diagnosis of

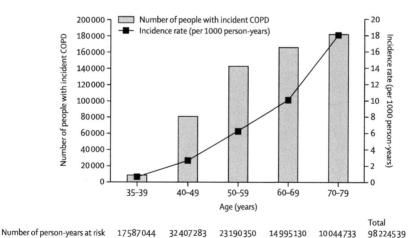

	35–39	40–49	50–59	60–69	70–79	Total
Number of person-years at risk	17 587 044	32 407 283	23 190 350	14 995 130	10 044 733	98 224 539

FIGURE 1.—Number of people with incident COPD, number of person-years at risk, and COPD incidence rate per 1000 person-years by age. COPD=chronic obstructive pulmonary disease. (Reprinted from The Lancet, Gershon AS, Warner L, Cascagnette P, et al. Lifetime risk of developing chronic obstructive pulmonary disease: a longitudinal population study. *Lancet.* 2011;378:991-996. © 2011, with permission from Elsevier.)

COPD to symptomatology (eg, shortness of breath) and record a diagnosis without objective confirmation. On the other hand, it is estimated that many people with actual COPD never have objective confirmation because the clinician does not order it. Which of these is most prevalent is unknown. At any rate, the study is thought-provoking and likely to achieve the authors' goal of increasing awareness.

J. R. Maurer, MD, MBA

Reference

1. Wise RA, Tashkin DP. Preventing chronic obstructive pulmonary disease: what is known and what needs to be done to make a difference to the patient? *Am J Med.* 2007;120:S14-S22.

Geographic Isolation and the Risk for Chronic Obstructive Pulmonary Disease—Related Mortality: A Cohort Study

Abrams TE, Vaughan-Sarrazin M, Fan VS, et al (Iowa City Veterans Affairs Med Ctr; Univ of Iowa; Veterans Affairs Puget Sound Health Care System and Univ of Washington, Seattle)
Ann Intern Med 155:80-86, 2011

Background.—Little is known about the possible differences in outcomes between patients with chronic obstructive pulmonary disease (COPD) who live in rural areas and those who live in urban areas of the United States.

Objective.—To determine whether COPD-related mortality is higher in persons living in rural areas, and to assess whether hospital characteristics influence any observed associations.

Design.—Retrospective cohort study.

Setting.—129 acute care Veterans Affairs hospitals.

Patients.—Hospitalized patients with a COPD exacerbation.

Measurements.—Patient rurality (primary exposure); 30-day mortality (primary outcome); and hospital volume and hospital rurality, defined as the mean proportion of hospital admissions coming from rural areas (secondary exposures).

Results.—18 809 patients (71% of the study population) lived in urban areas, 5671 (21%) in rural areas, and 1919 (7%) in isolated rural areas. Mortality was increased in patients living in isolated rural areas compared with urban areas (5.0% vs. 3.8%; $P = 0.002$). The increase in mortality associated with living in an isolated rural area persisted after adjustment for patient characteristics and hospital rurality and volume (odds ratio [OR], 1.42 [95% CI, 1.07 to 1.89]; $P = 0.016$). Adjusted mortality did not seem to be higher in patients living in nonisolated rural areas (OR, 1.09 [CI, 0.90 to 1.32]; $P = 0.47$). Results were unchanged in analyses assessing the influence of an omitted confounder on estimates.

Limitations.—The study population was limited to mostly male inpatients who were veterans. Results were based on administrative data.

Conclusion.—Patients with COPD living in isolated rural areas of the United States seem to be at greater risk for COPD exacerbation—related mortality than those living in urban areas, independent of hospital rurality and volume. Mortality was not increased for patients living in nonisolated rural areas.

▶ Over the last 20 years, many studies from The Dartmouth Atlas of Healthcare have documented a variety of health care disparities in the United States in the Medicare population. That particular entity uses administrative Medicare data to compare treatments, laboratory evaluation, and other components of health care delivery for various conditions and situations in different parts of the country. Its reports have detailed a dramatic level of disparity in the delivery of care for the same conditions or diseases in different geographic locations in the United States.[1] Abrams et al detail another type of disparity in a large Veterans Affairs population. This disparity is based on whether you live in rural areas versus those living in non-rural areas. The finding that COPD exacerbation—related mortality is increased only in isolated rural areas but not in other rural areas compared with urban areas is interesting. This differential mortality may be caused by either health care availability in the isolated areas or potentially by the type of person—including attitudes toward health care providers, socioeconomic level, etc—living in an isolated rural setting and his or her propensity to seek health care or when to seek health care. Which of these factors, or both, is at play here is unknown. This study, while intriguing, does have significant limitations in that its subjects were mostly male veterans and it used administrative data only.

J. R. Maurer, MD, MBA

Reference

1. Understanding of the Efficiency and Effectiveness of the Health Care System. http://www.dartmouthatlas.org/. Accessed December 29, 2011.

Lung Cancer in Patients with Chronic Obstructive Pulmonary Disease: Incidence and Predicting Factors

de Torres JP, Marín JM, Casanova C, et al (Clínica Universidad de Navarra, Pamplona, Spain; Hospital Universitario Miguel Servet, Zaragoza, Spain; Hospital Nuestra Sra de Candelaria, Tenerife, Spain; et al)
Am J Respir Crit Care Med 184:913-919, 2011

Rationale.—Little is known about the clinical factors associated with the development of lung cancer in patients with chronic obstructive pulmonary disease (COPD), although airway obstruction and emphysema have been identified as possible risk factors.

Objectives.—To explore incidence, histologic type, and factors associated with development of lung cancer diagnosis in a cohort of outpatients with COPD attending a pulmonary clinic.

Methods.—A cohort of 2,507 patients without initial clinical or radiologic evidence of lung cancer was followed a median of 60 months (30—90). At baseline, anthropometrics, smoking history, lung function, and body composition were recorded. Time to diagnosis and histologic type of lung cancer was then registered. Cox analysis was used to explore factors associated with lung cancer diagnosis.

Measurements and Main Results.—A total of 215 of the 2,507 patients with COPD developed lung cancer (incidence density of 16.7 cases per 1,000 person-years). The most frequent type was squamous cell carcinoma (44%). Lung cancer incidence was lower in patients with worse severity of airflow obstruction. Global Initiative for Chronic Obstructive Lung Disease Stages I and II, older age, lower body mass index, and lung diffusion capacity of carbon monoxide less than 80% were associated with lung cancer diagnosis.

Conclusions.—Incidence density of lung cancer is high in outpatients with COPD and occurs more frequently in older patients with milder airflow obstruction (Global Initiative for Chronic Obstructive Lung Disease Stages I and II) and lower body mass index. A lung diffusion capacity of carbon monoxide less than 80% is associated with cancer diagnosis. Squamous cell carcinoma is the most frequent histologic type. Knowledge of these factors may help direct efforts for early detection of lung cancer and disease management.

▶ It seems intuitively obvious that there would be a high likelihood that patients with more severe chronic obstructive pulmonary disease (COPD) are also particularly susceptible to lung cancer since tobacco is the primary risk factor in both diseases. Yet the data linking these disease entities are often not very detailed and somewhat contradictory.[1,2] One of the larger studies reported from registry data gave an incidence estimate in the population with moderate and severe obstruction followed over a median of 17.9 years but did not identify people with milder degrees of airway obstruction and therefore may underestimate the correlation between mild COPD and lung cancer.[3] The exclusion of patients with milder obstruction may be important, because other studies, including this one, identify a higher incidence of cancers in patients with milder obstructive disease, a seemingly paradoxical finding.[4,5] The authors provide speculation as to why this might be. The most intriguing reason hinges on immune function. The authors speculate that possibly smokers with mild disease that get cancer are relatively immune suppressed by their smoking and therefore have less immune-related lung destruction but also have a higher susceptibility to cancer because of immunosuppression. This study provides several valuable insights in addition to confirming the inverse relationship between airflow obstruction and development of lung cancer. In particular, because it was a study in which the patients were followed up clinically for a median of 5 years, other risk factors for lung cancer were observed: older age, lower body mass index, and diffusing capacity of the lung < 80%. Knowing the risk factors allows easier and less expensive monitoring of a specific subgroup and the potential for early diagnosis and improved outcomes.

J. R. Maurer, MD, MBA

References

1. Tockman MS, Anthonisen NR, Wright EC, Donithan MG. Airways obstruction and the risk for lung cancer. *Ann Intern Med.* 1987;106:512-518.
2. Van den Eeden SK, Friedman GD. Forced expiratory volume (1 second) and lung cancer incidence and mortality. *Epidemiology.* 1992;3:253-257.
3. Mannino DM, Aguayo SM, Petty TL, Redd SC. Low lung function and incident lung cancer in the United States: data from the First National Health and Nutrition Examination Survey follow-up. *Arch Intern Med.* 2003;163:1475-1480.
4. Caplin M, Festenstein F. Relation between lung cancer, chronic bronchitis, and airways obstruction. *Br Med J.* 1975;3:678-680.
5. Wilson DO, Weissfeld JL, Balkan A, et al. Association of radiographic emphysema and airflow obstruction with lung cancer. *Am J Respir Crit Care Med.* 2008;178:738-744.

Racial Differences in Quality of Life in Patients With COPD

Han MK, the COPDGene Investigators (Univ of Michigan Health System, Ann Arbor; et al)

Chest 140:1169-1176, 2011

Background.—Although COPD is associated with significant health-related quality-of-life (HRQL) impairment, factors influencing HRQL in patients with COPD are not well understood, particularly in African Americans. We hypothesized that HRQL in COPD differs by race and sought to identify factors associated with those differences.

Methods.—We analyzed 224 African American and 1,049 Caucasian subjects with COPD enrolled in the COPDGene (Genetic Epidemiology of COPD) Study whose conditions were classified as GOLD (Global Initiative for Chronic Obstructive Lung Disease) stages I to IV. HRQL and symptoms were compared using the St. George Respiratory Questionnaire (SGRQ) and the modified Medical Research Council Dyspnea (MMRC) scale. We constructed a mixed-effects linear regression model for SGRQ score.

Results.—African Americans were younger and reported fewer pack-years of smoking, more current smoking, and less attained education than Caucasians; MMRC scores were higher ($P = .02$) as were SGRQ scores (mean score difference, 8.4; $P < .001$). In a general linear model of SGRQ total score after adjusting for factors such as age, sex, and pack-years of smoking, SGRQ total score was similar for African Americans and Caucasians who reported no COPD exacerbations in the prior year. However, for subjects with exacerbations, SGRQ total score was increased to a greater relative extent for African Americans than for Caucasians (1.89 points for each exacerbation, $P = .006$). For hospitalized exacerbations, the effect on SGRQ total score also was greater for African Americans (4.19 points, $P = .04$). Furthermore, a larger percentage of African Americans reported having had at least one exacerbation that required hospitalization in the prior year (32% vs 16%, P < .001).

Conclusion.—In analyses that account for other variables that affect quality of life, HRQL is similar for African Americans and Caucasians with COPD without exacerbations but worse for African Americans who experience exacerbations, particularly hospitalized exacerbations.

▶ One of the most important benefits of the creation of large databases of victims of specific diseases is the ability to identify characteristics of the impact of the disease in specific subgroups of patients. For example, the large database from the National Emphysema Treatment Trial conducted at the turn of the century has been used to show differences in the pathophysiology and course of chronic obstructive pulmonary disease (COPD) in males and females.[1,2] The COPD Gene Study (Genetic Epidemiology of COPD) is a database of 10 000 COPD patients and, while focused initially on phenotypes of COPD, picks up and furthers the understanding of different phenotypes of COPD. This report describes differences in racial impact of the disease in terms of health-related quality of life. But, as the authors note, this may not be the whole story. In fact, this disease impact may relate to many factors that include, among others, social, economic, and education differences as well as differences in treatment available to African Americans. In fact, this type of report should be an initial foray into helping us better understand the multifactorial approaches necessary to improve health outcomes for everyone.

J. R. Maurer, MD, MBA

References

1. Martinez FJ, Curtis JL, Sciurba F, et al; National Emphysema Treatment Trial Research Group. Sex differences in severe pulmonary emphysema. *Am J Respir Crit Care Med.* 2007;176:243-252.
2. Fan VS, Ramsey SD, Giardino ND, et al; National Emphysema Treatment Trial (NETT) Research Group. Sex, depression, and risk of hospitalization and mortality in chronic obstructive pulmonary disease. *Arch Intern Med.* 2007;167:2345-2353.

Early-Onset Chronic Obstructive Pulmonary Disease Is Associated with Female Sex, Maternal Factors, and African American Race in the COPDGene Study

Foreman MG, the COPDGene Investigators (Morehouse School of Medicine, Atlanta, GA; et al)

Am J Respir Crit Care Med 184:414-420, 2011

Rationale.—The characterization of young adults who develop late-onset diseases may augment the detection of novel genes and promote new pathogenic insights.

Methods.—We analyzed data from 2,500 individuals of African and European ancestry in the COPDGene Study. Subjects with severe, early-onset chronic obstructive pulmonary disease (COPD) (n = 70, age < 55 yr,

FEV$_1$ < 50% predicted) were compared with older subjects with COPD (n = 306, age > 64 yr, FEV$_1$ < 50% predicted).

Measurements and Main Results.—Subjects with severe, early-onset COPD were predominantly females (66%), $P = 0.0004$. Proportionally, early-onset COPD was seen in 42% (25 of 59) of African Americans versus 14% (45 of 317) of non-Hispanic whites, $P < 0.0001$. Other risk factors included current smoking (56 vs. 17%, $P < 0.0001$) and self-report of asthma (39 vs. 25%, $P = 0.008$). Maternal smoking (70 vs. 44%, $P = 0.0001$) and maternal COPD (23 vs. 12%, $P = 0.03$) were reported more commonly in subjects with early-onset COPD. Multivariable regression analysis found association with African American race, odds ratio (OR), 7.5 (95% confidence interval [CI], 2.3—24; $P = 0.0007$); maternal COPD, OR, 4.7 (95% CI, 1.3—17; $P = 0.02$); female sex, OR, 3.1 (95% CI, 1.1—8.7; $P = 0.03$); and each pack-year of smoking, OR, 0.98 (95% CI, 0.96—1.0; $P = 0.03$).

Conclusions.—These observations support the hypothesis that severe, early-onset COPD is prevalent in females and is influenced by maternal factors. Future genetic studies should evaluate (*1*) gene-by-sex interactions to address sex-specific genetic contributions and (*2*) gene-by-race interactions.

▶ Chronic obstructive pulmonary disease (COPD) is well recognized in most cases as a primarily tobacco-caused disease with a loose dose-related relationship to the amount of tobacco used. Genetic studies are starting to identify innate susceptibilities to the effects of smoking. In recent years, the first large studies of populations with obstructive disease along with the collections of patients with advanced obstructive pathology in transplant centers and lung volume reduction programs has led to a better understanding of a complex array of disease features. One observation was that there exists a cohort of patients with early-onset disease. A report of a particular family cohort that did not have evidence of known hereditary alpha-1 antitrypsin disease but appeared to have onset of disease before the age of 52 noted that a large number of the family members with disease were women.[1] Another report from analysis of the database of the National Emphysema Treatment Trial (NETT) showed that the African-American participants appeared to have more severe and earlier-onset disease compared with whites with similar amounts of smoking.[2] With that background, Foreman et al looked at the first 2500 entrants into the COPDGene study in an attempt to more systematically confirm or disprove these findings. In addition to the propensity of women and African Americans to be victims of this disease, the authors found that maternal smoking and COPD were also influential. The "why" remains unknown. The good news is that the early-onset disease is a relatively rare phenotype of COPD in that only 70 participants were identified. However, those with early-onset disease had significantly lower levels of smoking than the general population of patients with COPD, suggesting that a dose response is not the primary factor in development of their disease. There is a significant limitation to this disease: it is not population based but rather a subanalysis of 2500 patients with COPD who voluntarily participate in a COPD database. This is, therefore, a self-selected population. Nevertheless, the description of this phenotype of COPD should help direct future genetic and molecular studies with, as the authors note, particular attention "to maternally inherited factors such as mitochondrial and X- chromosome genes as well as gene-by-sex and gene-by-race interactions." Only when we have the results of such studies will we be better able to understand the "why."

J. R. Maurer, MD, MBA

References

1. Silverman EK, Chapman HA, Drazen JM, et al. Genetic epidemiology of severe, early-onset chronic obstructive pulmonary disease. Risk to relatives for airflow obstruction and chronic bronchitis. *Am J Respir Crit Care Med.* 1998;157: 1770-1778.
2. Chatila WM, Hoffman EA, Gaughan J, Robinswood GB, Criner GJ. Advanced emphysema in African-American and white patients: do differences exist? *Chest.* 2006;130:108-118.

The Progression of Chronic Obstructive Pulmonary Disease Is Heterogeneous: The Experience of the BODE Cohort
Casanova C, de Torres JP, Aguirre-Jaíme A, et al (Hospital Universitario La Candelaria, Tenerife, Spain; Clínica Universitaria de Navarra, Pamplona, Spain; et al)
Am J Respir Crit Care Med 184:1015-1021, 2011

Rationale.—Chronic obstructive pulmonary disease (COPD) is thought to result in rapid and progressive loss of lung function usually expressed as mean values for whole cohorts.

Objectives.—Longitudinal studies evaluating individual lung function loss and other domains of COPD progression are needed.

Methods.—We evaluated 1,198 stable, well-characterized patients with COPD (1,100 males) recruited in two centers (Florida and Tenerife, Spain) and annually monitored their multidomain progression from 1997 to 2009. Patients were followed for a median of 64 months and up to 10 years. Their individual FEV_1 (L) and BODE index slopes, expressed as annual change, were evaluated using regression models for repeated measures. A total of 751 patients with at least three measurements were used for the analyses.

Measurements and Main Results.—Eighteen percent of patients had a statistically significant FEV_1 slope decline (−86 ml/yr; 95% confidence interval [CI], −32 to −278 ml/yr). Higher baseline FEV_1 (relative risk, 1.857; 95% CI, 1.322−2.610; $P < 0.001$) and low body mass index (relative risk, 1.071; 95% CI, 1.035−1.106; $P < 0.001$) were independently associated with FEV_1 decline. The BODE index had a statistically significant increase (0.55, 0.20−1.37 point/yr) in only 14% of patients and these had more severe baseline obstruction. Concordance between FEV_1 and BODE change was low (κ Cohen, 16%). Interestingly, 73% of patients had no significant slope change in FEV_1 or BODE. Only the BODE change was associated with mortality in patients without FEV_1 progression.

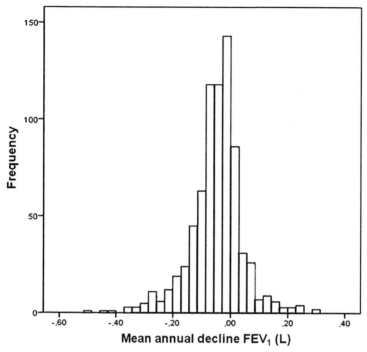

FIGURE 2.—Histogram of the mean annual FEV$_1$ decline (L) for the whole group. (Reprinted from Casanova C, de Torres JP, Aguirre-Jaíme A, et al. The progression of chronic obstructive pulmonary disease is heterogeneous: the experience of the BODE cohort. *Am J Respir Crit Care Med.* 2011;184:1015-1021. Official Journal of the American Thoracic Society © American Thoracic Society.)

Conclusions.—The progression of COPD is very heterogeneous. Most patients show no statistically significant decline of FEV$_1$ or increase in BODE. The multidimensional evaluation of COPD should offer insight into response to COPD management (Fig 2).

▶ The progression of chronic obstructive pulmonary disease (COPD) was initially documented by Fletcher and Peto in the 1970s.[1] Surprisingly, few longitudinal studies of patients with COPD have been done since that description of the natural history of airway obstruction, yet it has become very clear that COPD is a heterogeneous disease with many phenotypes. The studies that have been done have usually been in the context of drug treatment trials and included patients with specific characteristics that met the inclusion criteria of the study, which potentially limits the ability to capture varying courses of different phenotypes.[2,3] Clinical experience suggests that some patients may remain stable for long periods, whereas others may appear to progress rapidly. It would be natural to assume that different phenotypes behave differently and that progression may also be different. The study by Casanova et al sheds some light on this. The study reports follow up on a group of nearly 1200, mostly male, patients with COPD for a median of more than 5 years and up to 10 years. Progression was defined not only by change in FEV_1, but also by changes in the other parameters of the BODE index. During the follow-up period, most patients had neither a significant decrease in FEV_1 (Fig 2), or increase in BODE score. There was a small group that had a rapid progression of disease as measured by the BODE index but without a significant change in FEV_1. A third group had significant decreases in FEV_1 that was not related to their baseline level of obstruction. Vestbo et al,[4] reporting data from the ECLIPSE (Evaluation of COPD Longitudinally to Identify Predictive Surrogate Endpoints) trial, also noted large variability in the rate of decrease of FEV_1 and noted that the rate of decrease in smokers was greater than in nonsmokers and in patients with emphysema than those without.

These findings by Casanova et al led the authors to suggest that COPD should be thought of as having domains of both severity and activity. As COPD phenotype characteristics are better defined, categorizing by severity and activity—or using some other approach—may be helpful in tailoring therapy that is specific to the individual's needs.

J. R. Maurer, MD, MBA

References

1. Fletcher C, Peto R. The natural history of chronic airflow obstruction. *Br Med J.* 1977;1:1645-1648.
2. Anthonisen NR, Connett JE, Kiley JP, et al. Effects of smoking intervention and the use of an inhaled anticholinergic bronchodilator on the rate of decline of FEV1. The Lung Health Study. *JAMA.* 1994;272:1497-1505.
3. Celli BR, Thomas NE, Anderson JA, et al. Effect of pharmacotherapy on rate of decline of lung function in chronic obstructive pulmonary disease: results from the TORCH study. *Am J Respir Crit Care Med.* 2008;178:332-338.
4. Vestbo J, Edwards LD, Scanlon PD, et al; ECLIPSE investigators. Changes in forced expiratory volume in 1 second over time in COPD. *N Engl J Med.* 2011; 365:1184-1192.

The Chronic Bronchitic Phenotype of COPD: An Analysis of the COPDGene Study

Kim V, the COPDGene Investigators (Temple Univ School of Medicine, Philadelphia, PA; et al)

Chest 140:626-633, 2011

Background.—Chronic bronchitis (CB) in patients with COPD is associated with an accelerated lung function decline and an increased risk of respiratory infections. Despite its clinical significance, the chronic bronchitic phenotype in COPD remains poorly defined.

Methods.—We analyzed data from subjects enrolled in the Genetic Epidemiology of COPD (COPDGene) Study. A total of 1,061 subjects with GOLD (Global Initiative for Chronic Obstructive Lung Disease) stage II to IV were divided into two groups: CB (CB+) if subjects noted chronic cough and phlegm production for $\geq$ 3 mo/y for 2 consecutive years, and no CB (CB−) if they did not.

Results.—There were 290 and 771 subjects in the CB+ and CB− groups, respectively. Despite similar lung function, the CB+ group was younger (62.8 ± 8.4 vs 64.6 ± 8.4 years, $P = .002$), smoked more (57 ± 30 vs 52 ± 25 pack-years, $P = .006$), and had more current smokers (48% vs 27%, $P < .0001$). A greater percentage of the CB+ group reported nasal and ocular symptoms, wheezing, and nocturnal awakenings secondary to cough and dyspnea. History of exacerbations was higher in the CB 1 group (1.21 ± 1.62 vs 0.63 ± 1.12 per patient, $P < .027$), and more patients in the CB+ group reported a history of severe exacerbations (26.6% vs 20.0%, $P = .024$). There was no difference in percent emphysema or percent gas trapping, but the CB+ group had a higher mean percent segmental airway wall area (63.2% ± 2.9% vs 62.6% ± 3.1%, $P = .013$).

Conclusions.—CB in patients with COPD is associated with worse respiratory symptoms and higher risk of exacerbations. This group may need more directed therapy targeting chronic mucus production and smoking cessation not only to improve symptoms but also to reduce risk, improve quality of life, and improve outcomes.

Trial Registry.—ClinicalTrials.gov; No.: NCT00608764; URL: www. clinicaltrials.gov.

▶ The COPDGene Study is a National Heart, Lung, and Blood Institute—funded multicenter study that aims to find genetic predispositions to development of chronic obstructive pulmonary disease (COPD). Because the study has successfully enrolled its target of 10 000 patients, it is now in a unique position to fulfill one of its objectives of describing different COPD phenotypes. The study reported here included more than 1000 of the initial enrollees. Participants included 290 with classic symptoms that define chronic bronchitis and 771 controls who had obstruction but not symptoms of chronic bronchitis. Clinical data, including symptoms, exacerbation history, and quality-of-life assessment were collected primarily by questionnaires. The data on exacerbations were not verified by medical records, but the size of the populations included in the study minimizes the potential for significant error. Each patient did have pulmonary function studies, 6-minute walk test, and high-resolution computed tomography performed. This cross-sectional study revealed some interesting findings. Even though the chronic bronchitic group was, on average, about 2 years younger than the nonbronchitic group, they appear sicker both because of a higher rate of exacerbations and COPD symptomatology and because of more other medical comorbidities, such as angina, osteoporosis, diabetes, and poor-quality sleep. One area that unfortunately does not seem to have been addressed is whether the chronic bronchitic group had higher rates of depressive symptoms than the nonbronchitic group, although that seems highly likely given the higher level of pulmonary symptoms and other comorbidities. Although this is a cross-sectional observational study and, therefore, does not address outcomes, in general the findings suggest a need for a management strategy for this COPD phenotype. That strategy should include close coordination with the patient's primary care physician to ensure appropriate management of multiple medical conditions in addition to the pulmonary disease. More analysis of COPDGene Study participants will hopefully provide a better understanding of additional COPD phenotypes and enable directed management strategies.

J. R. Maurer, MD, MBA

Acute Exacerbations of Chronic Obstructive Pulmonary Disease: Identification of Biologic Clusters and Their Biomarkers

Bafadhel M, McKenna S, Terry S, et al (Univ of Leicester, UK; et al)
Am J Respir Crit Care Med 184:662-671, 2011

Rationale.—Exacerbations of chronic obstructive pulmonary disease (COPD) are heterogeneous with respect to inflammation and etiology.

Objectives.—Investigate biomarker expression in COPD exacerbations to identify biologic clusters and determine biomarkers that recognize clinical COPD exacerbation phenotypes, namely those associated with bacteria, viruses, or eosinophilic airway inflammation.

Methods.—Patients with COPD were observed for 1 year at stable and exacerbation visits. Biomarkers were measured in sputum and serum. Viruses and selected bacteria were assessed in sputum by polymerase chain reaction and routine diagnostic bacterial culture. Biologic phenotypes were explored using unbiased cluster analysis and biomarkers that differentiated clinical exacerbation phenotypes were investigated.

Measurements and Main Results.—A total of 145 patients (101 men and 44 women) entered the study. A total of 182 exacerbations were captured from 86 patients. Four distinct biologic exacerbation clusters were identified. These were bacterial-, viral-, or eosinophilic-predominant, and a fourth associated with limited changes in the inflammatory profile termed "pauciinflammatory." Of all exacerbations, 55%, 29%, and 28% were associated with bacteria, virus, or a sputum eosinophilia. The biomarkers that best identified these clinical phenotypes were sputum IL-1β, 0.89 (area under receiver operating characteristic curve) (95% confidence interval [CI], 0.83–0.95); serum CXCL10, 0.83 (95% CI, 0.70–0.96); and percentage peripheral eosinophils, 0.85 (95% CI, 0.78–0.93), respectively.

Conclusions.—The heterogeneity of the biologic response of COPD exacerbations can be defined. Sputum IL-1β, serum CXCL10, and peripheral eosinophils are biomarkers of bacteria-, virus-, or eosinophil-associated exacerbations of COPD. Whether phenotype-specific biomarkers can be applied to direct therapy warrants further investigation.

▶ Chronic obstructive pulmonary disease (COPD) exacerbations may appear similar clinically, but the underlying causes have been shown to be heterogeneous. Certain clinical features, eg, purulent sputum and laboratory tests such as cultures, have been used to help establish exacerbation phenotypes expressed in individual patients. In this study, the authors first assessed biologic phenotypes as bacterial, viral, or eosinophilic using culture, polymerase chain reaction, and eosinophil measurement and, in addition, performed biomarker analysis to try to associate specific biomarkers with the biologic data. Interestingly, in the study, etiology and inflammatory markers distinguished exacerbations; however, exacerbations were not clinically distinguishable. In the set of exacerbations, the following associations using the biologic and biomarker data were observed: bacteria alone, 37%; virus alone, 10%; sputum eosinophilia alone, 17%; bacteria plus virus, 12%; bacteria plus sputum eosinophilia, 6%; virus plus sputum eosinophilia, 3%; bacteria plus virus plus sputum eosinophilia, 1%; and no association (termed as *pauci-inflammatory*), 14%. Each exacerbation was placed in a category based on the predominant biologic and biomarker findings. Of note, the authors' bacterial and sputum eosinophilic, but not viral, exacerbations could be predicted from a stable state. Probably the most important result of this study was the ability to identify single specific biomarkers (sputum interleukin-1β, serum CXCL10, or peripheral eosinophilia) that are relatively sensitive and specific for different types of exacerbations. This type of information can potentially help target treatment and avoid shotgun approaches that might result in increased adverse events. Eosinophilic dominant exacerbations, for example, may respond to steroid alone. Another important question is whether outcomes can be predicted by better categorizing exacerbations. Is airway eosinophilia a prognostic marker?[1] Is the pauci-inflammatory cluster of exacerbations a real entity and if so, do they have prognostic value? As the authors note, their findings need to be prospectively tested in randomized studies of targeted therapy. We look forward to the results.

J. R. Maurer, MD, MBA

Reference

1. Hospers JJ, Schouten JP, Weiss ST, Rijcken B, Postma DS. Asthma attacks with eosinophilia predict mortality from chronic obstructive pulmonary disease in a general population sample. *Am J Respir Crit Care Med.* 1999;160:1869-1874.

Validation of a Novel Risk Score for Severity of Illness in Acute Exacerbations of COPD
Shorr AF, Sun X, Johannes RS, et al (Washington Hosp Ctr, DC; MedMined Services, Marlborough, MA)
Chest 140:1177-1183, 2011

Background.—Clinicians lack a validated tool for risk stratification in acute exacerbations of COPD (AECOPD). We sought to validate the BAP-65 (elevated BUN, altered mental status, pulse >109 beats/min, age >65 years) score for this purpose.

Methods.—We analyzed 34,699 admissions to 177 US hospitals (2007) with either a principal diagnosis of AECOPD or acute respiratory failure with a secondary diagnosis of AECOPD. Hospital mortality and need for mechanical ventilation (MV) served as co-primary end points. Length of stay (LOS) and costs represented secondary end points. We assessed the accuracy of BAP-65 via the area under the receiver operating characteristic curve (AUROC).

Results.—Nearly 4% of subjects died while hospitalized and approximately 9% required MV. Mortality increased with increasing BAP-65 class, ranging from < 1% in subjects in class I (score of 0) to >25% in those meeting all BAP-65 criteria (Cochran-Armitage trend test z = −38.48, P < .001). The need for MV also increased with escalating score (2% in the lowest risk cohort vs 55% in the highest risk group, Cochran-Armitage trend test z = −58.89, P < .001). The AUROC for BAP-65 for hospital mortality and/or need for MV measured 0.79 (95% CI, 0.78-0.80). The median LOS was 4 days, and mean hospital costs equaled $5,357. These also varied linearly with increasing BAP-65 score.

Conclusions.—The BAP-65 system captures severity of illness and represents a simple tool to categorize patients with AECOPD as to their risk for adverse outcomes. BAP-65 also correlates with measures of resource use. BAP-65 may represent a useful adjunct in the initial assessment of AECOPDs.

▶ Acute exacerbations of chronic obstructive pulmonary disease (COPD) contribute disproportionately to the morbidity and mortality of the disease. Despite the high rate of exacerbations in the disease, especially in moderately severe and severe disease, clinicians do not have a validated, easy-to-use tool to stratify exacerbation events according to severity or prognosis. Such a tool could improve treatment by assisting in making appropriate decisions early as well as providing much needed information about the epidemiology of COPD exacerbations. Similar tools have been useful to clinicians in the early management of community-acquired pneumonia[1,2] and pulmonary embolism.[3,4] In fact, clinicians may not even agree on what constitutes an exacerbation. Trappenburg et al[5] recently reviewed more than 50 articles assessing existing symptom-based algorithms to identify exacerbations. Most of the existing algorithms use a scoring system based on pulmonary symptoms. The authors found that not only were there "large inconsistencies in definitions, methods and accuracy to define symptom-based COPD exacerbations," they also found that minor changes in symptom criteria had large impacts on incidence and other features of exacerbations. Some investigators continue to pursue this approach; however, Jones et al[6] reported a possibly more sophisticated approach to pulmonary symptom assessment that tries to quantify symptoms to better characterize exacerbations. Unfortunately, this does not seem to meet the need for a useful tool to provide information on severity and prognosis. Shorr et al[7] have taken a different tack that is promising. They used an approach similar to that used in community-acquired pneumonia that relies on easily objectively measured systemic features of illness rather than specific qualitative or quantitative features of pulmonary symptoms. In this article, they validate retrospectively their previously reported scoring system in a very large cohort of patients who presented with COPD exacerbations. Of course, the patient requires a diagnosis of acute exacerbation before the tool can be applied. But the precise clinical changes an individual clinician uses to define an acute exacerbation may not be so important if this new tool can provide useful prognostic information once a diagnosis is made. The tool now requires validation prospectively over a large cohort of patients.

J. R. Maurer, MD, MBA

References

1. Fine MJ, Auble TE, Yealy DM, et al. A prediction rule to identify low-risk patients with community-acquired pneumonia. *N Engl J Med.* 1997;336:243-250.
2. Lim WS, van der Eerden MM, Laing R, et al. Defining community acquired pneumonia severity on presentation to hospital: an international derivation and validation study. *Thorax.* 2003;58:377-382.
3. Aujesky D, Obrosky DS, Stone RA, et al. Derivation and validation of a prognostic model for pulmonary embolism. *Am J Respir Crit Care Med.* 2005;172:1041-1046.
4. Sanchez O, Trinquart L, Caille V, et al. Prognostic factors for pulmonary embolism: the prep study, a prospective multicenter cohort study. *Am J Respir Crit Care Med.* 2010;181:168-173.
5. Trappenburg JC, van Deventer AC, Troosters T, et al. The impact of using different symptom-based exacerbation algorithms in patients with COPD. *Eur Respir J.* 2011;37:1260-1268.
6. Jones PW, Chen WH, Wilcox TK, Sethi S, Leidy NK, EXACT-PRO Study Group. Characterizing and quantifying the symptomatic features of COPD exacerbations. *Chest.* 2011;139:1388-1394.
7. Tabak YP, Sun X, Johannes RS, Gupta V, Shorr AF. Mortality and need for mechanical ventilation in acute exacerbations of chronic obstructive pulmonary disease: development and validation of a simple risk score. *Arch Intern Med.* 2009;169:1595-1602.

Effect of an action plan with ongoing support by a case manager on exacerbation-related outcome in patients with COPD: a multicentre randomised controlled trial

Trappenburg JCA, Monninkhof EM, Bourbeau J, et al (Univ Med Ctr Utrecht, The Netherlands; McGill Univ, Montreal, Quebec, Canada; et al)

Thorax 66:977-984, 2011

Background.—An individualised action plan (AP) is a potentially effective method of helping patients with chronic obstructive pulmonary disease (COPD) to recognise and anticipate early exacerbation symptoms. This multicentre randomised controlled trial evaluates the hypothesis that individualised APs reduce exacerbation recovery time.

Methods.—Two hundred and thirty-three patients with COPD (age 65 ± 10 years, forced expiratory volume in 1 s $56 \pm 21\%$ predicted) were randomised to receive either an individualised AP (n=111) or care as usual (n=122). The AP provides individualised treatment prescriptions (pharmaceutical and non-pharmaceutical) related to a colour-coded symptom status to enhance an adequate response to periods of symptom deterioration (reinforced at 1 and 4 months). Exacerbation onset was defined using the Anthonisen symptom diary card algorithm. Every 3 days the Clinical COPD Questionnaire (CCQ) was assessed to evaluate the longitudinal course of health status. The primary outcome was health status recovery in the event of an exacerbation.

Results.—During the 6-month follow-up period there was no difference in exacerbation rates and healthcare utilisation between the two groups. Cox-adjusted survival analysis including frailty showed enhanced health status recovery (HR 1.58; 95% CI 0.96 to 2.60) and reduced length of the exacerbation (HR 1.30; 95% CI 0.92 to 1.84). The mean difference in symptom recovery time was −3.68 days (95% CI −7.32 to −0.04). Mixed model repeated measure analysis showed that an AP decreased the impact of exacerbations on health status both in the prodromal and early post-onset periods. Between-group differences in CCQ scores were above the minimal clinically relevant difference of 0.4 points (3.0 ± 0.7 vs 3.4 ± 0.9; p≤0.01).

Conclusion.—This study shows that an individualised AP, including ongoing support by a case manager, decreases the impact of exacerbations on health status and tends to accelerate recovery. APs can be considered a key component of self-management programmes in patients with COPD.

▶ Increasing concerns about cost of management of patients with chronic illnesses like chronic obstructive pulmonary disease (COPD) as well as poor outcomes has focused attention on educating patients to take more responsibility for self-management. This approach is designed not only to hopefully reduce the use of expensive health care resources, but also to give patients a better sense of control over their illnesses, to initiate medication changes or other treatment interventions early when symptoms change, and to improve overall quality of life, including reducing depressive symptoms. Studies to date on the impact of self-management strategies have generally not shown a large impact in any of these areas.[1] However, many of these have been small and with relatively short follow-up, particularly in the context of a long-lived chronic condition. What is appealing in the self-management study by Trappenburg et al is that it focuses not on the ability to reduce the number of exacerbations (probably not something most patients have control over), but rather on achieving a better quality of life by reducing the impact of exacerbations that do occur. A great strength of the study is it is multicenter and it included a control arm. Because a very detailed diary approach to recording symptom changes was part of the study, it also provided better information about the day-to-day fluctuations of the disease. By the same token, a major limitation of this study is that it had only 6-month follow-up. The short follow-up probably is the reason that no impact on health care costs was seen as another recent randomized trial that had follow-up for 1 year did, in fact, show cost effectiveness of use of an action plan.[2] As more prospective studies using a variety of self-management approaches are published, we will hopefully be able to select strategies for individual patients that will not only improve lives but also reduce the cost of care.

J. R. Maurer, MD, MBA

References

1. Effing T, Monninkhof EM, van der Valk PD, et al. Self-management education for patients with chronic obstructive pulmonary disease. *Cochrane Database Syst Rev.* 2007;(4). CD002990.
2. Effing T, Kerstjens H, van der Valk P, Zielhuis G, van der Palen J. (Cost)-effectiveness of self-treatment of exacerbations on the severity of exacerbations in patients with COPD: the COPE II study. *Thorax.* 2009;64:956-962.

Azithromycin for Prevention of Exacerbations of COPD

Albert RK, for the COPD Clinical Research Network (Univ of Colorado Denver Health Sciences Ctr; et al)
N Engl J Med 365:689-698, 2011

Background.—Acute exacerbations adversely affect patients with chronic obstructive pulmonary disease (COPD). Macrolide antibiotics benefit patients with a variety of inflammatory airway diseases.

Methods.—We performed a randomized trial to determine whether azithromycin decreased the frequency of exacerbations in participants with COPD who had an increased risk of exacerbations but no hearing impairment, resting tachycardia, or apparent risk of prolongation of the corrected QT interval.

Results.—A total of 1577 subjects were screened; 1142 (72%) were randomly assigned to receive azithromycin, at a dose of 250 mg daily (570 participants), or placebo (572 participants) for 1 year in addition to their usual care. The rate of 1-year follow-up was 89% in the azithromycin group and 90% in the placebo group. The median time to the first exacerbation was 266 days (95% confidence interval [CI], 227 to 313) among participants receiving azithromycin, as compared with 174 days (95% CI, 143 to 215) among participants receiving placebo (P<0.001). The frequency of exacerbations was 1.48 exacerbations per patient-year in the azithromycin group, as compared with 1.83 per patient-year in the placebo group (P=0.01), and the hazard ratio for having an acute exacerbation of COPD per patient-year in the azithromycin group was 0.73 (95% CI, 0.63 to 0.84; P<0.001). The scores on the St. George's Respiratory Questionnaire (on a scale of 0 to 100, with lower scores indicating better functioning) improved more in the azithromycin group than in the placebo group (a mean [±SD] decrease of 2.8±12.8 vs. 0.6±11.4, P=0.004); the percentage of participants with more than the minimal clinically important difference of −4 units was 43% in the azithromycin group, as compared with 36% in the placebo group (P=0.03). Hearing decrements were more common in the azithromycin group than in the placebo group (25% vs. 20%, P=0.04).

Conclusions.—Among selected subjects with COPD, azithromycin taken daily for 1 year, when added to usual treatment, decreased the frequency of exacerbations and improved quality of life but caused hearing decrements in a small percentage of subjects. Although this intervention could change microbial resistance patterns, the effect of this change is not known. (Funded by the National Institutes of Health; ClinicalTrials.gov number, NCT00325897.)

▶ The COPD Clinical Research Network was first formed in 2003 to provide a mechanism through which multicenter clinical trials in chronic obstructive pulmonary disease (COPD) could be organized and executed. This mechanism has been very useful for not only COPD, but for other pulmonary diseases/conditions including asthma, pulmonary fibrosis, and adult respiratory distress syndrome in which there are rarely enough patients in single centers to conduct trials of adequate size in a reasonable period. The COPD Clinical Research Network has completed well-designed trials that assessed use of leukotriene inhibitors in COPD exacerbations and compared the immune response with pneumococcal capsular polysaccharide and protein conjugate vaccines in addition to the trial of azithromycin use reported here. The impetus for this trial came from some preliminary evidence that macrolides might be beneficial in reducing exacerbations. However, as is often the case, each of these previous trials had some methodologic issues that hampered interpretation of the results, eg, small numbers, lack of controls, and lack of blinding.[1-3] This trial included more than 1100 participants and had a placebo arm.

Approximately 80% of the participants in this study were already taking inhaled corticosteroids, so the considerable impact of azithromycin on reducing exacerbations (Fig 2 in the original article) appeared to be in addition to that of the steroids. The authors do note an increase in colonization with macrolide-resistant organisms (without an increase in infections) and a small increase in hearing loss in those patients in the active arm of the study. Since the study was continued for only a year, the negative impact of azithromycin beyond that period is unknown.

How should we apply the results of this trial? Acute exacerbations result in an increased risk of death, impaired quality of life, and more rapid loss of lung function. Thus, it seems appropriate to add azithromycin to the regimens of COPD patients who are at high risk of exacerbation; however, clinicians should avoid treating patients who are at high risk of complications from the drug and should reevaluate its use after a year. Those at risk of complications include patients with resting tachycardia, prolonged QTc intervals, hearing loss, and potentially those who colonize with macrolide-resistant organisms.

J. R. Maurer, MD, MBA

References

1. He ZY, Ou LM, Zhang JQ, et al. Effect of 6 months of erythromycin treatment on inflammatory cells in induced sputum and exacerbations in chronic obstructive pulmonary disease. *Respiration.* 2010;80:445-452.
2. Blasi F, Bonardi D, Aliberti S, et al. Long-term azithromycin use in patients with chronic obstructive pulmonary disease and tracheostomy. *Pulm Pharmacol Ther.* 2010;3:200-207.
3. Suzuki T, Yanai M, Yamaya M, et al. Erythromycin and common cold in COPD. *Chest.* 2001;120:730-733.

Mortality associated with tiotropium mist inhaler in patients with chronic obstructive pulmonary disease: systematic review and meta-analysis of randomised controlled trials

Singh S, Loke YK, Enright PL, et al (Johns Hopkins Univ School of Medicine, Baltimore, MD; Univ of East Anglia, Norwich, UK; Univ of Arizona, Tucson; et al)

BMJ 342:d3215, 2011

Objective.—To systematically review the risk of mortality associated with long term use of tiotropium delivered using a mist inhaler for symptomatic improvement in chronic obstructive pulmonary disease.

Data Sources.—Medline, Embase, the pharmaceutical company clinical trials register, the US Food and Drug Administration website, and ClinicalTrials.gov for randomised controlled trials from inception to July 2010.

Study Selection.—Trials were selected for inclusion if they were parallel group randomised controlled trials of tiotropium solution using a mist inhaler (Respimat Soft Mist Inhaler, Boehringer Ingelheim) versus placebo for chronic obstructive pulmonary disease; the treatment duration was more than 30 days, and they reported data on mortality. Relative risks of all cause mortality were estimated using a fixed effect meta-analysis, and heterogeneity was assessed with the I^2 statistic.

Results.—Five randomised controlled trials were eligible for inclusion. Tiotropium mist inhaler was associated with a significantly increased risk of mortality (90/3686 *v* 47/2836; relative risk 1.52, 95% confidence interval, 1.06 to 2.16; P=0.02; I^2=0%). Both 10 µg (2.15, 1.03 to 4.51; P=0.04; I^2=9%) and 5 µg (1.46, 1.01 to 2.10; P=0.04; I^2=0%) doses of tiotropium mist inhaler were associated with an increased risk of mortality. The overall estimates were not substantially changed by sensitivity analysis of the fixed effect analysis of the five trials combined using the random effects model (1.45, 1.02 to 2.07; P=0.04), limiting the analysis to three trials of one year's duration each (1.50, 1.05 to 2.15), or the inclusion of additional data on tiotropium mist inhaler from another investigational drug programme (1.42, 1.01 to 2.00). The number needed to treat for a year with the 5 µg dose to see one additional death was estimated to be 124 (95% confidence interval 52 to 5682) based on the average control event rate from the long term trials.

Conclusions.—This meta-analysis explains safety concerns by regulatory agencies and indicates a 52% increased risk of mortality associated with tiotropium mist inhaler in patients with chronic obstructive pulmonary disease.

▶ This systematic review adds a bit more detail to the growing body of data addressing significant side effects of anticholinergic agents. An increased risk of significant cardiovascular events has been reported in some reviews but not in others,[1,2] so the true impact remains controversial. The article by Singh et al is a systematic review of trials looking at mortality of patients using either tiotropium mist (delivered by Respimat Soft Mist Inhaler, not powder form) or placebo. The mist is not available in the United States but is available in many other countries. When delivered as the mist, tiotropium has been shown to achieve significantly higher plasma concentrations than delivery by the powder delivery system.[3] That has led to safety concerns that may be justified, as this review suggests a higher mortality rate with the tiotropium than with placebo. Cardiovascular events are not the only anticholinergic side effects receiving increased attention in the literature. Stephenson et al[4] did a Canadian population-based study of anticholinergic inhaler use in patients aged 66 or older and found that both long- and short-acting drugs resulted in increased rates of urinary retention compared with comparable populations not using the drugs. Men with benign prostatic hyperplasia were at greatest risk. Data from that same population showed that these older patients had fewer hospitalizations and emergency visits as well as better survival rates if they were prescribed long-acting beta agonists initially rather than anticholinergics.[5] While these findings are intriguing and concerning, we need to remember that these data come from large administrative databases and, therefore, have many limitations. Prospective studies that more carefully and specifically assess anticholinergic use in older populations are necessary.

J. R. Maurer, MD, MBA

References

1. Singh S, Loke YK, Furberg CD. Inhaled anticholinergics and risk of major adverse cardiovascular events in patients with chronic obstructive pulmonary disease: a systematic review and meta-analysis. *JAMA*. 2008;300:1439-1450.
2. Tashkin DP, Celli B, Senn S, et al; UPLIFT Study Investigators. A 4-year trial of tiotropium in chronic obstructive pulmonary disease. *N Engl J Med*. 2008;359:1543-1554.
3. van Noord JA, Cornelissen PJ, Aumann JL, Platz J, Mueller A, Fogarty C. The efficacy of tiotropium administered via Respimat Soft Mist Inhaler or Handihaler in COPD patients. *Respir Med*. 2009;103:22-29.
4. Stephenson A, Seitz D, Bell CM, et al. Inhaled anticholinergic drug therapy and the risk of acute urinary retention in chronic obstructive pulmonary disease: a population-based study. *Arch Intern Med*. 2011;171:914-920.
5. Gershon A, Croxford R, To T, et al. Comparison of inhaled long-acting-β-agonist and anticholinergic effectiveness in older patients with chronic obstructive pulmonary disease: a cohort study. *Ann Intern Med*. 2011;154:583-592.

Risk of fractures with inhaled corticosteroids in COPD: systematic review and meta-analysis of randomised controlled trials and observational studies
Loke YK, Cavallazzi R, Singh S (Univ of East Anglia, Norwich, UK; Univ of Louisville, KY; Johns Hopkins Univ School of Medicine, Baltimore, MD)
Thorax 66:699-708, 2011

Background.—The effect of inhaled corticosteroids (ICS) on fracture risk in patients with chronic obstructive pulmonary disease (COPD) remains uncertain. The aim of this study was to evaluate the association between ICS and fractures in COPD.

Methods.—MEDLINE, EMBASE, regulatory documents and company registries were searched up to August 2010. Randomised controlled trials (RCTs) of budesonide or fluticasone versus control treatment for COPD (≥24 weeks duration) and controlled observational studies reporting on fracture risk with ICS exposure vs no exposure in COPD were included. Peto OR meta-analysis was used for fracture risk from RCTs while ORs from observational studies were pooled using the fixed effect inverse variance method. Dose—response analysis was conducted using variance-weighted least squares regression in the observational studies. Heterogeneity was assessed using the I^2 statistic.

Results.—Sixteen RCTs (14 fluticasone, 2 budesonide) with 17 513 participants, and seven observational studies (n=69 000 participants) were included in the meta-analysis. ICSs were associated with a significantly increased risk of fractures (Peto OR 1.27; 95% CI 1.01 to 1.58; p=0.04; I^2=0%) in the RCTs. In the observational studies, ICS exposure was associated with a significantly increased risk of fractures (OR 1.21; 95% CI 1.12 to 1.32; p<0.001; I^2=37%), with each 500 µg increase in beclomethasone dose equivalents associated with a 9% increased risk of fractures, OR 1.09 (95% CI 1.06 to 1.12; p<0.001).

Conclusion.—Among patients with COPD, long-term exposure to fluticasone and budesonide is consistently associated with a modest but statistically significant increased likelihood of fractures (Fig 1).

▶ Inhaled corticosteroids (ICS), particularly in combination with bronchodilators, are now prescribed extensively in patients with chronic obstructive pulmonary disease (COPD). In fact, the GOLD (Global Initiative for Chronic Obstructive Lung Disease) Guidelines recommends this combination in patients

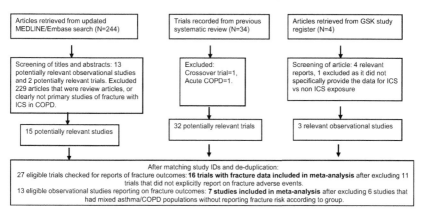

FIGURE 1.—Flow diagram of the process of article selection for meta-analysis. COPD, chronic obstructive pulmonary disease; ICS, inhaled corticosteroids. (Reproduced from Loke YK, Cavallazzi R, Singh S. Risk of fractures with inhaled corticosteroids in COPD: systematic review and meta-analysis of randomised controlled trials and observational studies. *Thorax.* 2011;66:699-708. Copyright 2011, with permission from BMJ Publishing Group Ltd.)

with severe (GOLD 3) or very severe (GOLD 4) disease to help reduce the frequency of exacerbations.[1] Yet studies in COPD populations have shown that even at therapeutic doses, ICS can have negative systemic effects. For example, COPD patients taking ICS have a higher incidence of pneumonia—although not clearly a higher mortality—than those who are not using the drug.[2,3] Another big concern is the impact on other organs, for example, cataract formation and osteoporosis (bone mineral density). Osteoporosis is not an unstudied area, but results of studies have been inconsistent. In part the data that have been collected, even in randomized controlled studies, on bone mineral density and fractures are incomplete because of inadequate follow-up and otherwise incomplete data collection.[4,5] Even meta-analyses have come to different conclusions.[6,7] The authors argue that these meta-analyses were underpowered and included patients with different diagnoses, thereby muddying the conclusions. They also note 2 Cochrane reviews that concluded that findings on the relationship of ICS to fractures in this population were inconclusive.[8,9] Thus, Loke and colleagues, aware of the methodological issues in these reports, set very specific parameters for their analysis (Fig 1). This allowed "consistency and similarity of the point estimates across randomized trials and observational study designs." In addition Loke et al feel that the ability to show a dose-response effect in this meta-analysis helps make their conclusions more credible. Although this may be a more plausible meta-analysis than those previously published, there remain significant limitations such as the following: many of the data came from unpublished (and therefore non—peer-reviewed) company trial results; temporal relationships of fractures and ICS use is often absent, as is a consistent way/requirement of reporting fractures; most participants were male, so direct application of results to mixed populations may not be accurate; concomitant use of bisphosphonates (or other osteoporosis drugs) was not controlled for in the randomized trials. So how important is the relatively small increased risk of fractures that this meta-analysis concludes exists in patients on ICS? That depends. In the sicker patients who are likely to use larger amounts of ICS over longer periods and who frequently have reduced bone mineral density for multifactorial reasons, it may be more of an issue than in other patient groups; however, the sicker patients also are the ones most likely to benefit from ICS. The most prudent approach is to consider and discuss the risk in the context of each individual's situation.

J. R. Maurer, MD, MBA

References

1. The Global Initiative for Chronic Obstructive Lung Disease Guidelines. GOLD 2011 Summary. http://www.goldcopd.org/guidelines-gold-summary-2011.html. Accessed December 26, 2011.
2. Calverley PM, Anderson JA, Celli B, et al; TORCH investigators. Salmeterol and fluticasone propionate and survival in chronic obstructive pulmonary disease. *N Engl J Med.* 2007;356:775-789.
3. Singanayagam A, Chalmers JD, Akram AR, Hill AT. Impact of inhaled corticosteroid use on outcome in COPD patients admitted with pneumonia. *Eur Respir J.* 2011;38:36-41.
4. Ferguson GT, Calverley PM, Anderson JA, et al. Prevalence and progression of osteoporosis in patients with COPD: results from the Towards a Revolution in COPD Health study. *Chest.* 2009;136:1456-1465.

5. Johnell O, Pauwels R, Löfdahl CG, et al. Bone mineral density in patients with chronic obstructive pulmonary disease treated with budesonide Turbuhaler. *Eur Respir J.* 2002;19:1058-1063.
6. Weatherall M, James K, Clay J, et al. Dose-response relationship for risk of non-vertebral fracture with inhaled corticosteroids. *Clin Exp Allergy.* 2008;1451-1458.
7. Drummond MB, Dasenbrook EC, Pitz MW, Murphy DJ, Fan E. Inhaled cortico-steroids in patients with stable chronic obstructive pulmonary disease: a systematic review and meta-analysis. *JAMA.* 2008;300:2407-2416.
8. Jones A, Fay JK, Burr M, Stone M, Hood K, Roberts G. Inhaled corticosteroid effects on bone metabolism in asthma and mild chronic obstructive pulmonary disease. *Cochrane Database Syst Rev.* 2002;(1). CD003537.
9. Yang IA, Fong KM, Sim EH, Black PN, Lasserson TJ. Inhaled corticosteroids for stable chronic obstructive pulmonary disease. *Cochrane Database Syst Rev.* 2007; (2). CD002991.

The Impact of Anxiety and Depression on Outcomes of Pulmonary Rehabilitation in Patients With COPD

von Leupoldt A, Taube K, Lehmann K, et al (Univ of Hamburg, Germany; Atem-Reha GmbH, Hamburg, Germany; et al)
Chest 140:730-736, 2011

Background.—Anxiety and depression are prevalent comorbidities in COPD and are related to a worse course of disease. The present study examined the impact of anxiety and depression on functional performance, dyspnea, and quality of life (QoL) in patients with COPD at the start and end of an outpatient pulmonary rehabilitation (PR) program.

Methods.—Before and after PR, 238 patients with COPD (mean FEV_1 % predicted = 54, mean age = 62 years) underwent a 6-min walking test (6MWT). In addition, anxiety, depression, QoL, and dyspnea at rest, after the 6MWT, and during activities were measured.

Results.—Except for dyspnea at rest, improvements were observed in all outcome measures after PR. Multiple regression analyses showed that before and after PR, anxiety and depression were significantly associated with greater dyspnea after the 6MWT and during activities and with reduced QoL, even after controlling for the effects of age, sex, lung function, and smoking status. Moreover, before and after PR, anxiety was related to greater dyspnea at rest, whereas depression was significantly associated with reduced functional performance in the 6MWT.

Conclusions.—This study demonstrates that anxiety and depression are significantly associated with increased dyspnea and reduced functional performance and QoL in patients with COPD. These negative associations remain stable over the course of PR, even when improvements in these outcomes are achieved during PR. The results underline the clinical importance of detecting and treating anxiety and depression in patients with COPD.

▶ Anxiety and depression are highly prevalent in all chronic conditions and often significantly complicate the management of those diseases by impacting adherence to treatment regimens as well as increasing the use of health care resources.[1,2] Unfortunately, clinicians often do not diagnose either anxiety or depression and, therefore, miss an important opportunity to improve the quality of life of the patient. Even when diagnosed, these mood issues may be difficult to manage—especially if the disease is progressive—and present an ongoing problem for the clinician. Complicating our ability to impact anxiety and depression in the chronic obstructive pulmonary disease (COPD) (or other chronic pulmonary) patient is our lack of knowledge about the specific ways in which these diagnoses affect the functioning and coping ability of the patients. The study by von Leupoldt et al is helpful in directly correlating the effect of these mood disorders on the ability of the patients to benefit from one of the most prescribed treatment regimens, pulmonary rehabilitation. In addition, the authors were able to help delineate specific areas of impairment by showing specific correlations between dyspnea and anxiety and 6-minute walk distance and depression. Dyspnea and reduced functional capacity have a major impact on quality of life for COPD patients. The findings of this study support the need for regular anxiety and depression screening in this population and the initiation of appropriate treatment or adjustment of existing treatment to provide the most relief possible for anxiety and depression.

J. R. Maurer, MD, MBA

References

1. Kalsekar ID, Madhavan SS, Amonkar MM, et al. Depression in patients with type 2 diabetes: impact on adherence to oral hypoglycemic agents. *Ann Pharmacother.* 2006;40:605-611.
2. Himelhoch S, Weller WE, Wu AW, Anderson GF, Cooper LA. Chronic medical illness, depression, and use of acute medical services among Medicare beneficiaries. *Med Care.* 2004;42:512-521.

Effect of β blockers in treatment of chronic obstructive pulmonary disease: a retrospective cohort study
Short PM, Lipworth SIW, Elder DHJ, et al (Univ of Dundee, Scotland, UK; Univ of St Andrews, Scotland, UK; et al)
BMJ 342:d2549, 2011

Objective.—To examine the effect of β blockers in the management of chronic obstructive pulmonary disease (COPD), assessing their effect on mortality, hospital admissions, and exacerbations of COPD when added to established treatment for COPD.

Design.—Retrospective cohort study using a disease specific database of COPD patients (TARDIS) linked to the Scottish morbidity records of acute hospital admissions, the Tayside community pharmacy prescription records, and the General Register Office for Scotland death registry.

Setting.—Tayside, Scotland (2001–2010).

Population.—5977 patients aged >50 years with a diagnosis of COPD.

Main Outcome Measures.—Hazard ratios for all cause mortality, emergency oral corticosteroid use, and respiratory related hospital admissions calculated through Cox proportional hazard regression after correction for influential covariates.

Results.—Mean follow-up was 4.35 years, mean age at diagnosis was 69.1 years, and 88% of β blockers used were cardioselective. There was a 22% overall reduction in all cause mortality with β blocker use. Furthermore, there were additive benefits of β blockers on all cause mortality at all treatment steps for COPD. Compared with controls (given only inhaled therapy with either short acting β agonists or short acting antimuscarinics), the adjusted hazard ratio for all cause mortality was 0.28 (95% CI 0.21 to 0.39) for treatment with inhaled corticosteroid, long acting β agonist, and long acting antimuscarinic plus β blocker versus 0.43 (0.38 to 0.48) without β blocker. There were similar trends showing additive benefits of β blockers in reducing oral corticosteroid use and hospital admissions due to respiratory disease. β blockers had no deleterious impact on lung function at all treatment steps when given in conjunction with either a long acting β agonist or antimuscarinic agent.

Conclusions.—β blockers may reduce mortality and COPD exacerbations when added to established inhaled stepwise therapy for COPD, independently of overt cardiovascular disease and cardiac drugs, and without adverse effects on pulmonary function (Fig 1).

▶ Smoking is a significant risk for both cardiovascular disease and chronic obstructive pulmonary disease (COPD), and the increased risk of cardiac issues is well recognized in COPD patients. Vanfleteren et al reported that undiagnosed cardiac disease is also common and is associated with increased symptoms such as dyspnea, decreased functional capacity, and increased markers of systemic inflammation.[1] Dalal et al recently noted that these comorbid patients have higher rates of exacerbations and consume many more health care resources.[2] It is also well established that beta blockers are critical drugs in managing coronary artery disease and, in fact, can reduce cardiac events and prolong life. However, these drugs are typically not prescribed for patients with comorbid cardiac disease

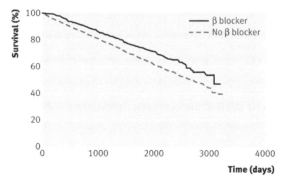

FIGURE 1.—Kaplan-Meier estimate of probability of survival among patients with COPD by use of β blockers. (Reproduced from Short PM, Lipworth SIW, Elder DHJ, et al. Effect of β blockers in treatment of chronic obstructive pulmonary disease: a retrospective cohort study. *BMJ.* 2011;342:d2549. Copyright 2011, with permission from BMJ Publishing Group Ltd.)

and COPD because of concerns that the beta-blocking effect will cause increased respiratory impairment. This approach is being reexamined. There is increasing evidence that death rates from cardiac disease are higher in patients comorbid with COPD who do not receive these drugs. Enriquez et al reported data from the Dynamic Registry, a large registry of the National Heart, Lung, and Blood Institute of the National Institutes of Health. In looking at patients undergoing percutaneous coronary interventions, the researchers found that patients with COPD did have more comorbidities than the general population but also received fewer of the class I drugs recommended for patients with coronary disease.[3] In the year after percutaneous intervention, these patients had higher risks of death, cardiac events, and need for repeat percutaneous intervention or revascularization. The data about use of beta blockers in patients with COPD are not well studied and results have been mixed. The study by Short et al, also retrospective, suggests a reduction in overall mortality in COPD patients that may be attributable to the impact of these drugs on cardiac disease but appeared to have an impact on survival independent of the cardiac effects (Fig 1). To be sure, there have been mixed results shown with beta blockers including a reduction in bronchodilator response and hypotension.[4,5] Nevertheless, the notion of potential benefit of beta blockers to treat airway disease and particularly the known impact on survival of patients with comorbid cardiac disease begs for prospective, well-designed trials to test these drugs in COPD populations.

J. R. Maurer, MD, MBA

References

1. Vanfleteren LE, Franssen FM, Uszko-Lencer NH, et al. Frequency and relevance of ischemic electrocardiographic findings in patients with chronic obstructive pulmonary disease. *Am J Cardiol*. 2011;108:1669-1674.
2. Dalal AA, Shah M, Lunacsek O, Hanania NA. Clinical and economic burden of patients diagnosed with COPD with comorbid cardiovascular disease. *Respir Med*. 2011;105:1516-1522.
3. Enriquez JR, Parikh SV, Selzer F, et al. Increased adverse events after percutaneous coronary intervention in patients with COPD: insights from the National Heart, Lung, and Blood Institute dynamic registry. *Chest*. 2011;140:604-610.
4. Lainscak M, Podbregar M, Kovacic D, Rozman J, von Haehling S. Differences between bisoprolol and carvedilol in patients with chronic heart failure and chronic obstructive pulmonary disease: a randomized trial. *Respir Med*. 2011;105:S44-S49.
5. Chang CL, Mills GD, McLachlan JD, Karalus NC, Hancox RJ. Cardio-selective and non-selective beta-blockers in chronic obstructive pulmonary disease: effects on bronchodilator response and exercise. *Intern Med J*. 2010;40:193-200.

Factors Associated With Bronchiectasis in Patients With COPD
Martínez-García MÁ, Soler-Cataluña JJ, Donat Sanz Y, et al (Requena General Hosp, Valencia, Spain; et al)
Chest 140:1130-1137, 2011

Background.—Previous studies have shown a high prevalence of bronchiectasis in patients with moderate to severe COPD. However, the factors associated with bronchiectasis remain unknown in these patients. The objective of this study is to identify the factors associated with bronchiectasis in patients with moderate to severe COPD.

Methods.—Consecutive patients with moderate (50% < FEV_1 ≤70%) or severe (FEV_1 ≤50%) COPD were included prospectively. All subjects filled out a clinical questionnaire, including information about exacerbations. Peripheral blood samples were obtained, and lung function tests were performed in all patients. Sputum samples were provided for monthly microbiologic analysis for 6 months. All the tests were performed in a stable phase for at least 6 weeks. High-resolution CT scans of the chest were used to diagnose bronchiectasis.

Results.—Ninety-two patients, 51 with severe COPD, were included. Bronchiectasis was present in 53 patients (57.6%). The variables independently associated with the presence of bronchiectasis were severe airflow obstruction (OR, 3.87; 95% CI, 1.38-10.5; $P =$ .001), isolation of a potentially pathogenic microorganism (PPM) (OR, 3.59; 95% CI, 1.3-9.9; $P =$ .014), and at least one hospital admission due to COPD exacerbations in the previous year (OR, 3.07; 95% CI, 1.07-8.77; $P =$ .037).

Conclusion.—We found an elevated prevalence of bronchiectasis in patients with moderate to severe COPD, and this was associated with severe airflow obstruction, isolation of a PPM from sputum, and at least one hospital admission for exacerbations in the previous year.

▶ The impact of concurrent bronchiectasis in the setting of emphysema or chronic bronchitis has not been well investigated. Radiologic studies have found that bronchiectasis is much more common in these diseases than previously recognized. Parr et al[1] identified bronchiectatic changes in 70 of 74 alpha-1 antitrypsin-deficient emphysema patients, and in 20 of those patients bronchiectatic symptoms were clinically significant. O'Brien et al[2] reported bronchiectatic changes on high-resolution computed tomography (HRCT) in 32 of 110 consecutive patients presenting with acute exacerbations of their chronic obstructive pulmonary disease (COPD). And Patel et al[3] were able to show that COPD patients with documented bronchiectatic changes on HRCT had more severe exacerbations, lower airway colonization, and higher levels of airway inflammatory cytokines. Martinez-Garcia and colleagues set out to better characterize the clinical characteristics of this COPD phenotype so that family practitioners or others who provide most of the care to these patients might be able to identify them without sophisticated or invasive studies. Like the findings of Patel et al,[3] the patients in this group had a high rate of bronchiectasis. Those with bronchiectasis were colonized with potentially pathogenic organisms and had a stronger history of exacerbations. The additional finding was that most had severe disease. Using these descriptors, it might be prudent in this phenotype of COPD patients to identify very early signs of exacerbation and treat aggressively. Another interesting focus for study might be the role/impact of inhaled corticosteroids (ICS) in this subgroup. On one hand, ICS reduce airway inflammation, potentially reducing exacerbations; on the other hand, ICS are associated with higher rates of pneumonia, which might be more likely in these highly colonized patients. Do ICS do more harm or good here?

J. R. Maurer, MD, MBA

References

1. Parr DG, Guest PG, Reynolds JH, Dowson LJ, Stockley RA. Prevalence and impact of bronchiectasis in alpha1-antitrypsin deficiency. *Am J Respir Crit Care Med.* 2007;176:1215-1221.
2. O'Brien C, Guest PJ, Hill SL, Stockley RA. Physiological and radiological characterisation of patients diagnosed with chronic obstructive pulmonary disease in primary care. *Thorax.* 2000;55:635-642.
3. Patel IS, Vlahos I, Wilkinson TM, et al. Bronchiectasis, exacerbation indices, and inflammation in chronic obstructive pulmonary disease. *Am J Respir Crit Care Med.* 2004;170:400-407.

3 Lung Cancer

Introduction

Lung cancer is the leading cause of cancer death worldwide, resulting in more than a million deaths annually.[1] In the United States, a projected 156 940 individuals will have succumbed to lung cancer in 2011.[2] While lung cancer mortality rates in men continue to decline and perhaps are beginning to also decrease in women, 5-year survival rates are still poor. More deaths in this country result from lung cancer than from breast, colorectal, and prostate cancers combined.[2]

Lung cancer screening was an important topic this year. Overall 5-year survival for lung cancer is only 16%. One of the major contributors to this dismal statistic is the fact that most patients are diagnosed at advanced stages, for which effective treatment options are limited. Survival with treated early-stage lung cancer is considerably better, so the imperative to achieve early detection is clear. In 2011, both the National Lung Screening Trial (NLST) and the Prostate, Lung, Colorectal, and Ovarian (PLCO) trial published their results, which will undoubtedly have an enormous effect on the field over the coming years.[3,4] The PLCO trial began in 1993 and is ongoing, evaluating the effect of screening interventions on mortality related to 4 solid tumors. The PLCO lung cancer screening intervention was an annual plain chest radiograph. After 13 years of monitoring, no difference was observed in lung cancer mortality between subjects receiving the screening intervention compared with subjects in the usual care (no screening) group. These results confirmed results of large studies done several decades ago, which demonstrated that lung cancer screening with chest radiography is not effective. In contrast, the NLST results demonstrate that screening for lung cancer with low-dose computed tomography (CT) scanning does result in a reduction in lung cancer mortality. The NLST began in 2002, enrolling over 50 000 subjects ages 55 to 74, with $\geq$ 30 pack-years of smoking history; individuals who had stopped smoking had to have quit within the previous 15 years. Study subjects were randomized to screening with low-dose CT (one baseline and two annual follow-up scans) or to usual care (no screening). Median follow-up was 6.5 years. The NLST was stopped early by its data-safety monitoring board as the primary endpoint, a 20% relative reduction in mortality from lung cancer with the screening intervention, was reached. The results of the NLST make it clear that for the population studied, lung cancer screening with low-dose CT scanning saves live.

The landmark findings of the NLST trial will influence clinical practice and health policy, but they leave us with an enormous question: what about screening for individuals who do not fulfill the NLST study subject criteria? Should we screen individuals with other lung cancer risks? It is unlikely that studies on the scale of the NLST for other at-risk groups (positive family history of lung cancer, personal history of other cancer, smoking history < 30 pack-years, asbestos, or other carcinogen exposure, etc) will be performed. This emphasizes the need for reliable methods of lung cancer risk stratification that would parallel models available, for example, for breast cancer. Several multivariable models for lung cancer risk prediction have been developed, including those recently published from the PLCO and the Liverpool Lung Project.[5,6] While none of these models have been validated for reliable clinic application as yet, they have the potential to be useful tools for evaluating individuals with the many defined lung cancer risks falling outside the strict definitions of the NLST.

The diagnostic evaluation for patients with lung cancer continues to evolve. Lababede and colleagues have created lung cancer staging charts incorporating all the changes of the current international lung cancer staging system, which would serve as user-friendly office or bronchoscopy suite references.[7] Annema and colleagues provide a large series evaluating the accuracy of endobronchial ultrasound-guided (EBUS) and endoscopic ultrasound-guided (EUS) evaluation of the mediastinum, demonstrating, as have others, that EBUS with or without EUS is at least as good as mediastinoscopy in properly trained hands.[8] We are reminded by Wiener and colleagues that diagnostic interventions are not without risk.[9] Their review of healthcare administrative data from 4 large states relating to complications from transthoracic needle biopsy for peripheral lung nodules demonstrated pneumothorax in 15%, requirement for chest tube placement in 6.6%, and hemorrhage in 1% of all biopsied patients. The balance of risk and benefit in clinical practice is further highlighted by the report by Stiles and colleagues evaluating radiation exposure from diagnostic imaging in 94 patients after curative intent surgical resection for non-small cell lung cancer (NSCLC).[10] In the 3 years subsequent to resection, approximately 40% of patients had accumulated radiation doses in excess of 100 mSv; this exceeds the regulated maximum allowed radiation exposure for healthcare and radiation workers over that time frame. This report emphasizes the fundamental imperative to thoughtfully evaluate the indications and necessity for imaging procedures, particularly those associated with substantial radiation exposure, and highlights the need for development and institution of tools that would facilitate monitoring of total radiation exposure for a given individual over time. This is particularly timely in light of the dramatic increase in the use of CT scanning and PET imaging over recent years—both potentially significant sources of diagnostic radiation exposure.[11]

Finally, advances continue to be made in the area of lung cancer treatment. Pao and Girard review the driver mutations currently recognized as potentially important in NSCLC.[12] These mutations encode proteins in signaling pathways controlling cellular proliferation and survival, which are integral to tumor formation and maintenance and which may serve as therapeutic targets. The best known driver mutations are those identified in the *EGFR* gene.[13] The *EML4-ALK* fusion oncogene, an activating mutation of the anaplastic lymphoma kinase (*ALK*) gene, is one of the newest identified molecular targets.[14,15] While a single driver mutation is typically present in only a small subset of patients, selectively targeted therapy may result in substantial benefit in survival for these patients. It is evident that many patients with lung cancer, particularly adenocarcinoma, harbor such mutations. Research directed at expanding our understanding of lung cancer biology on a molecular level should continue to improve our ability to develop better focused and less toxic therapies.

Lynn T. Tanoue, MD

References

1. Parkin DM, Bray F, Ferlay J, Pisani P. Global cancer statistics, 2002. *CA Cancer J Clin.* 2005;55:74-108.
2. Siegel R, Ward E, Brawley O, Jemal A. Cancer statistics, 2011: the impact of eliminating socioeconomic and racial disparities on premature cancer deaths. *CA Cancer J Clin.* 2011;61:212-236.
3. Oken MM, Hocking WG, Kvale PA, et al; PLCO Project Team. Screening by chest radiograph and lung cancer mortality: the Prostate, Lung, Colorectal, and Ovarian (PLCO) randomized trial. *JAMA.* 2011;306:1865-1873.
4. National Lung Screening Trial Research Team, Aberle DR, Adams AM, Berg CD, et al. Reduced lung-cancer mortality with low-dose computed tomographic screening. *N Engl J Med.* 2011;365:395-409.
5. Tammemagi CM, Pinsky PF, Caporaso NE, et al. Lung cancer risk prediction: Prostate, Lung, Colorectal and Ovarian Cancer Screening Trial models and validation. *J Natl Cancer Inst.* 2011;103:1058-1068.
6. Raji OY, Agbaje OF, Duffy SW, Cassidy A, Field JK. Incorporation of a genetic factor into an epidemiologic model for prediction of individual risk of lung cancer: the Liverpool Lung Project. *Cancer Prev Res (Phila).* 2010;3:664-669.
7. Lababede O, Meziane M, Rice T. Seventh edition of the cancer staging manual and stage grouping of lung cancer: quick reference chart and diagrams. *Chest.* 2011;139:183-189.
8. Annema JT, van Meerbeeck JP, Rintoul RC, et al. Mediastinoscopy vs endosonography for mediastinal nodal staging of lung cancer: a randomized trial. *JAMA.* 2010;304:2245-2252.
9. Wiener RS, Schwartz LM, Woloshin S, Welch HG. Population-based risk for complications after transthoracic needle lung biopsy of a pulmonary nodule: an analysis of discharge records. *Ann Intern Med.* 2011;155:137-144.
10. Stiles BM, Mirza F, Towe CW, et al. Cumulative radiation dose from medical imaging procedures in patients undergoing resection for lung cancer. *Ann Thorac Surg.* 2011;92:1170-1178.
11. Brenner DJ, Hall EJ. Computed tomography—an increasing source of radiation exposure. *N Engl J Med.* 2007;357:2277-2284.
12. Pao W, Girard N. New driver mutations in non-small-cell lung cancer. *Lancet Oncol.* 2011;12:175-180.
13. Cataldo VD, Gibbons DL, Pérez-Soler R, Quintás-Cardama A. Treatment of non-small-cell lung cancer with erlotinib or gefitinib. *N Engl J Med.* 2011;364:947-955.

14. Kwak EL, Bang YJ, Camidge DR, et al. Anaplastic lymphoma kinase inhibition in non-small-cell lung cancer. *N Engl J Med.* 2010;363:1693-1703.
15. Shaw AT, Solomon B. Targeting anaplastic lymphoma kinase in lung cancer. *Clin Cancer Res.* 2011;17:2081-2086.

Epidemiology of Lung Cancer

Cancer Statistics, 2011: The Impact of Eliminating Socioeconomic and Racial Disparities on Premature Cancer Deaths
Siegel R, Ward E, Brawley O, et al (American Cancer Society, Atlanta, GA)
CA Cancer J Clin 61:212-236, 2011

Each year, the American Cancer Society estimates the numbers of new cancer cases and deaths expected in the United States in the current year and compiles the most recent data on cancer incidence, mortality, and survival based on incidence data from the National Cancer Institute, the Centers for Disease Control and Prevention, and the North American Association of Central Cancer Registries and mortality data from the National Center for Health Statistics. A total of 1,596,670 new cancer cases and 571,950 deaths from cancer are projected to occur in the United

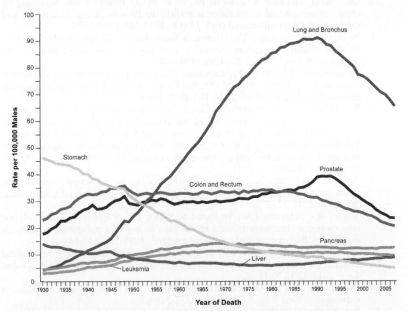

FIGURE 4.—Annual Age-Adjusted Cancer Death Rates* Among Males for Selected Cancers, United States, 1930 to 2007. *Rates are age adjusted to the 2000 US standard population. Due to changes in International Classification of Diseases (ICD) coding, numerator information has changed over time. Rates for cancers of the lung and bronchus, colon and rectum, and liver are affected by these changes. *Source:* US Mortality Volumes 1930 to 1959, US Mortality Data, 1960 to 2007. National Center for Health Statistics, Centers for Disease Control and Prevention. (Reprinted from Siegel R, Ward E, Brawley O, et al. Cancer statistics, 2011; the impact of eliminating socioeconomic and racial disparities on premature cancer deaths. *CA Cancer J Clin.* 2011;61:212-236, with permission from John Wiley and Sons (www.interscience.wiley.com).)

States in 2011. Overall cancer incidence rates were stable in men in the most recent time period after decreasing by 1.9% per year from 2001 to 2005; in women, incidence rates have been declining by 0.6% annually since 1998. Overall cancer death rates decreased in all racial/ethnic groups in both men and women from 1998 through 2007, with the exception of American Indian/Alaska Native women, in whom rates were stable. African American and Hispanic men showed the largest annual decreases in cancer death rates during this time period (2.6% and 2.5%, respectively). Lung cancer death rates showed a significant decline in women after continuously increasing since the 1930s. The reduction in the overall cancer death rates since 1990 in men and 1991 in women translates to the avoidance of about 898,000 deaths from cancer. However, this progress has not benefitted all segments of the population equally; cancer death rates for individuals with the least education are more than twice those of the most educated. The elimination of educational and racial disparities could potentially have avoided about 37% (60,370) of the premature cancer deaths among individuals aged 25 to 64 years in 2007 alone. Further progress can be accelerated by applying existing cancer control

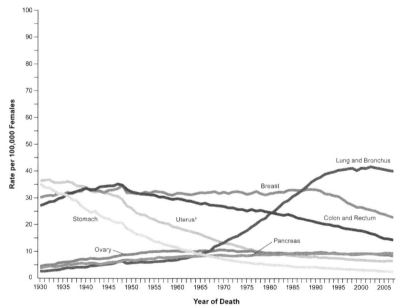

FIGURE 5.—Annual Age-Adjusted Cancer Death Rates* Among Females for Selected Cancers, United States, 1930 to 2007. *Rates are age adjusted to the 2000 US standard population. †Uterus indicates uterine cervix and uterine corpus. Due to changes in International Classification of Diseases (ICD) coding, numerator information has changed over time. Rates for cancers of the uterus, ovary, lung and bronchus, and colon and rectum are affected by these changes. *Source:* US Mortality Volumes 1930 to 1959, US Mortality Data, 1960 to 2007. National Center for Health Statistics, Centers for Disease Control and Prevention. (Reprinted from Siegel R, Ward E, Brawley O, et al. Cancer statistics, 2011; the impact of eliminating socioeconomic and racial disparities on premature cancer deaths. *CA Cancer J Clin.* 2011;61:212-236, with permission from John Wiley and Sons (www.interscience.wiley.com).)

knowledge across all segments of the population with an emphasis on those groups in the lowest socioeconomic bracket (Figs 4 and 5).

▶ Lung cancer is the leading cause of cancer death around the world, accounting for more than 1 million deaths annually.[1] In the United States, lung cancer has caused more deaths than breast cancer in women since 1987 and more deaths than prostate cancer in men since 1955. Age-adjusted annual cancer death rates among men and women in the United States from 1930 to 2007 are demonstrated in Figs 4 and 5. The American Cancer Society estimates that lung cancer will have caused death in 156 940 Americans in 2011, fewer persons than in 2010 but still more than the 3 next most common causes of cancer death combined (colorectal, breast, and prostate). These sobering statistics are a reminder of the challenges that remain in promoting prevention and improving treatment. The results of the National Lung Screening Trial indicate that early detection with low-dose CT screening in heavy smokers (> 30 pack-years) between the ages of 55 to 74 decreases lung cancer mortality.[2] What effect screening will have on overall incidence and mortality in the screening-eligible population as well as on outcomes in the general population will be a topic of intense scrutiny over the coming years.

L. T. Tanoue, MD

References

1. Parkin DM, Bray F, Ferlay J, Pisani P. Global cancer statistics, 2002. *CA Cancer J Clin*. 2005;55:74-108.
2. Aberle DR, Adams AM, Berg CD, et al. Reduced lung-cancer mortality with low-dose computed tomographic screening. *N Engl J Med*. 2011;365:395-409.

Lung Cancer Risk Prediction: Prostate, Lung, Colorectal and Ovarian Cancer Screening Trial Models and Validation
Tammemagi CM, Pinsky PF, Caporaso NE, et al (Brock Univ, Ontario, Canada; Natl Cancer Inst, Bethesda, MD; et al)
J Natl Cancer Inst 103:1058-1068, 2011

Introduction.—Identification of individuals at high risk for lung cancer should be of value to individuals, patients, clinicians, and researchers. Existing prediction models have only modest capabilities to classify persons at risk accurately.

Methods.—Prospective data from 70 962 control subjects in the Prostate, Lung, Colorectal, and Ovarian Cancer Screening Trial (PLCO) were used in models for the general population (model 1) and for a subcohort of ever-smokers (N = 38 254) (model 2). Both models included age, socioeconomic status (education), body mass index, family history of lung cancer, chronic obstructive pulmonary disease, recent chest x-ray, smoking status (never, former, or current), pack-years smoked, and smoking duration. Model 2 also included smoking quit-time (time in years since ever-smokers permanently quit smoking). External validation was performed with 44 223

PLCO intervention arm participants who completed a supplemental questionnaire and were subsequently followed. Known available risk factors were included in logistic regression models. Bootstrap optimism-corrected estimates of predictive performance were calculated (internal validation). Nonlinear relationships for age, pack-years smoked, smoking duration, and quit-time were modeled using restricted cubic splines. All reported *P* values are two-sided.

Results.—During follow-up (median 9.2 years) of the control arm subjects, 1040 lung cancers occurred. During follow-up of the external validation sample (median 3.0 years), 213 lung cancers occurred. For models 1 and 2, bootstrap optimism-corrected receiver operator characteristic area under the curves were 0.857 and 0.805, and calibration slopes (model-predicted probabilities vs observed probabilities) were 0.987 and 0.979, respectively. In the external validation sample, models 1 and 2 had area under the curves of 0.841 and 0.784, respectively. These models had high discrimination in women, men, whites, and nonwhites.

Conclusion.—The PLCO lung cancer risk models demonstrate high discrimination and calibration (Table 1).

▶ The Prostate, Lung, Colorectal and Ovarian (PLCO) Cancer Screening Trial enrolled over 150 000 subjects in the United States ages 55 to 74 years with the intent of assessing the benefit (or lack of benefit) related to screening interventions for the 4 cancers. The PLCO trial found no benefit in lung cancer mortality related to the lung cancer screening intervention, which consisted of 4 annual chest radiographs.[1] While this was a negative result, it was an important finding with respect to the National Lung Screening Trial (NLST), which found a reduction in lung cancer mortality with low-dose chest computed tomography screening.[2] Importantly, the PLCO trial resulted in a robust prospective database with a depth of clinical detail facilitating the construction of the lung cancer risk prediction models described in this report by Tammemagi and colleagues. Other lung cancer prediction models, including those published by Bach and colleagues,[3] Spitz and colleagues,[4,5] and the Liverpool Lung Project,[6,7] have to some extent been limited by a limited number of potential predictors and by being confined to smokers; none have performed consistently well enough to be useful in routine practice.[8]

Tammemagi and colleagues developed 2 models from the PLCO database, one for smokers and another for the general population. As demonstrated in Table 1, a large number of predictive variables were considered. Of note, variables available in the PLCO database included some predictors not included in other models but potentially important to lung cancer risk, including socioeconomic status (education), body mass index, history of recent chest radiograph, and chronic obstructive pulmonary disease. However, the PLCO models did not include several predictors that were useful in other models, including exposure to radon, asbestos, secondhand smoke, or occupational carcinogens or a history of adult pneumonia.

The NLST study subjects were 55 to 74 years of age with greater than 30 pack-years of smoking history; the decrease in lung cancer mortality demonstrated in the NLST with screening should be reproducible in the subset of the general population meeting these criteria. The challenge will be what to do with everyone

TABLE 1.—Distribution of Study Variables by Lung Cancer Status and Overall in the Model Development Sample*

Variable	No Lung Cancer[†] (n = 69 922)	Lung Cancer[†] (n = 1040)	P	Total[‡] (N = 70 962)
Sociodemographic				
Age, mean (SD), y	62.57 (5.35)	64.80 (5.09)	<.001[§]	62.60 (5.36)
Sex, No. (%)				
Women	34 994 (98.85)	408 (1.15)		35 402 (49.89)
Men	34 928 (98.22)	632 (1.78)	<.001[‖]	35 560 (50.11)
Race/ethnicity, No. (%)				
White, non-Hispanic	61 687 (98.52)	924 (1.48)	.017[‖]	62 611 (88.27)
Black, non-Hispanic	3606 (98.07)	71 (1.93)		3677 (5.18)
Hispanic	1336 (98.89)	15 (1.11)		1351 (1.90)
Asian	2675 (99.11)	24 (0.89)		2699 (3.81)
Pacific Islander	413 (99.04)	4 (0.96)		417 (0.59)
American Indian	172 (98.85)	2 (1.15)		174 (0.25)
Race–sex, No. (%)				
Black men	1590 (97.73)	37 (2.27)	.009[‖]	1627 (2.29)
Others	68 332 (97.73)	1003 (1.45)		69 335 (97.71)
Education, No. (%)				
High school and below	21 132 (98.03)	424 (1.97)	<.001[‖]	21 556 (30.49)
Greater than high school	48 519 (98.75)	613 (1.25)		49 132 (69.51)
Medical history				
Family history of lung cancer, No. (%)				
Absent	60 398 (98.67)	815 (1.33)	<.001[‖]	61 213 (87.00)
Present	8935 (97.67)	213 (2.33)		9148 (13.00)
COPD, No. (%)				
History absent	60 952 (98.75)	773 (1.25)	<.001[‖]	61 725 (92.81)
History present	4589 (95.92)	195 (4.08)		4784 (7.19)
Chest x-rays in past 3 y, No. (%)				
No	31 113 (98.97)	323 (1.03)	<.001[¶]	31 436 (46.10)
Yes, on one occasion	22 899 (98.41)	370 (1.59)		23 269 (34.12)
Yes, more than one occasion	13 186 (97.74)	305 (2.26)		13 491 (19.78)
Body mass index, mean (SD), kg/m^2	27.34 (5.01)	26.39 (4.51)	<.001[§]	27.32 (5.01)
Smoking history				
Smoking status, No. (%)				
Never-smoker	32 612 (99.77)	76 (0.23)	<.001[¶]	32 688 (46.08)
Former smoker	30 152 (98.32)	516 (1.68)		30 668 (43.23)
Current smoker	7138 (94.09)	448 (5.91)		7586 (10.69)
Smoking duration, mean (SD), y				
Former smokers	23.84 (12.48)	35.02 (11.18)	<.001[§]	24.03 (12.54)
Current smokers	42.02 (7.46)	45.68 (6.72)	<.001[§]	42.23 (7.47)
Quit-time in former smokers,[#] mean (SD), y	20.35 (12.02)	12.86 (10.65)	<.001[§]	20.23 (12.04)
Pack-years smoked,** mean (SD), y				
Former smokers	25.37 (24.91)	47.69 (30.90)	<.001[§]	25.75 (25.19)
Current smokers	40.10 (25.68)	52.40 (26.80)	<.001[§]	40.81 (25.90)

*Prostate, Lung, Colorectal, and Ovarian Cancer Screening Trial control arm. COPD = chronic obstructive pulmonary disease.
[†]Percentage values in parentheses are row percents for variable levels by lung cancer status. The row percents of lung cancer represent the cumulative incidence of lung cancer for that exposure (variable) level.
[‡]Percentage values in parentheses are column percents for variable totals.
[§]P value by two-sided Student t test.
[‖]P value by two-sided Fisher exact test.
[¶]P value by two-sided Wilcoxon rank-sum test.
[#]Time in years since ever-smokers permanently quit smoking.
**Pack-years is the average number of packages of cigarettes smoked per day times the number of years smoked.

else: individuals who smoke less, are younger or older, or have other lung cancer risk factors. What is clear is that a reliable lung cancer risk prediction strategy that can be applied to individual patients in both the smoking and general populations would be an invaluable clinical tool. Whether the PLCO models will eventually be refined and validated in a general population, or whether one or more of the existing models may be modified and made more robust by the addition of other predictive variables, such as molecular biomarkers, remains to be seen but is an area that merits much more research.

L. T. Tanoue, MD

References

1. Oken MM, Hocking WG, Kvale PA, et al. Screening by chest radiograph and lung cancer mortality: the Prostate, Lung, Colorectal, and Ovarian (PLCO) randomized trial. *JAMA*. 2011;306:1865-1873.
2. Aberle DR, Adams AM, Berg CD, et al. Reduced lung-cancer mortality with low-dose computed tomographic screening. *N Engl J Med*. 2011;365:395-409.
3. Bach PB, Kattan MW, Thornquist MD, et al. Variations in lung cancer risk among smokers. *J Natl Cancer Inst*. 2003;95:470-478.
4. Spitz MR, Hong WK, Amos CI, et al. A risk model for prediction of lung cancer. *J Natl Cancer Inst*. 2007;99:715-726.
5. Spitz MR, Etzel CJ, Dong Q, et al. An expanded risk prediction model for lung cancer. *Cancer Prev Res (Phila)*. 2008;1:250-254.
6. Cassidy A, Myles JP, van Tongeren M, et al. The LLP risk model: an individual risk prediction model for lung cancer. *Br J Cancer*. 2008;98:270-276.
7. Raji OY, Agbaje OF, Duffy SW, Cassidy A, Field JK. Incorporation of a genetic factor into an epidemiologic model for prediction of individual risk of lung cancer: the Liverpool Lung Project. *Cancer Prev Res (Phila)*. 2010;3:664-669.
8. D'Amelio AM Jr, Cassidy A, Asomaning K, et al. Comparison of discriminatory power and accuracy of three lung cancer risk models. *Br J Cancer*. 2010;103:423-429.

Incorporation of a Genetic Factor into an Epidemiologic Model for Prediction of Individual Risk of Lung Cancer: The Liverpool Lung Project

Raji OY, Agbaje OF, Duffy SW, et al (The Univ of Liverpool Cancer Res Centre, UK; Guy's Hosp, London, UK; Queen Mary Univ of London, UK)
Cancer Prev Res 3:664-669, 2010

The Liverpool Lung Project (LLP) has previously developed a risk model for prediction of 5-year absolute risk of lung cancer based on five epidemiologic risk factors. SEZ6L, a Met430IIe polymorphic variant found on 22q12.2 region, has been previously linked with an increased risk of lung cancer in a case-control population. In this article, we quantify the improvement in risk prediction with addition of SEZ6L to the LLP risk model. Data from 388 LLP subjects genotyped for SEZ6L single-nucleotide polymorphism (SNP) were combined with epidemiologic risk factors. Multivariable conditional logistic regression was used to predict 5-year absolute risk of lung cancer with and without this SNP. The improvement in the model associated with the SEZ6L SNP was assessed through pairwise comparison of the area under the receiver operating characteristic curve and the net reclassification improvements (NRI). The extended model showed better calibration compared with the baseline model. There was a statistically significant modest increase in the area under the receiver operating characteristic curve when SEZ6L was added into the baseline model. The NRI also revealed a statistically significant improvement of around 12% for the extended model; this improvement was better for subjects classified into the two intermediate-risk categories by the baseline model (NRI, 27%). Our results suggest that the addition of SEZ6L improved the performance of the LLP risk model, particularly for subjects whose initial absolute risks were unable to discriminate into "low-risk" or "high-risk" group. This work shows an approach to incorporate genetic biomarkers in risk models for predicting an individual's lung cancer risk.

▶ The Liverpool Lung Project (LLP) is a large, prospective, population-based lung cancer study in Liverpool, England. One of its primary goals is to develop and implement a molecular-epidemiologic risk assessment model for lung cancer, based on data obtained from incident lung cancer cases and matched controls in the Liverpool area. Over the past several years, the LLP has refined its lung cancer risk prediction model.[1] The components of the model include smoking duration, previous diagnosis of pneumonia, prior diagnosis of cancer, occupational exposure to asbestos, and family history of lung cancer. This report by Raji and colleagues describes improvement in the ability of the model to predict 5-year risk of lung cancer by the addition of a genetic factor. Single nucleotide polymorphisms in a region of chromosome 22q12.2 have been associated with significant differences between lung cancer cases and controls. One of these polymorphisms, located in the seizure 6-like (SEZ6L) gene, was incorporated into the LLP model, with significant improvement in the accuracy of lung cancer risk prediction. Combinations of molecular and epidemiologic information in lung cancer risk models are likely to become more extensive over time as more candidate molecular biomarkers are identified.

Risk assessment models have been developed for solid tumors including breast, colorectal, melanoma, ovarian, and bladder cancers. Several models, including the LLP, for lung cancer have been published, but none are robust enough yet for clinical use.[2-4] The ability to discuss individual lung cancer risk with a patient using such a predictive tool would have enormous impact on lifestyle modifications (including smoking cessation and diet), directing high-risk groups to screening, and potentially studying chemopreventive interventions.

L. T. Tanoue, MD

References

1. Cassidy A, Myles JP, van Tongeren M, et al. The LLP risk model: an individual risk prediction model for lung cancer. *Br J Cancer.* 2008;98:270-276.
2. Bach PB, Kattan MW, Thornquist MD, et al. Variations in lung cancer risk among smokers. *J Natl Cancer Inst.* 2003;95:470-478.
3. Spitz MR, Etzel CJ, Dong Q, et al. An expanded risk prediction model for lung cancer. *Cancer Prev Res (Phila).* 2008;1:250-254.
4. D'Amelio AM Jr, Cassidy A, Asomaning K, et al. Comparison of discriminatory power and accuracy of three lung cancer risk models. *Br J Cancer.* 2010;103:423-429.

Human Immunodeficiency Virus—Associated Primary Lung Cancer in the Era of Highly Active Antiretroviral Therapy: A Multi-Institutional Collaboration
D'Jaen GA, Pantanowitz L, Bower M, et al (Virginia Mason Med Ctr, Seattle, WA; Tufts Univ School of Medicine, Springfield, MA; Chelsea and Westminster Hosp, London, England; et al)
Clin Lung Cancer 11:396-404, 2010

Background.—Human immunodeficiency virus (HIV)-infected individuals are at increased risk for primary lung cancer (LC). We wished to compare the clinicopathologic features and treatment outcome of HIV-LC patients with HIV-indeterminate LC patients. We also sought to compare behavioral characteristics and immunologic features of HIV-LC patients with HIV-positive patients without LC.

Patients and Methods.—A database of 75 HIV-positive patients with primary LC in the HAART era was established from an international collaboration. These cases were drawn from the archives of contributing physicians who subspecialize in HIV malignancies. Patient characteristics were compared with registry data from the Surveillance Epidemiology and End Results program (SEER; n = 169,091 participants) and with HIV-positive individuals without LC from the Adult and Adolescent Spectrum of HIV-related Diseases project (ASD; n = 36,569 participants).

Results.—The median age at HIV-related LC diagnosis was 50 years compared with 68 years for SEER participants ($P < .001$). HIV-LC patients, like their SEER counterparts, most frequently presented with stage IIIB/IV cancers (77% vs. 70%), usually with adenocarcinoma (46% vs. 47%) or squamous carcinoma (35% vs. 25%) histologies. HIV-LC patients and ASD participants had comparable median nadir CD4+ cell counts (138 cells/µL vs. 160 cells/µL). At LC diagnosis, their median CD4+ count was 340 cells/µL and 86% were receiving HAART. Sixty-three HIV-LC patients (84%) received cancer-specific treatments, but chemotherapy-associated toxicity was substantial. The median survival for both HIV-LC patients and SEER participants with stage IIIB/IV was 9 months.

Conclusion.—Most HIV-positive patients were receiving HAART and had substantial improvement in CD4+ cell count at time of LC diagnosis. They were able to receive LC treatments; their tumor types and overall survival were similar to SEER LC participants. However, HIV-LC patients were diagnosed with LC at a younger age than their HIV-indeterminate counterparts. Future research should explore how screening, diagnostic and treatment strategies directed toward the general population may apply to HIV-positive patients at risk for LC.

▶ Human immunodeficiency virus (HIV) infection has become a chronic disease since the development of highly active antiretroviral therapy (HAART) in the late 1990s. Compared with 2 decades ago, opportunistic infections are less common in the developed world, and survival is substantially longer. In both HAART-treated and non-HAART-treated HIV-positive populations, it has become evident that patients with HIV have a higher incidence of cancer, both AIDS-defining malignancies (Kaposi's sarcoma, non-Hodgkin's lymphoma, invasive cervical carcinoma) as well as non-AIDS-defining malignancies.[1] Although the HIV virus is not directly oncogenic, it appears to promote the carcinogenic process. Longer survival with HAART provides opportunity for the development of malignancies, which are now a significant cause of mortality for HIV-infected patients.

It has long been observed that non-AIDS-defining malignancies appear to occur at higher rates and younger ages in HIV-positive patients and that these cancers tend to be of higher tumor grade with more aggressive clinical behavior. The HIV-positive population may also be at increased risk for lung cancer related to higher smoking prevalence. A 2- to 4-fold increase in lung cancer incidence has been reported in HIV-positive patients compared with age- and gender-matched cohorts.[2] This report describes a series of 75 cases of primary lung cancer in HIV-positive patients from the United States and the United Kingdom and compares their clinical presentation and outcomes with non-HIV lung cancer patients in the Surveillance Epidemiology and End Results (SEER) database. There was no difference between the 2 groups in the distribution of lung cancer stage at presentation; 77% of HIV-positive patients presented with advanced disease (Stages IIIB and IV) compared with 70% in the SEER group. A significant difference in age at lung cancer diagnosis was demonstrated, with a median age at diagnosis of 50 years in the HIV-positive group compared with 68 years in the SEER group. In contrast to prior reports, there were no differences between the 2 groups in receipt of treatment or in outcomes; median overall survival for both groups was 9 months. Based on these observations, the threshold for consideration of a lung cancer diagnosis in HIV-positive patients should be low, and preventive strategies, most importantly smoking cessation, are of particular importance.

L. T. Tanoue, MD

References

1. Spano JP, Costagliola D, Katlama C, Mounier N, Oksenhendler E, Khayat D. AIDS-related malignancies: state of the art and therapeutic challenges. *J Clin Oncol.* 2008;26:4834-4842.
2. Pakkala S, Ramalingam SS. Lung cancer in HIV-positive patients. *J Thorac Oncol.* 2010;5:1864-1871.

Serum B Vitamin Levels and Risk of Lung Cancer

Johansson M, Relton C, Ueland PM, et al (International Agency for Research on Cancer (IARC), Lyon, France; Newcastle Univ, UK; Univ of Bergen, Norway; et al)
JAMA 303:2377-2385, 2010

Context.—B vitamins and factors related to 1-carbon metabolism help to maintain DNA integrity and regulate gene expression and may affect cancer risk.

Objective.—To investigate if 1-carbon metabolism factors are associated with onset of lung cancer.

Design, Setting, and Participants.—The European Prospective Investigation into Cancer and Nutrition (EPIC) recruited 519 978 participants from 10 countries between 1992 and 2000, of whom 385 747 donated blood. By 2006, 899 lung cancer cases were identified and 1770 control participants were individually matched by country, sex, date of birth, and date of blood collection. Serum levels were measured for 6 factors of 1-carbon metabolism and cotinine.

Main Outcome Measure.—Odds ratios (ORs) of lung cancer by serum levels of 4 B vitamins (B_2, B_6, folate [B_9], and B_{12}), methionine, and homocysteine.

Results.—Within the entire EPIC cohort, the age-standardized incidence rates of lung cancer (standardized to the world population, aged 35-79 years) were 6.6, 44.9, and 156.1 per 100 000 person-years among never, former, and current smokers for men, respectively. The corresponding incidence rates for women were 7.1, 23.9, and 100.9 per 100 000 person years, respectively. After accounting for smoking, a lower risk for lung cancer was seen for elevated serum levels of B_6 (fourth vs first quartile OR, 0.44; 95% confidence interval [CI], 0.33-0.60; P for trend <.000001), as well as for serum methionine (fourth vs first quartile OR, 0.52; 95% CI, 0.39-0.69; P for trend <.000001). Similar and consistent decreases in risk were observed in never, former, and current smokers, indicating that results were not due to confounding by smoking. The magnitude of risk was also constant with increasing length of follow-up, indicating that the associations were not explained by preclinical disease. A lower risk was also seen for serum folate (fourth vs first quartile OR, 0.68; 95% CI, 0.51-0.90; P for trend = .001), although this was apparent only for former and current smokers. When participants were classified by median levels of serum methionine and B_6, having above-median levels of both was associated with a lower lung cancer risk overall (OR, 0.41; 95% CI, 0.31-0.54), as well as separately among never (OR, 0.36; 95% CI, 0.18-0.72), former (OR, 0.51; 95% CI, 0.34-0.76), and current smokers (OR, 0.42; 95% CI, 0.27-0.65).

Conclusion.—Serum levels of vitamin B_6 and methionine were inversely associated with risk of lung cancer.

▶ The B vitamins (B2 [riboflavin], B6 [pyridoxal 5-phosphate], folate, and B12 [cobalamin]) and related compounds (methionine and homocysteine) are essential for DNA synthesis and repair. Reports that supplementation with folate and other B vitamins may actually increase cancer risk are in striking contrast to reports associating supplementation with a reduction in the risk of colorectal cancer.[1,2] Folate has probably received the most attention in this regard because of mandated fortification of grain products to reduce the incidence of neural tube birth defects.

This report by Johansson and colleagues comes out of the European Prospective Investigation into Cancer and Nutrition (EPIC) project, which prospectively monitored more than 500 000 Europeans in 10 countries after an extensive baseline intake between 1992 and 2000. This particular report is a case-control study of vitamin B intake and serum levels in 1592 EPIC subjects in whom lung cancer developed during the observation period. No vitamin supplementation was undertaken; subjects had vitamin B levels and food frequency questionnaires administered on entry to the study. After stratifying for smoking status, a lower risk for lung cancer was observed for increasing levels of B6 as well as methionine in current and former smokers and nonsmokers, as demonstrated in Fig 1 in the original article. A similar decrease in lung cancer risk was observed for increasing levels of folate in current and former smokers only. Subjects who had high levels of B6 and methionine had a reduction of more than 50% in their risk of lung cancer.

The effect of diet on cancer risk is a topic that has been challenging to study because of the large numbers of subjects and the long duration of monitoring required to eventually obtain meaningful results. As evident in this report, particular interest in the chemopreventive properties of vitamins is a topic of ongoing interest. This study reflects the effect of the baseline diet of its subjects on lung cancer risk as opposed to the effect of supplementation. As yet, no study of vitamin supplementation has shown benefit; in fact, there have been trials notoriously showing harm, including 2 studies showing increased lung cancer mortality with beta carotene supplementation.[3] The takeaway message for patients remains the same: eat a healthy diet.

L. T. Tanoue, MD

References

1. Stevens VL, McCullough ML, Sun J, Jacobs EJ, Campbell PT, Gapstur SM. High levels of folate from supplements and fortification are not associated with increased risk of colorectal cancer. *Gastroenterology.* 2011;141:98-105.
2. Ebbing M, Bønaa KH, Nygård O, et al. Cancer incidence and mortality after treatment with folic acid and vitamin B12. *JAMA.* 2009;302:2119-2126.
3. Omenn GS. Chemoprevention of lung cancers: lessons from CARET, the beta-carotene and retinol efficacy trial, and prospects for the future. *Eur J Cancer Prev.* 2007;16:184-191.

Tobacco-Related Issues

Quitting Smoking Among Adults — United States, 2001–2010

Centers for Disease Control and Prevention (CDC)
MMWR Morb Mortal Wkly Rep 60:1513-1519, 2011

Quitting smoking is beneficial to health at any age, and cigarette smokers who quit before age 35 years have mortality rates similar to those who never smoked. From 1965 to 2010, the prevalence of cigarette smoking among adults in the United States decreased from 42.4% to 19.3%, in part because of an increase in the number who quit smoking. Since 2002, the number of former U.S. smokers has exceeded the number of current smokers. Mass media campaigns, increases in the prices of tobacco products, and smoke-free policies have been shown to increase smoking cessation. In addition, brief cessation advice by health-care providers; individual, group, and telephone counseling; and cessation medications are effective cessation treatments. To determine the prevalence of 1) current interest in quitting smoking, 2) successful recent smoking cessation, 3) recent use of cessation treatments, and 4) trends in quit attempts over a 10-year period, CDC analyzed data from the 2001—2010 National Health Interview Surveys (NHIS). This report summarizes the results of that analysis, which found that, in 2010, 68.8% of adult smokers wanted to stop smoking, 52.4% had made a quit attempt in the past year, 6.2% had recently quit, 48.3% had been advised by a health professional to quit, and 31.7% had used counseling and/or medications when they tried to quit. The prevalence of quit attempts increased during 2001—2010 among smokers aged 25—64 years, but not among other age groups. Health-care providers should identify smokers and offer them brief cessation advice at each visit; counseling and medication should be offered to patients willing to make a quit attempt.

▶ Tobacco control is hailed as one of the 10 great public health achievements in the United States over the last decade.[1] Despite significant gains, it is estimated that cigarette smoking and second-hand smoke exposure still result in approximately 443 000 premature deaths and $193 billion in health care costs and productivity losses annually.[2] This report from the Centers for Disease Control and its accompanying editorial provide a comprehensive look at the various aspects of smoking cessation, both its successes and its continued challenges, in the United States from 2001 to 2010. Data were obtained from the National Health Interview Surveys (NHIS) over that period of time. Overall, approximately 61% of surveyed individuals responded to the NHIS questionnaire. In 2010, 68.8% of current cigarette smokers said they would like to completely quit. A total of 52.4% had tried to quit within the previous year, but only 31.7% had used medications and/or received counseling. Only 48.3% of those who had visited a health care provider within that year reported receiving smoking cessation counseling.

Smoking cessation counseling by a health professional and the use of pharmacotherapy are individually effective in increasing the likelihood of smoking cessation and are more effective when used together. Clinical guidelines for treating tobacco use and dependence are available through the US Department of Health and Human Services at http://www.surgeongeneral.gov/tobacco/treating_tobacco_use08.pdf.[3] Medicare now compensates health care providers for time spent in tobacco cessation counseling. Effective pharmacotherapies as well as a number of nicotine replacement therapies are readily available. Every state now has a cessation quitline (national toll-free number 1-800-QUIT NOW). Since approximately 20% of all adult Americans continue to be habitual tobacco users, all of these resources should be used to help enable our patients to quit smoking.

L. T. Tanoue, MD

References

1. Centers for Disease Control and Prevention (CDC). Ten great public health achievements—United States, 2001—2010. *MMWR Morb Mortal Wkly Rep.* 2011; 60:619-623.

2. Centers for Disease Control and Prevention (CDC). Smoking-attributable mortality, years of potential life lost, and productivity losses—United States, 2000–2004. *MMWR Morb Mortal Wkly Rep.* 2008;57:1226-1228.
3. Fiore M, Jaen C, Baker T, et al. *Treating Tobacco Use and Dependence: 2008 Update. Clinical Practice Guideline.* Rockville, MD: US Department of Health and Human Services, Public Health Service; 2008. http://www.surgeongeneral. gov/tobacco/treating_tobacco_use08.pdf. Accessed January 2, 2012.

Treating Smokers in the Health Care Setting

Fiore MC, Baker TB (Univ of Wisconsin School of Medicine and Public Health, Madison)

N Engl J Med 365:1222-1231, 2011

Background.—Smoking prevalence has fallen dramatically in the United States, but recently prevalence rates have been concentrated among persons with low incomes, low educational levels, and psychiatric conditions. However, these persons benefit from the same treatments that help other smokers, so clinicians should be vigilant about offering help and guidance for smoking cessation.

Clinical Effects of Smoking.—Within 10 seconds of each inhalation, nicotine is carried by tar particles into lung alveoli, then to the brain. It binds to nicotinic cholinergic receptors in the brain and triggers the release of neurotransmitters that augment the attractiveness of smoking and reinforce smoking cues. Tolerance develops with long-term smoking, leading to the proliferation of nicotinic receptors and higher levels of self-administered nicotine. If nicotine is unavailable to bind to receptors, through reduced smoking or smoking cessation, withdrawal symptoms such as craving, negative moods, and restlessness develop. These symptoms prompt the person to return to smoking. About half of phenotypic variance in tobacco dependence is the result of genetic influences.

Challenges to Clinical Treatment.—Many clinicians fail to consistently offer smoking cessation treatments to smokers. Only about 20% of smokers are ready to quit at any given time, and smokers often choose unaided methods of quitting, which fail in 95% of cases. The success of smoking cessation is less likely with nonadherence to medications and counseling, but this nonadherence is common. Typically, patients take about half of the recommended doses of medication and attend fewer than half of their counseling appointments.

Evidence-Based Treatments and Strategies.—At every health care visit, smokers should be encouraged to quit and asked if they are willing to do so. Patients who are initially unwilling can be approached using motivational interviewing, which involves the use of nonconfrontational counseling to resolve the patient's ambivalence and encourages choices consistent with the patient's long-term goals. Motivational interviewing increases 6-month cessation rates, especially if smokers receive two or more sessions that last at least 20 minutes. "Five R's" counseling focuses on personally relevant reasons to quit, risks associated with continued smoking, rewards for

TABLE 3.—Medications for Smoking Cessation

Medication	Dose	Instructions	Cautions and Warnings	Side Effects	Availability
Sustained-release bupropion	Days 1–3: 150 mg each morning; day 4–end: 150 mg twice daily	Start 1–2 wk before quit date; use for 2–6 mo	Do not use with monoamine oxidase inhibitors or bupropion in any other form or in patients with a history of seizures or eating disorders; see FDA black-box warning on serious mental health events: www.fda.gov/News Events/Newsroom/PressAnnounce ments/ucm170100.htm	Insomnia, dry mouth, vivid or abnormal dreams	Prescription only; generic or brandname drugs (Zyban, Wellbutrin SR)
Nicotine gum	1 piece every 1–2 hr initially, then taper; up to 24 pieces/day; 2 mg if patient smokes ≤24 cigarettes/day and 4 mg if patient smokes ≥25 cigarettes/day	Use up to 12 weeks	Patients with dentures should use with caution; patients should not eat or drink 15 min before or during use	Mouth soreness, heartburn	Over-the-counter only; generic or brand-name drug (Nicorette)
Nicotine inhaler	6–16 cartridges/day; inhale 80 times/cartridge	Use up to 6 mo; taper at end	May irritate mouth and throat	Mouth and throat irritation	Prescription only (Nicotrol inhaler)
Nicotine lozenges	1 piece every 1–2 hr initially, then taper; 2 mg if patient smokes 30 min or more after waking and 4 mg if patient smokes <30 min after waking	Use 3–6 mo	Patients should not eat or drink 15 min before or during use	Hiccups, cough, heartburn	Over-the-counter only; generic or brand-name drug (Commit)
Nicotine nasal spray	1 dose is 1 squirt/nostril; 1–2 doses/hr; up to 40 doses/day	Use 3–6 mo	Not for patients with asthma; may irritate nose; may cause dependence	Nasal irritation	Prescription only (Nicotrol NS)
Nicotine patch	If patient smokes ≥10 cigarettes/day, 21 mg/day for 4 wk, then 14 mg/day for 2 wk, then 7 mg/day for 2 wk; if patient smokes <10 cigarettes/day, start with 14 mg/day for 6 wk, then 7 mg/day for 2 wk	Use new patch every morning for 8–12 wks	Do not use if patient has severe eczema or psoriasis; patch can be removed at night if sleep is disrupted	Local skin reaction, insomnia	Over-the-counter or prescription; generic or brand-name drugs (Nicoderm CQ, Nicotrol)

(Continued)

TABLE 3.—(*Continued*)

Medication	Dose	Instructions	Cautions and Warnings	Side Effects	Availability
Varenicline	Days 1–3: 0.5 mg every morning; days 4–7: 0.5 mg twice daily; days 8–end: 1 mg twice daily	Start 1 wk before quit date; use 3–6 mo	Use with caution in patients with clinically significant renal impairment, patients undergoing dialysis, and patients with serious psychiatric illness; see FDA Web sites for black-box warning on serious mental health events and statement on risk of cardiovascular adverse events among patients with cardiovascular disease: www.fda.gov/NewsEvents/Newsroom/Press Announcements/ucm170100.htm and www.fda.gov/Drugs/DrugSafety/ucm259161.htm	Nausea, insomnia, vivid or abnormal dreams	Prescription only (Chantix)
Combination therapies*					
Patch plus bupropion	Follow instructions for individual medications above	Follow instructions for individual medications above	See information for individual medications above	See information for individual medications above	See above
Patch plus gum, inhalers, or lozenges	Follow instructions for individual medications above	Follow instructions for individual medications above	See information for individual medications above	See information for individual medications above	See above

*Only the nicotine patch plus bupropion is currently approved by the Food and Drug Administration.

quitting, and roadblocks to successful quitting, with repetition of the counseling at each clinic visit. Counseling using these approaches plus the offer of nicotine-replacement therapy is associated with a higher quit rate among smokers. Patients unwilling to quit can be encouraged to reduce their smoking and use nicotine-replacement therapy for at least several months. Patients who are willing to quit should be provided with practical advice on avoiding smoking triggers and encouraged to use available resources for smoking cessation. These include adjuvant counseling, online resources, or both. Clinicians should explain the benefits and risks associated with medications and clarify any misconceptions the patient may have.

Conclusions.—The use of motivational interviewing, counseling, and smoking reduction is in line with the clinical practice guidelines of the US Public Health Service. Nicotine-replacement therapy is a useful alternative for smokers reluctant to take on smoking cessation. Adhering to the use of these medications shows a strong link to successful outcomes (Table 3).

▶ Smoking rates have decreased dramatically in the United States since the publication of the first Surgeon General's report on the health consequences of smoking in 1964. However, smoking rates over the last decade among the adult American population have plateaued at approximately 20%, still unacceptably high. This concise and practical review by Fiore and Baker summarizes many of the points of the clinical practice guideline of the US Public Health Service, "Treating Tobacco Use and Dependence."[1] On average, smokers incur $1600 more in annual health care costs than nonsmokers.[2] From the perspectives of both disease prevention and health economics, smoking cessation must be a priority. Strong and positive interventions can be highly effective in the health care setting. Seventy percent of smokers in the United States see a primary care physician each year, providing substantial opportunity for intervention. While higher smoking prevalence correlates with lower income, lower levels of education, and the presence of psychiatric illness, smoking cessation interventions that are effective in general have been demonstrated to be of benefit in these populations. Fiore and Baker clearly and succinctly describe the interventions that can and should be made by health care providers, particularly motivational interviewing and counseling for the patient willing to quit as well as the patient unwilling to quit, and outlines strategies for nicotine replacement and pharmacotherapy (Table 3). This useful and practical reference should be a must read for all physicians.

L. T. Tanoue, MD

References

1. Fiore M, Jaen C, Baker T, et al. *Treating Tobacco Use and Dependence: 2008 Update. Clinical Practice Guideline.* Rockville, MD: US Department of Health and Human Services, Public Health Service; 2008.
2. Centers for Disease Control and Prevention (CDC). Annual smoking-attributable mortality, years of potential life lost, and economic costs—United States, 1995–1999. *MMWR Morb Mortal Wkly Rep.* 2002;51:300-303.

Lung Cancer Screening

Reduced Lung-Cancer Mortality with Low-Dose Computed Tomographic Screening

The National Lung Screening Trial Research Team (Univ of California at Los Angeles; Brown Univ, Providence, RI; Natl Cancer Inst, Bethesda, MD; et al)
N Engl J Med 365:395-409, 2011

Background.—The aggressive and heterogeneous nature of lung cancer has thwarted efforts to reduce mortality from this cancer through the use of screening. The advent of low-dose helical computed tomography (CT) altered the landscape of lung-cancer screening, with studies indicating that low-dose CT detects many tumors at early stages. The National Lung Screening Trial (NLST) was conducted to determine whether screening with low-dose CT could reduce mortality from lung cancer.

Methods.—From August 2002 through April 2004, we enrolled 53,454 persons at high risk for lung cancer at 33 U.S. medical centers. Participants were randomly assigned to undergo three annual screenings with either low-dose CT (26,722 participants) or single-view posteroanterior chest radiography (26,732). Data were collected on cases of lung cancer and deaths from lung cancer that occurred through December 31, 2009.

Results.—The rate of adherence to screening was more than 90%. The rate of positive screening tests was 24.2% with low-dose CT and 6.9% with radiography over all three rounds. A total of 96.4% of the positive screening results in the low-dose CT group and 94.5% in the radiography group were false positive results. The incidence of lung cancer was 645 cases per 100,000 person-years (1060 cancers) in the low-dose CT group, as compared with 572 cases per 100,000 person-years (941 cancers) in the radiography group (rate ratio, 1.13; 95% confidence interval [CI], 1.03 to 1.23). There were 247 deaths from lung cancer per 100,000 person-years in the low-dose CT group and 309 deaths per 100,000 person-years in the radiography group, representing a relative reduction in mortality from lung cancer with low-dose CT screening of 20.0% (95% CI, 6.8 to 26.7; $P = 0.004$). The rate of death from any cause was reduced in the low-dose CT group, as compared with the radiography group, by 6.7% (95% CI, 1.2 to 13.6; $P = 0.02$).

Conclusions.—Screening with the use of low-dose CT reduces mortality from lung cancer. (Funded by the National Cancer Institute; National Lung Screening Trial ClinicalTrials.gov number, NCT00047385.)

▶ The results of the National Lung Screening Trial presented in this report demonstrate that screening for lung cancer with low-dose CT scanning reduces mortality from lung cancer. This is a landmark study. No prior study of lung cancer screening by any modality has ever demonstrated a mortality benefit. As shown in Fig 1 in the original article, low-dose CT screening resulted in an increase in the number of lung cancers diagnosed as well as a decrease in the number of deaths from lung cancer when compared with screening with chest radiography. The Prostate,

Lung, Colorectal, and Ovarian (PLCO) Cancer Randomized Trial demonstrated that chest radiography as a lung cancer screening intervention is no better than usual care (ie, no systematic screening).[1] Although no direct comparison of low-dose CT versus usual care is available, the negative finding of the PLCO is integral to the interpretation and application of the NLST.

Several key points should be noted regarding application of the results of the NLST. First, the study population was clearly defined and included only individuals aged 55 to 74 with relatively heavy smoking history (> 30 pack-years, currently smoking or if former smokers, having quit within the previous 15 years). Generalizing the NLST results to other populations is problematic. Specifically, the NLST does not address individuals with other lung cancer risk factors, such as positive family history, domestic or occupational carcinogen exposure, underlying pulmonary diseases such as chronic obstructive pulmonary disease, interstitial lung disease, for example, or individuals who smoked less than 30 pack-years. The question of whether screening would be of benefit in these other populations remains unanswered. Second, as with prior studies of low-dose CT screening, the NLST had a very high rate of false-positive findings.[2,3] Approximately 25% of all subjects had an abnormality identified on screening each year of the study, of which 96% were false positives. The health care and emotional costs of these false-positive findings have as yet to be measured but will undoubtedly be substantial. Third, the issue of overdiagnosis, specifically cancers diagnosed by screening that are not destined to cause death, is still a concern, as it has been with prior studies evaluating screening with either chest radiography or low-dose CT.[4] Fourth, both the medical and lay communities are increasingly aware of the potential carcinogenic risks associated with diagnostic radiation. The NLST investigators estimated that the radiation incurred from serial screening studies in 55-year-old smokers would result in 1 to 3 new lung cancer deaths per 10 000 screened and 0.3 new breast cancers deaths per 10 000 screened. Strict adherence to radiation dosing protocols at sites providing screening CT studies will be necessary and should be monitored. Fifth, the population who would potentially be screening candidates is large, even by the strict criteria of the NLST, consisting of an estimated 7 million Americans. An even larger number, 94 million American adults, are either current or former smokers. The costs of a broadly applied screening program would be staggering. Publication of a health care cost analysis of the NLST is anticipated soon.

Despite the many questions that remain, the NLST demonstrates that screening for lung cancer with low-dose CT saves lives. The current 5-year survival rate for lung cancer is a dismal 16%.[5] The need for an intervention that will improve our ability to detect lung cancer early is clearly pressing. Although many advances have been made in treatment for lung cancer, the fact remains that the majority of patients are diagnosed at advanced stage, when cure is unlikely and improvements in survival related to treatment are measured in months, not years. Further work of the NLST investigators is anticipated regarding cost-effectiveness of screening and the increases in heath care utilization that seem inevitable, as well as the impact of screening on smoking behavior and quality of life. The results of these studies are likely to inform any major changes in health care policy on a national level.

L. T. Tanoue, MD

References

1. Oken MM, Hocking WG, Kvale PA, et al. Screening by chest radiograph and lung cancer mortality: the Prostate, Lung, Colorectal, and Ovarian (PLCO) randomized trial. *JAMA.* 2011;306:1865-1873.
2. Swensen SJ, Jett JR, Hartman TE, et al. CT screening for lung cancer: five-year prospective experience. *Radiology.* 2005;235:259-265.
3. Henschke CI, Naidich DP, Yankelevitz DF, et al. Early lung cancer action project: initial findings on repeat screenings. *Cancer.* 2001;92:153-159.
4. Marcus PM, Bergstralh EJ, Zweig MH, Harris A, Offord KP, Fontana RS. Extended lung cancer incidence follow-up in the Mayo Lung Project and overdiagnosis. *J Natl Cancer Inst.* 2006;98:748-756.
5. Siegel R, Ward E, Brawley O, Jemal A. Cancer statistics, 2011: the impact of eliminating socioeconomic and racial disparities on premature cancer deaths. *CA Cancer J Clin.* 2011;61:212-236.

Screening by Chest Radiograph and Lung Cancer Mortality: The Prostate, Lung, Colorectal, and Ovarian (PLCO) Randomized Trial

Oken MM, for the PLCO Project Team (Univ of Minnesota, Minneapolis; et al)
JAMA 306:1865-1873, 2011

Context.—The effect on mortality of screening for lung cancer with modern chest radiographs is unknown.

Objective.—To evaluate the effect on mortality of screening for lung cancer using radiographs in the Prostate, Lung, Colorectal, andOvarian (PLCO) Cancer Screening Trial.

Design, Setting, and Participants.—Randomized controlled trial that involved 154 901 participants aged 55 through 74 years, 77 445 of whom were assigned to annual screenings and 77 456 to usual care at 1 of 10 screening centers across the United States between November 1993 and July 2001. The data from a subset of eligible participants for the National Lung Screening Trial (NLST), which compared chest radiograph with spiral computed tomographic (CT) screening, were analyzed.

Intervention.—Participants in the intervention group were offered annual posteroanterior view chest radiograph for 4 years. Diagnostic follow-up of positive screening results was determined by participants and their health care practitioners. Participants in the usual care group were offered no interventions and received their usual medical care. All diagnosed cancers, deaths, and causes of death were ascertained through the earlier of 13 years of follow-up or until December 31, 2009.

Main Outcome Measures.—Mortality from lung cancer. Secondary outcomes included lung cancer incidence, complications associated with diagnostic procedures, and all-cause mortality.

Results.—Screening adherence was 86.6% at baseline and 79% to 84% at years 1 through 3; the rate of screening use in the usual care group was 11%. Cumulative lung cancer incidence rates through 13 years of follow-up were 20.1 per 10 000 person-years in the intervention group and 19.2 per 10 000 person-years in the usual care group (rate ratio [RR]; 1.05, 95% CI, 0.98-1.12). A total of 1213 lung cancer deaths were observed in the intervention group compared with 1230 in usual care group through 13 years (mortality RR, 0.99; 95% CI, 0.87-1.22). Stage and histology were similar between the 2 groups. The RR of mortality for the subset of participants eligible for the NLST, over the same 6-year follow-up period, was 0.94 (95% CI, 0.81-1.10).

Conclusion.—Annual screening with chest radiograph did not reduce lung cancer mortality compared with usual care.

Trial Registration.—clinicaltrials.gov Identifier: NCT00002540.

▶ The Prostate, Lung, Colorectal, and Ovarian (PLCO) Cancer Screening Trial was initiated in 1993, eventually enrolling more than 154 000 subjects aged 55 to 74 years in the United States. The intent of the PLCO trial was to evaluate the effect of a package of screening interventions on prevention of death from 4 cancers. The PLCO participants were enrolled from 10 centers across the country, representing a geographically and ethnically diverse population. There was no eligibility requirement for smoking. Subjects in the lung cancer arm were randomized to either usual care (ie, no screening) or to a lung cancer screening intervention, which consisted of a baseline chest radiograph with 3 annual follow-up studies. Subjects were then monitored over 13 years. As demonstrated in Fig 2 in the original article, there was no difference in cumulative lung cancer incidence in the usual care group compared with the intervention group (19.2 per 10 000 person-years in the usual care group vs 20.1 per 10 000 person-years in the intervention group). As demonstrated in Fig 3 in the original article, there was also no difference in lung cancer mortality (relative risk of mortality in the usual care vs intervention group 0.99; 95% confidence interval, 0.87—1.22). Similar negative results were reported more than 20 years ago in several lung cancer screening trials evaluating chest radiography as a screening intervention.[1,2] The PLCO trial robustly confirms that lung cancer screening with chest radiography is not effective.

The PLCO trial results are of great significance in the context of the National Lung Screening Trial (NLST), which did not include an arm with chest radiography as a screening intervention. Of note, approximately 21% of subjects in the PLCO trial met the more than 30 pack-year smoking entry requirement for the NLST.[3] It is particularly pertinent to note that, in a subset analysis, this group also did not demonstrate any decrease in lung cancer mortality with chest radiography as the screening intervention compared with the benefit in mortality demonstrated with low-dose chest CT scanning in the NLST. The findings of the PLCO are thus fundamentally important to the interpretation of the NLST and to health policy recommendations that should inevitably evolve from the results of the 2 trials.

L. T. Tanoue, MD

References

1. Melamed MR, Flehinger BJ, Zaman MB, Heelan RT, Perchick WA, Martini N. Screening for early lung cancer. Results of the Memorial Sloan-Kettering study in New York. *Chest.* 1984;86:44-53.
2. Fontana RS, Sanderson DR, Woolner LB, Taylor WF, Miller WE, Muhm JR. Lung cancer screening: the Mayo program. *J Occup Med.* 1986;28:746-750.
3. Aberle DR, Adams AM, Berg CD, et al. Reduced lung-cancer mortality with low-dose computed tomographic screening. *N Engl J Med.* 2011;365:395-409.

Baseline Characteristics of Participants in the Randomized National Lung Screening Trial

The National Lung Screening Trial Research Team (David Geffen School of Medicine at UCLA; Brown Univ, Providence, RI; Natl Cancer Inst, Bethesda, MD; et al)

J Natl Cancer Inst 102:1771-1779, 2010

Background.—The National Lung Screening Trial (NLST), a randomized study conducted at 33 US sites, is comparing lung cancer mortality among persons screened with reduced dose helical computerized tomography and among persons screened with chest radiograph. In this article, we present characteristics of the study population.

Methods.—Eligible participants were aged 55–74 years and were current or former smokers with a cigarette smoking history of at least 30 pack-years. Randomization was stratified by site, sex, and age. To assess representativeness of the study population, demographic characteristics of individuals from the general population who met NLST age and smoking history inclusion criteria were obtained from the Tobacco Use Supplement of the US Census Bureau Current Population Surveys.

Results.—The NLST enrolled 53 456 persons, with 26 733 randomly assigned to chest radiograph screening and 26 723 to computerized tomography screening. Characteristics of the participants were as follows: 31 533 (59%) were men, 39 234 (73%) were younger than 65 years, 25 779 (48%) were current smokers, and 16 839 (32%) had a college or higher degree. Median cigarette exposure was 48 pack-years. Among Tobacco Use Supplement respondents who met NLST age and smoking history criteria, 59% were men, 65% were younger than 65 years, and 57% were current smokers. Median cigarette exposure among this group was 47 pack-years, and 14% had a college degree or higher.

Conclusion.—The NLST cohort has a distribution of sex and pack-year history that is similar to the component of the general US population that meets the major NLST eligibility criteria; however, NLST participants are younger, better educated, and less likely to be current smokers.

▶ Even with more than 50 000 individuals enrolled in the National Lung Screening Trial (NLST), it is necessary to evaluate the generalizability of the results to the population at large.[1] The baseline characteristics of the study population, as described in this report by the NLST Research Team, are critical to the applicability of the results of the trial. The NLST study population consisted of men and women ages 55 to 74, with more than 30 pack-years of smoking, currently smoking, or having quit within the prior 15 years. These individuals were very heavy smokers (median 48 pack-years in current and 50 pack-years in former smokers). There were several differences between the NLST population and the general US population who would have been eligible for the trial. The NLST population was younger (73% of the NLST cohort was < 65 years old compared with 65% of the general population), were more educated (32% of the NLST cohort had at least a college degree compared with 14% of the general population), were more likely to be married (67% compared with 60%, respectively), and were less likely to be current smokers (48% vs 57%, respectively). These differences do not affect the interpretation of the NLST itself but may have an impact on our ability to generalize the NLST findings to the US population at large, as younger age, more years of education, and married status are factors that may positively impact overall health and disease outcomes. This is perhaps not surprising because research participants are often healthier than the general populations they represent ("healthy volunteer effect"). However, one could speculate that the benefit of lung cancer screening in the population at large might actually be even greater than in the study population of the NLST.

L. T. Tanoue, MD

Reference

1. Aberle DR, Adams AM, Berg CD, et al. Reduced lung-cancer mortality with low-dose computed tomographic screening. *N Engl J Med.* 2011;365:395-409.

Identification of Chronic Obstructive Pulmonary Disease in Lung Cancer Screening Computed Tomographic Scans

Mets OM, Buckens CFM, Zanen P, et al (Univ Med Ctr Utrecht, The Netherlands; et al)

JAMA 306:1775-1781, 2011

Context.—Smoking is a major risk factor for both cancer and chronic obstructive pulmonary disease (COPD). Computed tomography (CT)—based lung cancer screening may provide an opportunity to detect additional individuals with COPD at an early stage.

Objective.—To determine whether low-dose lung cancer screening CT scans can be used to identify participants with COPD.

Design, Setting, and Patients.—Single-center prospective cross-sectional study within an ongoing lung cancer screening trial. Prebronchodilator pulmonary function testing with inspiratory and expiratory CT on the same day was obtained from 1140 male participants between July 2007 and September 2008. Computed tomographic emphysema was defined as percentage of voxels less than −950 Hounsfield units (HU), and CT air trapping was defined as the expiratory:inspiratory ratio of mean lung density. Chronic obstructive pulmonary disease was defined as the ratio of forced expiratory volume in the first second to forced vital capacity (FEV_1/FVC) of less than 70%. Logistic regression was used to develop a diagnostic prediction model for airflow limitation.

Main Outcome Measures.—Diagnostic accuracy of COPD diagnosis using pulmonary function tests as the reference standard.

Results.—Four hundred thirty-seven participants (38%) had COPD according to lung function testing. A diagnostic model with CT emphysema, CT air trapping, body mass index, pack-years, and smoking status corrected for overoptimism (internal validation) yielded an area under the receiver operating characteristic curve of 0.83 (95% CI, 0.81-0.86). Using the point of optimal accuracy, the model identified 274 participants with COPD with 85 false-positives, a sensitivity of 63% (95% CI, 58%-67%), specificity of 88% (95% CI, 85%-90%), positive predictive value of 76% (95% CI, 72%-81%); and negative predictive value of 79% (95% CI, 76%-82%). The diagnostic model showed an area under the receiver operating characteristic curve of 0.87 (95% CI, 0.86-0.88) for participants with symptoms and 0.78 (95% CI, 0.76-0.80) for those without symptoms.

Conclusion.—Among men who are current and former heavy smokers, low-dose inspiratory and expiratory CT scans obtained for lung cancer screening can identify participants with COPD, with a sensitivity of 63% and a specificity of 88%.

▶ Chronic obstructive pulmonary disease (COPD) is one of the major health consequences of cigarette smoking and is associated with substantial morbidity and mortality. COPD is typically underdiagnosed; patients often present with advanced and symptomatic disease after a long period of insidious progression. As is true with lung cancer, early detection of COPD may allow interventions that can improve outcomes and, in particular, may be important in encouraging smoking cessation and avoidance of other tobacco-related health issues. This study by Mets and colleagues was performed within the ongoing Dutch and Belgian randomized lung cancer computed tomography (CT) screening trial (NELSON trial).[1] NELSON participants included 1800 men between the ages of 50 to 75 with greater than 16.5 pack-years of smoking. In addition to the lung cancer CT screening examination, 1140 subjects in this study received pulmonary function testing (PFT) as well as an expiratory CT scan. A total of 3.6% of participants self-reported physician-diagnosed emphysema, whereas 38% were identified with COPD based on PFT demonstrating forced expiratory volume in the first second to forced vital capacity of less than 70%. Automated analysis of the screening and expiratory CT scans was performed to evaluate attenuation for quantifying emphysema and air trapping severity. Logistic regression was used to develop a multivariable model incorporating 5 variables found to be independently associated with COPD: (1) emphysema on CT scan; (2) air trapping seen on expiratory CT scan; (3) body mass index; (4) pack-years smoked; and (5) current smoking status. The model had a 76% positive predictive value and a 79% negative predictive value.

Based on the results of the National Lung Screening Trial, low-dose screening CT scanning may be implemented for individuals who are heavy smokers.[2] This study by Mets and colleagues suggests that detection of COPD may be feasible using clinical prediction models incorporating data obtained from CT screening, even in the absence of symptoms. Since COPD has enormous adverse health care consequences, early disease identification using such a model could have important potential benefit. Alternatively, if the rate of COPD is very high in a population that will qualify for screening, one could argue that PFT, or at least simple spirometry, should be strongly considered in any patient undergoing lung cancer screening.

L. T. Tanoue, MD

References

1. van Iersel CA, de Koning HJ, Draisma G, et al. Risk-based selection from the general population in a screening trial: selection criteria, recruitment and power for the Dutch-Belgian randomised lung cancer multi-slice CT screening trial (NELSON). *Int J Cancer.* 2007;120:868-874.
2. Aberle DR, Adams AM, Berg CD, et al. Reduced lung-cancer mortality with low-dose computed tomographic screening. *N Engl J Med.* 2011;365:395-409.

Diagnostic Evaluation

Seventh Edition of the Cancer Staging Manual and Stage Grouping of Lung Cancer: Quick Reference Chart and Diagrams

Lababede O, Meziane M, Rice T (Cleveland Clinic, OH)
Chest 139:183-189, 2011

Lung cancer remains the most common cause of cancer-related death in the United States. TNM staging, which is an important guide to the prognosis and treatment of lung cancer, has been revised recently. In this article, we propose a quick reference chart and diagrams that consolidate TNM staging information in a simple format. The current classification of lymph node stations and zones is illustrated as well (Fig 1).

▶ The TNM cancer staging system provides an anatomic framework for consistent and reproducible descriptions of solid tumors, including lung cancer. The current 7th edition of the TNM staging classification for lung cancer reflects a remarkable decade of work by the International Association for the Study of Lung Cancer (IASLC), culminating in endorsement by the International Union Against Cancer and the American Joint Committee on Cancer in 2009, and subsequent implementation into clinical practice.[1-4] The IASLC also adopted a new international lymph node map, resolving differences between previous mapping strategies.[5] The descriptors for the primary tumor (T), lymph node involvement (N), and distant metastasis (M) contain a great deal of detail that can be challenging to remember. Lababede and colleagues offer a user-friendly staging chart for clinicians, which concisely incorporates much of this detail

M1a
- Satellite (separate) tumor nodule(s) in contralateral lung
- Pleural nodules or malignant pleural or pericardial effusion

M1b
Distant metastasis

Stage IV (Any T, Any N, M1)

(Distant metastasis present)

M1

DISTANT METASTASIS (M)

M0

(No distant metastasis)

◄ Explanation of lymph node staging:

- For any N category, one or more of the groups marked by ● must be involved and the involvement of all groups marked by ⊟ should be absent

- The presence or absence of involvement in groups marked by ▨ does not alter N staging in the corresponding category.

LYMPH NODE (N)

Columns: Scalene (ipsi./contralateral) | Supraclavicular | Hilar | Mediastinal [Contralateral] | Subcarinal | Mediastinal | Hilar [Ipsilateral] | Peribronchial

N	Scalene	Supraclav	Hilar(C)	Med(C)	Subcarinal	Med(I)	Hilar(I)	Peribronch	Stage
N3	●	●	●	●	▨				Stage III B
N2	–	–	–	–	●	●	▨		Stage III A
N1	–	–	–	–	–	–	●	●	Stage II A / II B
N0	–	–	–	–	–	–	–	–	Stage I A / I B / II A / II B

PRIMARY TUMOR (T) ▷

		T1a	T1b	T2a	T2b	T3	T4
Stage 0 (Tis N0 M0) Tis: Carcinoma in situ	**1- Size**	≤2 cm	>2 cm ≤3 cm	>3 cm ≤5 cm; Any size ≤7 cm if 1 or more of the criteria of extent are present *	>5 cm ≤7 cm	>7 cm or Any size if 1 or more of the criteria of extent are present	Any size if 1 or more of the criteria of extent are present
Occult Carcinoma (Tx N0 M0) Tx: Tumor is proven histopathologically (+ Cytology) but not detected by imaging or bronchoscopy	**Endo-bronchial Location**	No extension proximal to the lobar bronchus **		Main bronchus ≥ 2 cm distal to the carina **; Vs. Atelectasis or obstructive pneumonitis extending to the hilum but not involving the entire lung		Main bronchus < 2 cm distal to the carina **; Vs. Atelectasis or obstructive pneumonitis involving the entire lung	Involvement of the carina
The 2009 TNM staging system applies to non-small cell lung carcinoma as well as to small cell carcinoma and carcinoid tumor of the lung	**Local Invasion**	None; the tumor is surrounded by lung or visceral pleura		Visceral pleura		Chest wall ***, diaphragm, phrenic nerve, mediastinal pleura and/or parietal pericardium	Mediastinum, trachea, heart, great vessels, recurrent laryngeal nerve, esophagus, vertebral body
	Satellite Nodule(s)	None		None		Separate tumor nodule(s) in the same lobe	Separate tumor nodule(s) in a different ipsilateral lobe

(Rows under "2- Criteria of Extent")

* : A tumor with these features is classified as T2a if ≤ 5 cm in size and T2b if > 5 cm and ≤ 7 cm
** : The uncommon superficial spreading tumor with invasion limited to the bronchial wall is considered T1a regardless of size and extension to the main bronchus
*** : Including superior sulcus tumors

FIGURE 1.—Reference chart for 2009 TNM staging system of lung cancer. M = metastases; N = regional lymph node involvement; T = tumor. (Reprinted from Lababede O, Meziane M, Rice T. Seventh edition of the cancer staging manual and stage grouping of lung cancer: quick reference chart and diagrams. *Chest*. 2011;139:183-189, © American College of Chest Physicians.)

(Fig 1). The accompanying tables and diagrams should serve as useful references in the office or bronchoscopy suite.

L. T. Tanoue, MD

References

1. Goldstraw P, Crowley J, Chansky K, et al; International Association for the Study of Lung Cancer International Staging Committee, Participating Institutions. The IASLC Lung Cancer Staging Project: proposals for the revision of the TNM stage groupings in the forthcoming (seventh) edition of the TNM classification of malignant tumours. *J Thorac Oncol.* 2007;2:706-714.
2. Postmus PE, Brambilla E, Chansky K, et al; International Association for the Study of Lung Cancer International Staging Committee, Cancer Research and Biostatistics, Observers to the Committee, Participating Institutions. The IASLC Lung Cancer Staging Project: proposals for revision of the M descriptors in the forthcoming (seventh) edition of the TNM classification of lung cancer. *J Thorac Oncol.* 2007;2:686-693.
3. Rusch VW, Crowley J, Giroux DJ, et al; International Association for the Study of Lung Cancer International Staging Committee, Cancer Research and Biostatistics, Observers to the Committee, Participating Institutions. The IASLC Lung Cancer Staging Project: proposals for the revision of the N descriptors in the forthcoming seventh edition of the TNM classification for lung cancer. *J Thorac Oncol.* 2007;2: 603-612.
4. Rami-Porta R, Ball D, Crowley J, et al; International Association for the Study of Lung Cancer International Staging Committee, Cancer Research and Biostatistics, Observers to the Committee, Participating Institutions. The IASLC Lung Cancer Staging Project: proposals for the revision of the T descriptors in the forthcoming (seventh) edition of the TNM classification for lung cancer. *J Thorac Oncol.* 2007; 2:593-602.
5. Rusch VW, Asamura H, Watanabe H, Giroux DJ, Rami-Porta R, Goldstraw P; Members of IASLC Staging Committee. The IASLC lung cancer staging project: a proposal for a new international lymph node map in the forthcoming seventh edition of the TNM classification for lung cancer. *J Thorac Oncol.* 2009;4:568-577.

Mediastinoscopy vs Endosonography for Mediastinal Nodal Staging of Lung Cancer: A Randomized Trial

Annema JT, van Meerbeeck JP, Rintoul RC, et al (Leiden Univ Med Ctr, the Netherlands; Ghent Univ Hosp, Belgium; Papworth Hosp, Cambridge, UK; et al)
JAMA 304:2245-2252, 2010

Context.—Mediastinal nodal staging is recommended for patients with resectable non—small cell lung cancer (NSCLC). Surgical staging has limitations, which results in the performance of unnecessary thoracotomies. Current guidelines acknowledge minimally invasive endosonography followed by surgical staging (if no nodal metastases are found by endosonography) as an alternative to immediate surgical staging.

Objective.—To compare the 2 recommended lung cancer staging strategies.

Design, Setting, and Patients.—Randomized controlled multicenter trial (Ghent, Leiden, Leuven, Papworth) conducted between February 2007 and April 2009 in 241 patients with resectable (suspected) NSCLC in whom mediastinal staging was indicated based on computed or positron emission tomography.

Intervention.—Either surgical staging or endosonography (combined transesophageal and endobronchial ultrasound [EUS-FNA and EBUS-TBNA]) followed by surgical staging in case no nodal metastases were found at endosonography. Thoracotomy with lymph node dissection was performed when there was no evidence of mediastinal tumor spread.

Main Outcome Measures.—The primary outcome was sensitivity for mediastinal nodal (N2/N3) metastases. The reference standard was surgical pathological staging. Secondary outcomes were rates of unnecessary thoracotomy and complications.

Results.—Two hundred forty-one patients were randomized, 118 to surgical staging and 123 to endosonography, of whom 65 also underwent surgical staging. Nodal metastases were found in 41 patients (35%; 95% confidence interval [CI], 27%-44%) by surgical staging vs 56 patients (46%; 95% CI, 37%-54%) by endosonography ($P=.11$) and in 62 patients (50%; 95% CI, 42%-59%) by endosonography followed by surgical staging ($P=.02$). This corresponded to sensitivities of 79% (41/52; 95% CI, 66%-88%) vs 85% (56/66; 95% CI, 74%-92%) ($P=.47$) and 94% (62/66; 95% CI, 85%-98%) ($P=.02$). Thoracotomy was unnecessary in 21 patients (18%; 95% CI, 12%-26%) in the mediastinoscopy group vs 9 (7%; 95% CI, 4%-13%) in the endosonography group ($P=.02$). The complication rate was similar in both groups.

Conclusions.—Among patients with (suspected) NSCLC, a staging strategy combining endosonography and surgical staging compared with surgical staging alone resulted in greater sensitivity for mediastinal nodal metastases and fewer unnecessary thoracotomies.

Trial Registration.—clinicaltrials.gov Identifier: NCT00432640.

▶ Endosonographic approaches (endobronchial ultrasound [EBUS] and endoscopic ultrasound [EUS]) to mediastinal staging in lung cancer are becoming more widely available, but the question of whether these techniques are as reliable and accurate as surgical mediastinoscopy continues to be debated. In this large study, 241 patients with known or suspected potentially resectable non—small cell lung cancer in whom concern for malignant involvement of the mediastinal nodes was raised based on abnormal computed tomography or positron emission tomography imaging were randomly assigned to either cervical mediastinoscopy or combined EBUS and EUS. Patients with confirmed mediastinal (N2) cancer involvement by either approach did not proceed to surgical resection. Patients with negative EBUS/EUS went on to mediastinoscopy, as would be standard practice in many institutions, based on the concern for malignancy raised by the abnormal noninvasive imaging studies. Patients with negative mediastinoscopy or negative EBUS/EUS/mediastinoscopy underwent subsequent cancer resection with systematic mediastinal lymph node dissection. The sensitivities of mediastinoscopy, EBUS/EUS, and EBUS/EUS/mediastinoscopy were 79%, 85%, and 94%, respectively. Unnecessary thoracotomies (defined loosely as the identification of N2 nodal metastasis at surgical resection in patients with negative minimally invasive evaluation) were more frequent in the mediastinoscopy group than in the EBUS/EUS/mediastinoscopy group.

In this study, the sensitivity of combined EBUS/EUS for mediastinal staging in patients with lung cancer and radiographically abnormal mediastinal nodes, while still high, was lower than described elsewhere. In properly trained hands, there is little question that the accuracy of EBUS with or without EUS in mediastinal staging for lung cancer is at least as good as mediastinoscopy.[1,2] Decisions relating to the choice of staging procedures will inevitably reflect institutional availability and expertise in the various diagnostic modalities but should include the considerations that endosonographic mediastinal lymph node staging may be more cost effective than mediastinoscopy and, with appropriate planning, can yield adequate material for molecular mutational analysis in addition to usual histologic examination.[3-5]

L. T. Tanoue, MD

References

1. Wallace MB, Pascual JM, Raimondo M, et al. Minimally invasive endoscopic staging of suspected lung cancer. *JAMA*. 2008;299:540-546.
2. Herth FJ, Krasnik M, Kahn N, Eberhardt R, Ernst A. Combined endoscopic-endobronchial ultrasound-guided fine-needle aspiration of mediastinal lymph nodes through a single bronchoscope in 150 patients with suspected lung cancer. *Chest*. 2010;138:790-794.
3. Nakajima T, Yasufuku K, Nakagawara A, Kimura H, Yoshino I. Multigene mutation analysis of metastatic lymph nodes in non-small cell lung cancer diagnosed by endobronchial ultrasound-guided transbronchial needle aspiration. *Chest*. 2010; 140:1319-1324.
4. Nakajima T, Yasufuku K. How I do it—optimal methodology for multidirectional analysis of endobronchial ultrasound-guided transbronchial needle aspiration samples. *J Thorac Oncol*. 2011;6:203-206.
5. Steinfort DP, Liew D, Conron M, Hutchinson AF, Irving LB. Cost-benefit of minimally invasive staging of non-small cell lung cancer: a decision tree sensitivity analysis. *J Thorac Oncol*. 2010;5:1564-1570.

Population-Based Risk for Complications After Transthoracic Needle Lung Biopsy of a Pulmonary Nodule: An Analysis of Discharge Records

Wiener RS, Schwartz LM, Woloshin S, et al (Boston Univ School of Medicine, MA; Edith Nourse Rogers Memorial Veterans Affairs Hosp, Bedford, MA; Veterans Affairs Outcomes Group, White River Junction, VT; et al)
Ann Intern Med 155:137-144, 2011

Background.—Because pulmonary nodules are found in up to 25% of patients undergoing computed tomography of the chest, the question of whether to perform biopsy is becoming increasingly common. Data on complications after transthoracic needle lung biopsy are limited to case series from selected institutions.

Objective.—To determine population-based estimates of risks for complications after transthoracic needle biopsy of a pulmonary nodule.

Design.—Cross-sectional analysis.

Setting.—The 2006 State Ambulatory Surgery Databases and State Inpatient Databases for California, Florida, Michigan, and New York from the Healthcare Cost and Utilization Project.

Patients.—15 865 adults who had transthoracic needle biopsy of a pulmonary nodule.

Measurements.—Percentage of biopsies complicated by hemorrhage, any pneumothorax, or pneumothorax requiring a chest tube, and adjusted odds ratios for these complications associated with various biopsy characteristics, calculated by using multivariate, population-averaged generalized estimating equations.

Results.—Although hemorrhage was rare, complicating 1.0% (95% CI, 0.9% to 1.2%) of biopsies, 17.8% (CI, 11.8% to 23.8%) of patients with hemorrhage required a blood transfusion. In contrast, the risk for any pneumothorax was 15.0% (CI, 14.0% to 16.0%), and 6.6% (CI, 6.0% to 7.2%) of all biopsies resulted in pneumothorax requiring a chest tube. Compared with patients without complications, those who experienced hemorrhage or pneumothorax requiring a chest tube had longer lengths of stay ($P < 0.001$) and were more likely to develop respiratory failure requiring mechanical ventilation ($P = 0.020$). Patients aged 60 to 69 years (as opposed to younger or older patients), smokers, and those with chronic obstructive pulmonary disease had higher risk for complications.

Limitations.—Estimated risks may be inaccurate if coding of complications is incomplete. The analyzed databases contain little clinical detail (such as information on nodule characteristics or biopsy pathology) and cannot indicate whether performing the biopsy produced useful information.

Conclusion.—Whereas hemorrhage is an infrequent complication of transthoracic needle lung biopsy, pneumothorax is common and often necessitates chest tube placement. These population-based data should help patients and physicians make more informed choices about whether to perform biopsy of a pulmonary nodule.

▶ Transthoracic needle aspiration or biopsy is a common diagnostic intervention for suspicious peripheral lung nodules. The yield for small peripheral nodules by bronchoscopy is relatively low, particularly for nodules less than 2 cm in diameter. While this is improved with the use of radial ultrasound scan or electromagnetic navigational bronchoscopy, these techniques are not widely available. Small pulmonary nodules are found in approximately 25% of patients undergoing low-dose screening chest computed tomography scanning.[1] With the decrease in lung cancer mortality seen in the National Lung Screening Trial, it seems likely that increasing numbers of such nodules will be identified as screening is implemented, and it will be even more important to appreciate the risks of diagnostic interventions that will ensue, including transthoracic needle lung biopsy.[1] Wiener and colleagues examined national health care administrative databases from the states of California, Florida, Michigan, and New York, representing 28.2% of the 2006 United States population. A total of 15 865 patients who had a single transthoracic needle lung biopsy of a pulmonary nodule were identified, and the databases were examined for the occurrence of procedure-related complications. Complications were surprisingly common, particularly pneumothorax, which occurred in 15% of all patients and required chest tube placement in 6.6% of all patients. While hemorrhage occurred in only 1% of patients, 17.8% of these were severe enough to require transfusion.

Balancing risk and benefit is an inevitable challenge in the practice of medicine. If the evaluation of a peripheral pulmonary nodule results in a decision that a biopsy is necessary, then transthoracic needle biopsy will often be the procedure of choice. In all cases, the benefit of the information obtained from the procedure should outweigh the inevitable accompanying risks, and both benefit and risks should be included in a thorough discussion with the patient.

L. T. Tanoue, MD

Reference

1. Aberle DR, Adams AM, Berg CD, et al. Reduced lung-cancer mortality with low-dose computed tomographic screening. *N Engl J Med.* 2011;365:395-409.

Cumulative Radiation Dose From Medical Imaging Procedures in Patients Undergoing Resection for Lung Cancer
Stiles BM, Mirza F, Towe CW, et al (New York Presbyterian Hosp; Mount Sinai School of Medicine, NY)
Ann Thorac Surg 92:1170-1179, 2011

Background.—Radiation dose from diagnostic imaging procedures is not monitored in patients undergoing surgery for lung cancer. Evidence suggests an increased lifetime risk of malignancy of 1.0% per 100 millisieverts (mSv). As such, recommendations are to restrict healthcare and radiation workers to a maximum dose of 50 mSv per year or to 100 mSv over a three-year period. The purpose of this study was to estimate cumulative effective doses of radiation in patients undergoing lung cancer resection and to determine predictors of increased exposure.

Methods.—We identified 94 consecutive patients undergoing resection for non-small cell lung cancer. Radiologic procedures performed from one year prior to resection until two years postresection were recorded. Estimates of effective doses (mSv) were obtained from published literature and institutional records. Predictors of dose greater than 50 mSv per year and greater than 100 mSv per three years were examined statistically.

Results.—The majority of patients (median age = 67 years) had stage IA cancer (52%). In the three-year period, patients had 1,958 radiologic studies (20.8/patient) including 398 computed tomographic (CT) scans (4.23/patient) and 211 positron emission tomography (PET) scans (2.24 per patient). The three-year median estimated radiation dose was 84.0 mSv (interquartile range, 44.1 to 123.2 mSv). The highest dose was in the preoperative year. In any one year, 66% of patients received more than 50 mSv, while 19% received over 100 mSv. Over the three-year period, 43.6% of patients exceeded 100 mSv. The majority of the radiation (89.8%) was from CT or PET scans. On multivariate analysis, a history of previous malignancy (odds ratio [OR] 3.8; confidence interval [CI] 1.14 to 12.7), postoperative complications (OR 6.16; CI 1.42 to 26.6), and postoperative surveillance with PET-CT (OR 13.2; CI 4.34 to 40.3) predicted exposure greater than 100 mSv over the three-year period.

Conclusions.—This study demonstrates that lung cancer patients often receive a higher dose of radiation than that considered safe for healthcare and radiation workers. The median cumulative dose reported in this study could potentially increase the individual estimated lifetime cancer risk by as much as 0.8%. Although risk-benefit considerations are clearly different between these groups, strategies should be in place to decrease radiation doses during the preoperative workup and postoperative period (Fig 2).

▶ Physicians and patients are increasingly aware of the potential hazards of diagnostic radiation.[1] The frequency of use of imaging studies resulting in radiation exposure to patients, particularly computed tomography (CT) and positron emission tomography (PET), has increased rapidly over the last 2 decades.[2] There is great controversy surrounding cancer risk related to low-dose radiation exposure related to diagnostic studies. Most of the information available relating to radiation-associated cancer risk derives from the Japanese atomic bomb survivor cohort, whose radiation exposure obviously occurred acutely, compared with the cumulative exposure over time associated with medical imaging. Nonetheless, the BEIR VII (Seventh Biologic Effects of Ionizing Radiation) report lifetime risk model predicts that approximately 1 in 100 persons exposed to a radiation dose of 100 mSv would be expected to develop a radiation-induced cancer. As a frame of reference, average radiation exposure from a regular chest computed tomography (CT) scan is approximately 8 mSv, from a low-dose chest CT scan approximately 2 mSv, and from a PET scan approximately 25 mSv, although wide ranges of radiation doses for these studies have been reported.[3]

Stiles and colleagues retrospectively reviewed 94 consecutive patients with non—small cell lung cancer (NSCLC) who underwent surgical resection for NSCLC during 2006 and had at least 2 years of follow-up. The number of diagnostic imaging studies and the associated effective radiation doses over the 3-year period were calculated. The median estimated radiation dose was 84 mSv. A total of 43.6% of patients had a cumulative dose in excess of 100 mSv over 3 years, which exceeds the regulated maximum allowed exposure for health care and radiation workers over that time span. Fig 2 shows the distribution of individual imaging procedures (A) as well as the contribution of those procedures to the total estimated radiation dose (B).

Seventy-five percent of the patients in this study had stage I NSCLC and would therefore be expected to have good long-term survival after curative resection. For all lung cancer patients, and most particularly for this group, the risks and benefits of diagnostic imaging studies need to be carefully weighed, particularly as radiation exposure is cumulative over time. The results of this study indicate that our utilization of imaging studies that expose patients to radiation needs to be more closely monitored. Radiation dose can be calculated for any given study; that information should be readily available to both radiologist

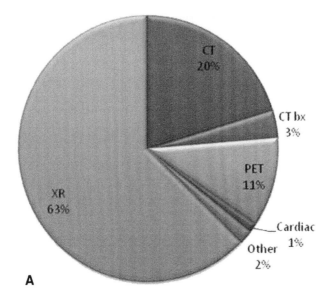

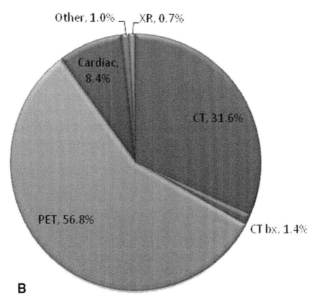

FIGURE 2.—(A) Contribution of individual imaging procedure to total number of studies. (B) Contribution of individual imaging procedures to total estimated radiation dose (mSv). (CT = computed tomography; PET = positron emission tomography; XR = X-ray.) (This article was published in The Annals of Thoracic Surgery, Stiles BM, Mirza F, Towe CW, et al. Cumulative radiation dose from medical imaging procedures in patients undergoing resection for lung cancer. *Ann Thorac Surg.* 2011;92:1170-1179, © The Society of Thoracic Surgeons 2011.)

and clinician but typically is not. Real-time documentation and monitoring of cumulative radiation exposure for an individual patient should be considered as we develop quality and safety metrics in lung cancer care as well as medical care in general.

L. T. Tanoue, MD

References

1. Berrington de González A, Mahesh M, Kim KP, et al. Projected cancer risks from computed tomographic scans performed in the United States in 2007. *Arch Intern Med.* 2009;169:2071-2077.
2. Brenner DJ, Hall EJ. Computed tomography—an increasing source of radiation exposure. *N Engl J Med.* 2007;357:2277-2284.
3. Smith-Bindman R, Lipson J, Marcus R, et al. Radiation dose associated with common computed tomography examinations and the associated lifetime attributable risk of cancer. *Arch Intern Med.* 2009;169:2078-2086.

International Association for the Study of Lung Cancer/American Thoracic Society/European Respiratory Society International Multidisciplinary Classification of Lung Adenocarcinoma
Travis WD, Brambilla E, Noguchi M, et al (Memorial Sloan Kettering Cancer Ctr, NY)
J Thorac Oncol 6:244-285, 2011

Introduction.—Adenocarcinoma is the most common histologic type of lung cancer. To address advances in oncology, molecular biology, pathology, radiology, and surgery of lung adenocarcinoma, an international multidisciplinary classification was sponsored by the International Association for the Study of Lung Cancer, American Thoracic Society, and European Respiratory Society. This new adenocarcinoma classification is needed to provide uniform terminology and diagnostic criteria, especially for bronchioloalveolar carcinoma (BAC), the overall approach to small nonresection cancer specimens, and for multidisciplinary strategic management of tissue for molecular and immunohistochemical studies.

Methods.—An international core panel of experts representing all three societies was formed with oncologists/pulmonologists, pathologists, radiologists, molecular biologists, and thoracic surgeons. A systematic review was performed under the guidance of the American Thoracic Society Documents Development and Implementation Committee. The search strategy identified 11,368 citations of which 312 articles met specified eligibility criteria and were retrieved for full text review. A series of meetings were held to discuss the development of the new classification, to develop the recommendations, and to write the current document. Recommendations for key questions were graded by strength and quality of the evidence according to the Grades of Recommendation, Assessment, Development, and Evaluation approach.

Results.—The classification addresses both resection specimens, and small biopsies and cytology. The terms BAC and mixed subtype adenocarcinoma are no longer used. For resection specimens, new concepts are introduced such as adenocarcinoma in situ (AIS) and minimally invasive adenocarcinoma (MIA) for small solitary adenocarcinomas with either pure lepidic growth (AIS) or predominant lepidic growth with ≤5 mm invasion (MIA) to define patients who, if they undergo complete resection, will have 100% or near 100% disease-specific survival, respectively. AIS and MIA are usually nonmucinous but rarely may be mucinous. Invasive adenocarcinomas are classified by predominant pattern after using comprehensive histologic subtyping with lepidic (formerly most mixed subtype tumors with nonmucinous BAC), acinar, papillary, and solid patterns; micropapillary is added as a new histologic subtype. Variants include invasive mucinous adenocarcinoma (formerly mucinous BAC), colloid, fetal, and enteric adenocarcinoma. This classification provides guidance for small biopsies and cytology specimens, as approximately 70% of lung cancers are diagnosed in such samples. Non-small cell lung carcinomas (NSCLCs), in patients with advanced-stage disease, are to be classified into more specific types such as adenocarcinoma or squamous cell carcinoma, whenever possible for several reasons: (1) adenocarcinoma or NSCLC not otherwise specified should be tested for epidermal growth factor receptor (*EGFR*) mutations as the presence of these mutations is predictive of responsiveness to EGFR tyrosine kinase inhibitors, (2) adenocarcinoma histology is a strong predictor for improved outcome with pemetrexed therapy compared with squamous cell carcinoma, and (3) potential life-threatening hemorrhage may occur in patients with squamous cell carcinoma who receive bevacizumab. If the tumor cannot be classified based on light microscopy alone, special studies such as immunohistochemistry and/or mucin stains should be applied to classify the tumor further. Use of the term NSCLC not otherwise specified should be minimized.

Conclusions.—This new classification strategy is based on a multidisciplinary approach to diagnosis of lung adenocarcinoma that incorporates clinical, molecular, radiologic, and surgical issues, but it is primarily based on histology. This classification is intended to support clinical practice, and research investigation and clinical trials. As *EGFR* mutation is a validated predictive marker for response and progression-free survival with EGFR tyrosine kinase inhibitors in advanced lung adenocarcinoma, we recommend that patients with advanced adenocarcinomas be tested for *EGFR* mutation. This has implications for strategic management of tissue, particularly for small biopsies and cytology samples, to maximize high-quality tissue available for molecular studies. Potential impact for tumor, node, and metastasis staging include adjustment of the size T factor according to only the invasive component (1) pathologically in invasive tumors with lepidic areas or (2) radiologically by measuring the solid component of part-solid nodules.

▶ Adenocarcinoma is now the most common lung cancer histology. It is increasingly appreciated that different adenocarcinoma subtypes may be associated with distinct molecular characteristics and that they may portend different clinical outcomes. For example, the presence of signet ring cells is unusual in lung adeno-carcinoma but, when present, may herald the presence of a fusion mutation in the anaplastic lymphoma kinase (ALK) gene, for which there is potentially a specific and effective biologically targeted therapy.[1] This new evidence-based classification for lung adenocarcinoma was sponsored by the International Association for the Study of Lung Cancer, the European Respiratory Society, and the American Thoracic Society. It redefines the adenocarcinoma hierarchy. The new classification recommends that the pathologic evaluation include an assessment of whether a lung adenocarcinoma has an invasive component and, if so, the type and extent. One important change is the proposal that the term "bronchoalveolar carcinoma" be replaced by the term "adenocarcinoma in situ", a change that should be acknowledged when implemented to avoid confusion with the term "carcinoma in situ". From a practical standpoint, it also provides a pathologic algorithm for tumor immunostaining and molecular analysis, with specific acknowledgement of the clinical relevance of driver mutations, which have the potential to influence the treatment approach beyond traditional TNM staging. It will be very important for physicians caring for lung cancer patients, both pathologists and clinicians, to be cognizant of the changes proposed, as the consistency of the language used to describe tumor histology is critical to the consistency of patient care.

L. T. Tanoue, MD

Reference

1. Shaw AT, Solomon B. Targeting anaplastic lymphoma kinase in lung cancer. *Clin Cancer Res.* 2011;17:2081-2086.

Trends in Stage Distribution for Patients with Non-small Cell Lung Cancer: A National Cancer Database Survey

Morgensztern D, Ng SH, Gao F, et al (Washington Univ School of Medicine, St Louis, MO)
J Thorac Oncol 5:29-33, 2010

Introduction.—We examined the recent changes in stage distribution in newly diagnosed patients with non-small cell lung cancer (NSCLC) using a national database to assess the impact of recent advances in imaging modalities.

Methods.—We searched the National Cancer Database for patients with NSCLC diagnosed between the calendar years 1998 and 2006 for which staging information was available.

Results.—Among the 877,518 patients diagnosed with NSCLC during the study period, staging information was available for 813,302 patients (92.6%). We observed a change in stage distribution between the years 2000 and 2001, with a decrease in stage I, from 27.5 to 24.8%, and a corresponding increase in stage IV, from 35.4 to 38.8%. No significant changes in stage distribution were noted after 2002.

Conclusion.—Our study showed a recent and significant stage migration in patients with NSCLC. It is likely that increased acceptance and widespread use of [18]fluorodeoxyglucose-positron emission tomography scan and routine brain imaging could account for these changes.

▶ Over the past several decades, changes have been seen in the epidemiology of non—small cell lung cancer (NSCLC) in the United States. For example, the distribution of histology now demonstrates a predominance of adenocarcinoma with fewer squamous cell carcinomas, and the absolute number of lung cancers in women is approaching the number in men.[1] Unfortunately, little change has been seen in 5-year survival, which at 16% reflects the reality that the majority of patients with NSCLC have advanced (Stage IIB or IV) disease at the time of diagnosis.[1,2] This report by Morgansztern and colleagues is even more sobering; their analysis of more than 800 000 patients with NSCLC in the National Cancer Database between 1998 and 2006 indicates that over that period, the relative number of patients with Stage IV (metastatic) disease actually increased from 35.4% to 38.8%. They suggest that this reflects more accurate noninvasive staging with increased use of positron emission tomography and, to a lesser degree, brain imaging, rather than an actual change in the distribution of disease. They point out that correctly staging patients with advanced disease may result in the "Will Rogers phenomenon"—specifically, redistributing patients with previously undetected metastatic disease from early stage to advanced stage may increase the measured survival in the early-stage group, while conversely moving patients with occult metastatic disease and less tumor burden to the advanced-stage group may also increase that group's overall prognosis. This underscores the importance of accurate staging in the interpretation of interventions affecting survival.

L. T. Tanoue, MD

References

1. Siegel R, Ward E, Brawley O, Jemal A. Cancer statistics, 2011: the impact of eliminating socioeconomic and racial disparities on premature cancer deaths. *CA Cancer J Clin.* 2011;61:212-236.
2. Goldstraw P, Crowley J, Chansky K, et al; International Association for the Study of Lung Cancer International Staging Committee, Participating Institutions. The IASLC Lung Cancer Staging Project: proposals for the revision of the TNM stage groupings in the forthcoming (seventh) edition of the TNM Classification of malignant tumours. *J Thorac Oncol.* 2007;2:706-714.

Variability of Lung Tumor Measurements on Repeat Computed Tomography Scans Taken Within 15 Minutes
Oxnard GR, Zhao B, Sima CS, et al (Memorial Sloan-Kettering Cancer Ctr, NY)
J Clin Oncol 29:3114-3119, 2011

Purpose.—We use changes in tumor measurements to assess response and progression, both in routine care and as the primary objective of clinical trials. However, the variability of computed tomography (CT) —based tumor measurement has not been comprehensively evaluated. In this study, we assess the variability of lung tumor measurement using repeat CT scans performed within 15 minutes of each other and discuss the implications of this variability in a clinical context.

Patients and Methods.—Patients with non–small-cell lung cancer and a target lung lesion ≥1 cm consented to undergo two CT scans within a period of minutes. Three experienced radiologists measured the diameter of the target lesion on the two scans in a side-by-side fashion, and differences were compared.

Results.—Fifty-seven percent of changes exceeded 1 mm in magnitude, and 33% of changes exceeded 2 mm. Median increase and decrease in tumor measurements were +4.3% and −4.2%, respectively, and ranged from 23% shrinkage to 31% growth. Measurement changes were within ± 10% for 84% of measurements, whereas 3% met criteria for progression according to Response Evaluation Criteria in Solid Tumors (RECIST; ≥20% increase). Smaller lesions had greater variability of percent measurement change $(P = .005)$.

Conclusion.—Apparent changes in tumor diameter exceeding 1 to 2 mm are common on immediate reimaging. Increases and decreases less than 10% can be a result of the inherent variability of reimaging. Caution should be exercised in interpreting the significance of small changes in lesion size in the care of individual patients and in the interpretation of clinical trial results (Table 2).

▶ The measurement of a lung nodule by computed tomography (CT) is the means by which nodule growth, stability, or regression is typically defined. These characteristics are the primary data-informing concern relating to the likelihood of malignancy, which in turn drives medical decision making regarding invasive intervention, continued watchful monitoring, or discontinuation of follow-up. In patients undergoing lung cancer treatment, CT measurements also are relied on for determination of response to therapy or lack thereof. In many situations, we may base these crucial decisions on changes in nodule or tumor dimension of only a few millimeters. This report from Oxnard and colleagues examined the variability of CT-based tumor measurement in patients with non–small cell lung cancer with target lung lesions greater than 1 cm in diameter (mean, 3.7 cm). Thirty-three patients underwent 2 consecutive CT scans; the median time between scans was 8 minutes (range, 5 to 14 minutes). As demonstrated in

TABLE 2.—Frequency of Different Magnitude Changes Found on Repeat Computed Tomography Scans Performed Within 15 Minutes of Each Other

Magnitude of Change (Positive or Negative, mm)	Frequency (%)
≥1.0	57
≥2.0	33
≥3.0	20
≥4.0	10
≥5.0	4

Table 2, differences in tumor size between the 2 scans were common. Thirty-three percent of patients had a difference of magnitude of greater than 2 mm, whereas 10% of patients had a difference of magnitude of greater than 4 mm. Furthermore, relative changes in tumor measurements ranged from 23% shrinkage to 31% growth between the first and second scans, with this effect more pronounced in tumors less than 3 cm in diameter. Six percent of this latter group had changes that met Response Evaluation Criteria in Solid Tumors criteria, which would have been interpreted as response or lack of response to treatment.

These results show the inevitable variability associated with CT measurements, particularly in small lesions. In the patient population in the study, this underscores the fact that the clinical evaluation of response to therapy should not depend solely on such measurements. As an increasing number of small pulmonary nodules are incidentally identified on CT scans done for other purposes or on CT scans done for lung cancer screening, this variability has important implications for scan interpretation and decision making relating to clinical intervention.

L. T. Tanoue, MD

Lung Cancer Treatment

Anaplastic Lymphoma Kinase Inhibition in Non–Small-Cell Lung Cancer

Kwak EL, Bang Y-J, Camidge DR, et al (Massachusetts General Hosp Cancer Ctr, Boston; Seoul Natl Univ College of Medicine, Korea; Univ of Colorado Cancer Ctr, Aurora; et al)
N Engl J Med 363:1693-1703, 2010

Background.—Oncogenic fusion genes consisting of *EML4* and anaplastic lymphoma kinase (*ALK*) are present in a subgroup of non–small-cell lung cancers, representing 2 to 7% of such tumors. We explored the therapeutic efficacy of inhibiting ALK in such tumors in an early-phase clinical trial of crizotinib (PF-02341066), an orally available small-molecule inhibitor of the ALK tyrosine kinase.

Methods.—After screening tumor samples from approximately 1500 patients with non–small-cell lung cancer for the presence of *ALK* rearrangements, we identified 82 patients with advanced *ALK*-positive disease who were eligible for the clinical trial. Most of the patients had received previous treatment. These patients were enrolled in an expanded cohort study instituted after phase 1 dose escalation had established a recommended crizotinib dose of 250 mg twice daily in 28-day cycles. Patients were assessed for adverse events and response to therapy.

Results.—Patients with *ALK* rearrangements tended to be younger than those without the rearrangements, and most of the patients had little or no exposure to tobacco and had adenocarcinomas. At a mean treatment duration of 6.4 months, the overall response rate was 57% (47 of 82 patients, with 46 confirmed partial responses and 1 confirmed complete response); 27 patients (33%) had stable disease. A total of 63 of 82 patients (77%) were continuing to receive crizotinib at the time of data cutoff, and the

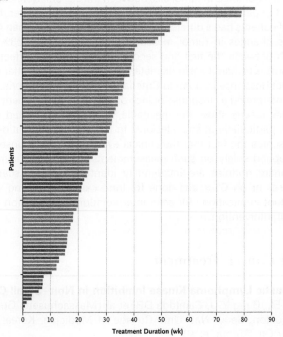

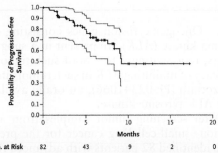

FIGURE 4.—Duration of Treatment and Estimated Progression-free Survival. Panel A shows the duration of treatment for the 82 patients, with blue bars indicating patients who were continuing to receive crizotinib by data cutoff. Red bars indicate 19 patients who discontinued treatment (13 because of disease progression, 1 because of crizotinib-related adverse events, 1 because of unrelated adverse events, 2 because of death from unrelated causes, and 2 because of other reasons). Panel B shows a Kaplan—Meier curve of estimated progression-free survival, with the lighter curves above and below the Kaplan—Meier curve representing 95% Hall—Wellner confidence limits. For interpretation of the references to color in this figure legend, the reader is referred to web version of this article. (Reprinted from Kwak EL, Bang Y-J, Camidge DR, et al. Anaplastic lymphoma kinase inhibition in non—small-cell lung cancer. *N Engl J Med.* 2010;363:1693-1703, © 2010 Massachusetts Medical Society.)

estimated probability of 6-month progression-free survival was 72%, with no median for the study reached. The drug resulted in grade 1 or 2 (mild) gastrointestinal side effects.

Conclusions.—The inhibition of ALK in lung tumors with the *ALK* rearrangement resulted in tumor shrinkage or stable disease in most patients. (Funded by Pfizer and others; ClinicalTrials.gov number, NCT00585195.) (Fig 4).

▶ Activating mutations of the anaplastic lymphoma kinase gene (*ALK*) have been associated with several solid tumors. It is estimated that the *EML4-ALK* fusion rearrangement is present in 2% to 7% of non—small cell lung cancers (NSCLC). This investigation by Kwak and colleagues began as a dose-escalation study in patients with any solid tumor refractory to standard therapy for the purpose of determining safety and maximum tolerated dose of crizotinib, an oral small-molecule tyrosine kinase inhibitor. The study was expanded to enroll a cohort of 82 patients identified with NSCLC and *ALK* rearrangement based on the observation of benefit in 2 such patients. This cohort tended to be of younger age with a history of never smoking or light smoking, and 96% had tumors with adenocarcinoma histology. Fig 4 demonstrates progression-free survival (PFS) in this cohort; median PFS was 6.4 months, with an overall response rate (partial and complete responses) of 57%. This is impressive, considering that the expected response rate with second-line chemotherapy for relapsed or refractory NSCLC is approximately 10%. Other small molecule *ALK* inhibitors are currently under investigation. This report underscores the feasibility and importance of prospective genotyping, particularly for patients with clinical and pathologic characteristics suggesting a higher likelihood of identifying a driver mutation.

L. T. Tanoue, MD

Targeting Anaplastic Lymphoma Kinase in Lung Cancer
Shaw AT, Solomon B (Massachusetts General Hosp Cancer Ctr, Boston; Peter MacCallum Cancer Centre, Melbourne, Australia)
Clin Cancer Res 17:2081-2086, 2011

Several decades of cancer research have revealed a pivotal role for tyrosine kinases as key regulators of signaling pathways, controlling cell growth and differentiation. Deregulation of tyrosine kinase—mediated signaling occurs frequently in cancer and is believed to drive the initiation and progression of disease. Chromosomal rearrangements involving the tyrosine kinase anaplastic lymphoma kinase (*ALK*) occur in a variety of human malignancies including non—small cell lung cancer (NSCLC), anaplastic large cell lymphomas, and inflammatory myofibroblastic tumors. The aberrant activation of ALK signaling leads to "oncogene addiction" and marked sensitivity to ALK inhibitors such as crizotinib (PF-02341066). This review focuses on *ALK* rearrangements in NSCLC, starting with the discovery of the *EML4-ALK* fusion oncogene, and culminating in the recent validation of ALK as a therapeutic target in patients with ALK-rearranged NSCLC. Current efforts seek to expand the role of ALK kinase inhibition in lung and other cancers and to address the molecular basis for the development of resistance.

▶ The EML4-ALK fusion oncogene is one of the newest molecular targets in lung cancer. Chromosomal aberrations in the anaplastic lymphoma kinase (*ALK*) gene have been identified in anaplastic large cell lymphomas, inflammatory myofibroblastic tumors, and neuroblastomas. The fusion of *ALK* to the echinoderm microtubule associated protein-like 4 (*EML4*) gene occurs in several variations, and is the most common of a number of variants of *ALK* fusions identified in lung tumors. Like epidermal growth factor receptor (EGFR), *ALK* is a receptor tyrosine kinase. The majority of lung tumors demonstrating *EML4-ALK* fusion mutations are adenocarcinomas. Of note, the *EML4-ALK* mutation is more likely than other driver mutations to be associated with adenocarcinoma histology in a solid pattern with abundant signet ring cells, a feature relatively uncommon in lung cancer.[1,2] Clinical characteristics in the subset of *EML4-ALK*–positive lung cancers include younger median age at diagnosis and a history of never or light smoking, characteristics that are also associated with *EGFR* mutations. As *EGFR* and *ALK* (as well as *KRAS*) mutations appear to be mutually exclusive, an evaluation for *ALK* rearrangement mutations should be strongly considered in patients with these features who have negative *EGFR* mutational analysis, as targeted therapy with *ALK* inhibitors is available in clinical trials.

L. T. Tanoue, MD

References

1. Rodig SJ, Mino-Kenudson M, Dacic S, et al. Unique clinicopathologic features characterize ALK-rearranged lung adenocarcinoma in the western population. *Clin Cancer Res.* 2009;15:5216-5223.
2. Kwak EL, Bang YJ, Camidge DR, et al. Anaplastic lymphoma kinase inhibition in non-small-cell lung cancer. *N Engl J Med.* 2010;363:1693-1703.

Treatment of Non–Small-Cell Lung Cancer with Erlotinib or Gefitinib
Cataldo VD, Gibbons DL, Pérez-Soler R, et al (Louisiana State Univ Health Sciences Ctr and Hematology–Oncology Clinic, Baton Rouge; Univ of Texas MD Anderson Cancer Ctr, Houston; Albert Einstein College of Medicine, Bronx, NY)
N Engl J Med 364:947-955, 2011

A 64-year-old woman who has never smoked receives the diagnosis of stage I adenocarcinoma of the lung and undergoes right upper lobectomy. One year later, bone and liver metastases develop. She is treated with carboplatin, paclitaxel, and bevacizumab, but progressive bone metastases are noted after 6 weeks of therapy. An oncologist recommends the initiation of erlotinib therapy.

▶ The clinical success of imatinib for chronic myelocytic leukemia in 1998 was a landmark achievement in drug discovery. Since then, the search for biologically targeted therapies has resulted in the identification of potentially targetable abnormalities in signaling pathways that are important to tumor genesis and maintenance in other malignancies, including the epidermal growth factor receptor (EGFR) signaling pathway in lung cancer. This synopsis by Cataldo and colleagues succinctly reviews the biology of the EGFR signaling pathway, discusses the clinical trials that provide the evidence base demonstrating benefit of EGFR inhibition in lung cancer treatment, reviews the indications for use as well as adverse effects of erlotinib and gefitinib, and summarizes guideline recommendations. Inhibitors of EGFR can clearly be of benefit in the treatment of patients with advanced adenocarcinoma of the lung and are now incorporated into treatment algorithms endorsed by the major oncology groups.[1] This article is written for clinicians, for whom a working knowledge of EGFR inhibitors is important because it is increasingly common to encounter medical issues related to ambulatory-based oncologic treatments as more oral targeted agents such as erlotinib are developed and used and as the longevity of patients with advanced lung cancer improves.

L. T. Tanoue, MD

Reference

1. NCCN Clinical Practice Guidelines in Oncology (NCCN Guidelines). *Non-Small Cell Lung Cancer. Version 2.2012.* National Comprehensive Cancer Network; 2012.

Survival Following Lobectomy and Limited Resection for the Treatment of Stage I Non-small Cell Lung Cancer ≤1 cm in Size: A Review of SEER Data
Kates M, Swanson S, Wisnivesky JP (Mount Sinai School of Medicine, NY; Brigham and Women's Hosp, Boston, MA)
Chest 139:491-496, 2011

Background.—Although lobectomy is the standard treatment for stage I non-small cell lung cancer (NSCLC), recent studies have suggested that limited resection may be a viable alternative for small-sized tumors. The objective of this study was to compare survival after lobectomy and limited resection among patients with stage IA tumors ≤1 cm by using a large, US-based cancer registry.

Methods.—Using the Surveillance, Epidemiology, and End Results (SEER) registry, we identified 2,090 patients with stage I NSCLC ≤1 cm in size who underwent lobectomy or limited resection (segmentectomy or wedge resection). We used propensity score analysis to adjust for potential differences in the baseline characteristics of patients in the two treatment groups. Overall and lung cancer-specific survival rates of patients undergoing lobectomy vs limited resection were compared in stratified and adjusted analyses, controlling for propensity scores.

Results.—Overall, 688 (33%) patients underwent limited resection. For the entire cohort, we were not able to identify a difference in outcomes among patients treated with lobectomy vs limited resection, as demonstrated by an adjusted hazard ratio (HR) for overall survival (1.12; 95% CI, 0.93-1.35) and lung cancer-specific survival (HR, 1.24; 95% CI, 0.95-1.61). Similarly, when the cohort was divided into propensity score quintiles, we did not find a difference in survival rate between the two groups.

Conclusions.—Limited resection and lobectomy may lead to equivalent survival rates among patients with stage I NSCLC tumors ≤1 cm in size. If confirmed in prospective studies, limited resection may be preferable for the treatment of small tumors because it may be associated with fewer complications and better postoperative lung function.

▶ For patients with stage I and II non—small cell lung cancer (NSCLC) who are medically fit for surgical resection, lobectomy is the best treatment.[1] Less extensive sublobar resections are generally recommended only in cases in which lobectomy would not be medically tolerated, most commonly elderly patients, those with limited pulmonary function, or patients with competing medical comorbidities.[1] However, several studies have suggested that limited sublobar resection may have survival outcomes equivalent to full lobectomy for patients with small (< 2 cm) stage IA NSCLC.[2-5]

The issue of lobectomy versus sublobar resection for early-stage NSCLC is addressed in this report by Kates and colleagues. Their analysis of 2090 patients with stage IA NSCLC from the Surveillance, Epidemiology, and End Results (SEER) program database included 688 patients who had undergone limited as opposed to lobar resection. All patients included in this study had small tumors, less than 1 cm in size. Of note, this analysis included a large number of patients younger than 60 years, for whom the question of long-term survival after a limited resection for lung cancer is particularly pertinent, given the likelihood of their long-term survival otherwise. No difference was seen in either overall survival or lung cancer—specific survival between patients receiving limited resection or lobectomy, regardless of age.

With widespread and increasing use of computed tomography (CT) scanning, it is clear that we identify many more small pulmonary nodules, some of which are lung cancers. We know that earlier cancer stage and smaller cancer size correlate with better prognosis. Excellent long-term survival has been reported in patients with very small NSCLC discovered by CT screening and treated surgically.[6] The question of whether patients with small early-stage NSCLC can have equally good outcomes with sublobar resection compared with full lobectomy is increasingly relevant in light of the results of the National Lung Screening Trial and the likelihood that lung cancer screening with low-dose CT scanning will be recommended in the future.[7] Ideally, this question should be addressed by a randomized, controlled trial, as the answer has implications not only for the surgical treatment of older patients or those with limited lung function but also for younger patients in whom lung preservation for future years of life will be important.

L. T. Tanoue, MD

References

1. Scott WJ, Howington J, Feigenberg S, Movsas B, Pisters K; American College of Chest Physicians. Treatment of non-small cell lung cancer stage I and stage II: ACCP evidence-based clinical practice guidelines (2nd edition). *Chest*. 2007;132: 234S-242S.
2. El-Sherif A, Gooding WE, Santos R, et al. Outcomes of sublobar resection versus lobectomy for stage I non-small cell lung cancer: a 13-year analysis. *Ann Thorac Surg*. 2006;82:408-415.
3. Nakamura H, Kawasaki N, Taguchi M, Kabasawa K. Survival following lobectomy vs limited resection for stage I lung cancer: a meta-analysis. *Br J Cancer*. 2005;92:1033-1037.
4. Wisnivesky JP, Henschke CI, Swanson S, et al. Limited resection for the treatment of patients with stage IA lung cancer. *Ann Surg*. 2010;251:550-554.
5. Miller DL, Rowland CM, Deschamps C, et al. Surgical treatment of non-small cell lung cancer 1 cm or less in diameter. *Ann Thorac Surg*. 2002;73:1545-1550.
6. Henschke CI, Yankelevitz DF, Libby DM, et al. Survival of patients with stage I lung cancer detected on CT screening. *N Engl J Med*. 2006;355:1763-1771.
7. Aberle DR, Adams AM, Berg CD, et al. Reduced lung-cancer mortality with low-dose computed tomographic screening. *N Engl J Med*. 2011;365:395-409.

Lung Cancer in Chronic Obstructive Pulmonary Disease: Enhancing Surgical Options and Outcomes

Raviv S, Hawkins KA, DeCamp MM Jr, et al (Northwestern Univ Feinberg School of Medicine, Chicago, IL)
Am J Respir Crit Care Med 183:1138-1146, 2011

Patients with chronic obstructive pulmonary disease (COPD) are at increased risk for both the development of primary lung cancer, as well as poor outcome after lung cancer diagnosis and treatment. Because of existing impairments in lung function, patients with COPD often do not meet traditional criteria for tolerance of definitive surgical lung cancer therapy. Emerging information regarding the physiology of lung resection in COPD indicates that postoperative decrements in lung function may be less than anticipated by traditional prediction tools. In patients with COPD, more inclusive consideration for surgical resection with curative intent may be appropriate as limited surgical resections or nonsurgical therapeutic options provide inferior survival. Furthermore, optimizing perioperative COPD medical care according to clinical practice guidelines including smoking cessation can potentially minimize morbidity and improve functional status in this often severely impaired patient population.

▶ The American Thoracic Society has begun a useful series of concise clinical reviews on topics important in the practice of pulmonary and critical care medicine, including this article by Raviv and colleagues addressing surgical options and outcomes in patients with lung cancer and chronic obstructive pulmonary disease (COPD). COPD is the fourth leading cause of death in the United States, and lung cancer is the leading cause of cancer death, with the obvious shared etiologic influence of cigarette smoking. COPD is a recognized risk factor for lung cancer, independent of cigarette smoking and presumably related to chronic inflammation of the airway epithelium.[1,2] The interaction between the 2 diseases is complex beyond etiologic concerns; the severity of COPD influences operability, the optimization of patients for lung cancer treatment—both surgical and medical—requires treatment of underlying COPD, and the overall prognosis for patients with lung cancer and COPD is worse than that for patients with lung cancer and without COPD.[3] This useful review discusses mechanistic associations, limited resection with or without concomitant lung volume reduction surgery, operative preparation, and prognostic factors in patients with COPD and lung cancer.

L. T. Tanoue, MD

References

1. Malkinson AM. Role of inflammation in mouse lung tumorigenesis: a review. *Exp Lung Res.* 2005;31:57-82.
2. Young RP, Hopkins RJ, Christmas T, Black PN, Metcalf P, Gamble GD. COPD prevalence is increased in lung cancer, independent of age, sex and smoking history. *Eur Respir J.* 2009;34:380-386.
3. Kiri VA, Soriano J, Visick G, Fabbri L. Recent trends in lung cancer and its association with COPD: an analysis using the UK GP Research Database. *Prim Care Respir J.* 2010;19:57-61.

Surgeon Specialty and Long-Term Survival After Pulmonary Resection for Lung Cancer

Farjah F, Flum DR, Varghese TK Jr, et al (Univ of Washington, Seattle)
Ann Thorac Surg 87:995-1006, 2009

Background.—Long-term outcomes and processes of care in patients undergoing pulmonary resection for lung cancer may vary by surgeon type. Associations between surgeon specialty and processes of care and long-term survival have not been described.

Methods.—A cohort study (1992 through 2002, follow-up through 2005) was conducted using Surveillance, Epidemiology, and End-Results-Medicare data. The American Board of Thoracic Surgery Diplomates list was used to differentiate board-certified thoracic surgeons from general surgeons (GS). Board-certified thoracic surgeons were designated as cardiothoracic surgeons (CTS) if they performed cardiac procedures and as general thoracic surgeons (GTS) if they did not.

Results.—Among 19,745 patients, 32% were cared for by GTS, 45% by CTS, and 24% by GS. Patient age, comorbidity index, and resection type did not vary by surgeon specialty (all $p > 0.10$). Compared with GS and CTS, GTS more frequently used positron emission tomography (36% versus 26% versus 26%, respectively; $p = 0.005$) and lymphadenectomy (33% versus 22% versus 11%, respectively; $p < 0.001$). After adjustment for patient, disease, and management characteristics, hospital teaching status, and surgeon and hospital volume, patients treated by GTS had an 11%

lower hazard of death compared with those who underwent resection by GS (hazard ratio, 0.89; 99% confidence interval, 0.82 to 0.97). The risks of death did not vary significantly between CTS and GS (hazard ratio, 0.94; 99% confidence interval, 0.88 to 1.01) or GTS and CTS (hazard ratio, 0.94; 99% confidence interval, 0.87 to 1.03).

Conclusions.—Lung cancer patients treated by GTS had higher long-term survival rates than those treated by GS. General thoracic surgeons performed preoperative and intraoperative staging more often than GS or CTS.

▶ Primary surgical resection is the recommended therapy for early-stage non—small cell lung cancer (NSCLC), followed by adjuvant chemotherapy for stage IB, IIA, and IIB disease. Prior studies examining surgeon specialty and operative mortality with lung resection found that board certification is associated with lower operative mortality rates.[1,2] This provocative report by Farjah and colleagues, using the Surveillance, Epidemiology, and End Results (SEER)-Medicare database, found a significant difference in long-term outcomes associated with the specialty of the operating surgeon. In particular, 5-year lung cancer cause-specific survival rate after lung resection for early stage (I and II) NSCLC was 70% when performed by thoracic surgeons who performed only thoracic surgery, compared with 63% when performed by general surgeons and 67% when performed by cardiothoracic surgeons who performed both cardiac and thoracic surgery (*P* < .001). Short-term outcomes also varied by surgeon specialty; 30-day mortality rate after lung cancer surgery performed by general thoracic surgeons was 4.4%, compared with 6.0% when performed by general surgeons and 5.0% when performed by cardiothoracic surgeons (*P* = .005). The reasons for these differences merit investigation. General thoracic surgeons used preoperative positron emission tomography and performed lymphadenectomy more frequently, raising the likelihood that these patients had their disease staged more accurately, which would contribute to better observed survival. Access to general thoracic or cardiothoracic surgeons might be limited in some regions, and the volume of cases in rural areas or smaller hospitals may limit the expertise of the rest of the medical-surgical team and hospital. Addressing these issues must take into account limitations imposed by the workforce of general thoracic surgeons, regional variations in access and volume, and the availability and cost of resources for the infrastructure requirements of multidisciplinary teams. In the SEER-Medicare patient database examined, only 24% of patients underwent surgery by general thoracic surgeons; it seems unlikely that all lung cancer surgeries in the country could be performed by this group without a substantive increase in manpower. Similarly, limiting lung cancer care to large regional centers would impose a geographic and potential economic burden on patients needing to travel distances to obtain care. Nonetheless, the differences noted in short- and long-term survival associated with surgeon specialty are significant enough to warrant further study with the goal of improving the quality of thoracic surgical care.

L. T. Tanoue, MD

References

1. Silvestri GA, Handy J, Lackland D, Corley E, Reed CE. Specialists achieve better outcomes than generalists for lung cancer surgery. *Chest*. 1998;114:675-680.
2. Goodney PP, Lucas FL, Stukel TA, Birkmeyer JD. Surgeon specialty and operative mortality with lung resection. *Ann Surg*. 2005;241:179-184.

Molecular Approach to Lung Cancer

New driver mutations in non-small-cell lung cancer

Pao W, Girard N (Vanderbilt-Ingram Cancer Ctr, Nashville, TN; Claude-Bernard Univ, Lyon, France)
Lancet Oncol 12:175-180, 2011

Treatment decisions for patients with lung cancer have historically been based on tumour histology. Some understanding of the molecular composition of tumours has led to the development of targeted agents, for which initial findings are promising. Clearer understanding of mutations in relevant genes and their effects on cancer cell proliferation and survival, is, therefore, of substantial interest. We review current knowledge about molecular subsets in non-small-cell lung cancer that have been identified as potentially having clinical relevance to targeted therapies. Since mutations in *EGFR* and *KRAS* have been extensively reviewed elsewhere, here, we discuss subsets defined by so-called driver mutations in *ALK*, *HER2* (also known as *ERBB2*), *BRAF*, *PIK3CA*, *AKT1*, *MAP2K1*, and *MET*. The adoption of treatment tailored according to the genetic make-up of individual tumours would involve a paradigm shift, but might lead to substantial therapeutic improvements (Fig 1).

▶ Our increasing ability to identify driver mutations in non–small cell lung cancer is leading to the identification of new targets for treatment. These mutations in genes encoding proteins integral to signaling pathways controlling cellular proliferation and survival can potentially drive tumor formation and maintenance. Although the majority of human cancers are not associated with such mutations, an increasing number of mutations associated with lung cancer, particularly adenocarcinomas, have been identified. About 10% of all lung adenocarcinomas harbor an activating epidermal growth factor receptor (EGFR) mutation. In subpopulations "enriched" for known risk characteristics (women, nonsmokers, Asian descent), the prevalence of EGFR mutations is higher.[1] For these patients, effective targeted therapies can substantively improve outcomes. Two prospective, randomized trials in patients with untreated metastatic adenocarcinoma and EGFR mutant tumors have shown longer progression-free survival with first-line gefitinib compared with conventional platinum-based doublet chemotherapy.[2,3] This review by Pao and Girard discusses several gene mutations other than EGFR with documented or potential relevance to NSCLC, some of which already have available targeted therapies. The figure demonstrates the evolution of knowledge relating to the identification of driver mutations in NSCLC. Currently, molecular analysis can identify mutations in more than half

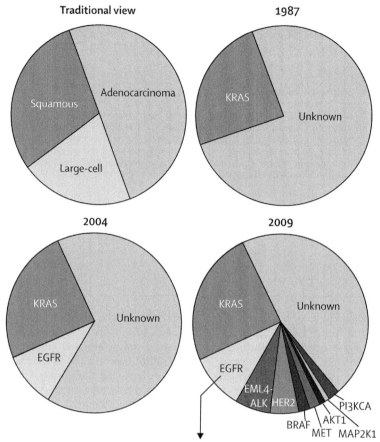

- **Mutations associated with drug sensitivity**
  EGFR Gly719X, exon 19 deletion, Leu858Arg, Leu861Gln
- **Mutations associated with primary drug resistance**
  EGFR exon 20 insertions
- **Mutations associated with acquired drug resistance**
  EGFR Thr790Met, Asp761Tyr, Leu747Ser, Thr854Ala

FIGURE 1.—Evolution of knowledge in non-small-cell lung cancer. Traditionally, non-small-cell lung cancers have been classified according to histological features. Various driver mutations have been associated with these cancers over time. The mutations are mutually exclusive, except for those in *PIK3CA*. (Reprinted from Lancet Oncol Pao W, Girard N. New driver mutations in non-small-cell lung cancer. *Lancet Oncol.* 2011;12:175-180. © 2011, with permission from Elsevier.)

of all lung adenocarcinomas. Not all mutations are associated with successful targeted therapies, in particular *KRAS*, but the success seen with *EGFR* inhibitors has energized research in molecular-targeted therapies. As with *EGFR*, mutations in *EML4-ALK* fusion genes, *HER2, PIK3CA, AKT, BRAF, MAP2K1*, and *MET* are present in only a small percentage of patients with NSCLC. These mutations were originally identified in association with other solid tumors. The development of targeted agents for those tumors will likely provide a wealth of potential therapies to be studied in clinical trials in lung cancer in the near future.

L. T. Tanoue, MD

References

1. Maemondo M, Inoue A, Kobayashi K, et al. Gefitinib or chemotherapy for non-small-cell lung cancer with mutated EGFR. *N Engl J Med.* 2010;362:2380-2388.
2. Mok TS, Wu YL, Thongprasert S, et al. Gefitinib or carboplatin-paclitaxel in pulmonary adenocarcinoma. *N Engl J Med.* 2009;361:947-957.
3. Mitsudomi T, Morita S, Yatabe Y, et al; West Japan Oncology Group. Gefitinib versus cisplatin plus docetaxel in patients with non-small-cell lung cancer harbouring mutations of the epidermal growth factor receptor (WJTOG3405): an open label, randomised phase 3 trial. *Lancet Oncol.* 2009;11:121-128.

Frequency of *EGFR* and *KRAS* Mutations in Lung Adenocarcinomas in African Americans
Reinersman JM, Johnson ML, Riely GJ, et al (Memorial Sloan-Kettering Cancer Ctr, NY; et al)
J Thorac Oncol 6:28-31, 2011

Introduction.—The detection of mutations in the epidermal growth factor receptor (*EGFR*) gene, which predict sensitivity to treatment with *EGFR* tyrosine kinase inhibitors, represents a major advance in the treatment of lung adenocarcinoma. *KRAS* mutations confer resistance to *EGFR*-tyrosine kinase inhibitors. The prevalence of these mutations in African American patients has not been thoroughly investigated.

Methods.—We collected formalin-fixed, paraffin-embedded material from resected lung adenocarcinomas from African American patients at three institutions for DNA extraction. The frequencies of *EGFR* exon 19 deletions, exon 21 L858R substitutions, and *KRAS* mutations in tumor specimens from African American patients were compared with data in white patients ($n = 476$).

Results.—*EGFR* mutations were detected in 23 of the 121 specimens from African American patients (19%, 95% confidence interval [CI]: 13–27%), whereas *KRAS* mutations were found in 21 (17%, 95% CI: 12–25%). There was no significant difference between frequencies of *EGFR* mutations comparing African American and white patients, 19% versus 13% (61/476, 95% CI: 10–16%; $p = 0.11$). *KRAS* mutations were more likely among whites, 26% (125/476, 95% CI: 23–30%; $p = 0.04$).

Conclusions.—This is the largest study to date examining the frequency of mutations in lung adenocarcinomas in African Americans. Although *KRAS* mutations were somewhat less likely, there was no difference between the frequencies of *EGFR* mutations in African American patients, when compared with whites. These results suggest that all patients with advanced lung adenocarcinomas should undergo mutational analysis before initiation of therapy.

▶ The prevalence of epidermal growth factor receptor (*EGFR*) mutations in lung adenocarcinomas varies by population. As many as 50% of lung adenocarcinomas in East Asian patients harbor *EGFR* mutations, compared with approximately 15% in heterogeneous populations in North America and Europe.[1,2] The often positive and sometimes dramatic responses seen when patients with advanced *EGFR*-mutant lung cancers are treated with *EGFR*-tyrosine kinase inhibitors justifies mutational analysis in populations in which *EGFR* mutations are observed more commonly, typically nonsmokers, women, and individuals of East Asian descent. In this study, *EGFR* mutational analysis was performed in a cohort of 121 African American patients with lung adenocarcinomas from 3 institutions and compared with an analysis of a cohort of 476 white patients from 1 of those institutions. To date, this is the largest such series reported in African Americans. *EGFR* exon 19 deletions or exon 21 mutations were identified in 19% of the African American patients, compared with 13% in the white population. This is in contrast to previous reports in smaller series in which the frequency of *EGFR* mutations in African Americans was reported as considerably lower.[3,4] These data suggest that *EGFR* mutations occur as frequently in African American patients as in white patients. The frequency of mutation is high enough to support the approach that all patients with advanced lung adenocarcinoma, regardless of race, should have genetic analysis performed for the presence of *EGFR* mutations.

L. T. Tanoue, MD

References

1. Mok TS, Wu YL, Thongprasert S, et al. Gefitinib or carboplatin-paclitaxel in pulmonary adenocarcinoma. *N Engl J Med.* 2009;361:947-957.
2. Rosell R, Moran T, Queralt C, et al. Screening for epidermal growth factor receptor mutations in lung cancer. *N Engl J Med.* 2009;361:958-967.
3. Yang SH, Mechanic LE, Yang P, et al. Mutations in the tyrosine kinase domain of the epidermal growth factor receptor in non-small cell lung cancer. *Clin Cancer Res.* 2005;11:2106-2110.
4. Leidner RS, Fu P, Clifford B, et al. Genetic abnormalities of the *EGFR* pathway in African American patients with non-small-cell lung cancer. *J Clin Oncol.* 2009;27:5620-5626.

Prognostic and Predictive Gene Signature for Adjuvant Chemotherapy in Resected Non—Small-Cell Lung Cancer
Zhu C-Q, Ding K, Strumpf D, et al (Univ Health Network, Toronto, Ontario, Canada; Univ of Toronto, Ontario, Canada; Queen's Univ, Kingston, Ontario, Canada; et al)
J Clin Oncol 28:4417-4424, 2010

Purpose.—The JBR.10 trial demonstrated benefit from adjuvant cisplatin/vinorelbine (ACT) in early-stage non—small-cell lung cancer (NSCLC). We hypothesized that expression profiling may identify stage-independent subgroups who might benefit from ACT.

Patients and Methods.—Gene expression profiling was conducted on mRNA from 133 frozen JBR.10 tumor samples (62 observation [OBS], 71 ACT). The minimum gene set that was selected for the greatest separation of good and poor prognosis patient subgroups in OBS patients was identified. The prognostic value of this gene signature was tested in four independent published microarray data sets and by quantitative reverse-transcriptase polymerase chain reaction (RT-qPCR).

Results.—A 15-gene signature separated OBS patients into high-risk and low-risk subgroups with significantly different survival (hazard ratio [HR], 15.02; 95% CI, 5.12 to 44.04; $P < .001$; stage I HR, 13.31; $P < .001$; stage II HR, 13.47; $P < .001$). The prognostic effect was verified in the same 62 OBS patients where gene expression was assessed by qPCR. Furthermore, it was validated consistently in four separate microarray data sets (total 356 stage IB to II patients without adjuvant treatment) and additional JBR.10 OBS patients by qPCR (n = 19). The signature was also predictive of improved survival after ACT in JBR.10 high-risk patients (HR, 0.33; 95% CI, 0.17 to 0.63; $P = .0005$), but not in low-risk patients (HR, 3.67; 95% CI, 1.22 to 11.06; $P = .0133$; interaction $P < .001$). Significant interaction between risk groups and ACT was verified by qPCR.

Conclusion.—This 15-gene expression signature is an independent prognostic marker in early-stage, completely resected NSCLC, and to our knowledge, is the first signature that has demonstrated the potential to select patients with stage IB to II NSCLC most likely to benefit from adjuvant chemotherapy with cisplatin/vinorelbine.

▶ It is clear that considerable heterogeneity in outcomes exists within the stages of the non–small cell lung cancer (NSCLC) TNM classification system, but our ability to identify patients with better or worse prognosis within a given stage is lacking. Even with surgical resection, 5-year survival is achieved in only approximately 60% of patients with stage I NSCLC, and survival is even shorter in patients with stage II disease.[1] If we had the ability to identify patients who were destined to relapse, we would likely offer them further treatment for presumed occult local or distant disease. Conversely, adjuvant chemotherapy should be avoided in cases in which relapse is very unlikely, to avoid unnecessary toxicity. A number of studies have attempted to predict prognosis for resected early-stage NSCLC patients by identifying tumor gene expression "signatures" that stratify patient outcomes.[2-4] This report by Zhu and colleagues extends this work to patients with resected early-stage NSCLC enrolled in the JBR.10 randomized, controlled trial of adjuvant vinorelbine/cisplatin versus observation.[5] They developed a prognostic 15-gene signature in patients with stage IB and II NSCLC who had not received adjuvant chemotherapy. As demonstrated in Fig 1 in the original article, the signature was able to discriminate between patient subgroups at high or low risk for relapse. The signature was validated in 4 other cohorts of patients with stage IB or II NSCLC, as shown in Fig 2 in the original article.

Zhu and colleagues also found that when the signature was applied to the JBR.10 patient subgroup that had received adjuvant chemotherapy, survival of high-risk patients was prolonged by adjuvant chemotherapy, while survival of low-risk patients was not. These findings are important in light of several facts: (1) adjuvant chemotherapy is not a standard part of therapy for NSCLC patients with stage IA, even though a significant number of these patients will eventually relapse; (2) adjuvant chemotherapy for stage IB disease is controversial; and (3) adjuvant chemotherapy is the standard of care for stage II disease, but not all these patients are destined to relapse. A prognostic tool, such as the gene signature reported here, would be very useful in identifying individual patients with completely resected early-stage NSCLC who would or would not benefit from adjuvant chemotherapy.

L. T. Tanoue, MD

References

1. Goldstraw P, Crowley J, Chansky K, et al; International Association for the Study of Lung Cancer International Staging Committee, Participating Institutions. The IASLC Lung Cancer Staging Project: proposals for the revision of the TNM stage groupings in the forthcoming (seventh) edition of the TNM Classification of malignant tumours. *J Thorac Oncol.* 2007;2:706-714.
2. Chen HY, Yu SL, Chen CH, et al. A five-gene signature and clinical outcome in non-small-cell lung cancer. *N Engl J Med.* 2007;356:11-20.
3. Herbst RS, Lippman SM. Molecular signatures of lung cancer—toward personalized therapy. *N Engl J Med.* 2007;356:76-78.
4. Raponi M, Zhang Y, Yu J, et al. Gene expression signatures for predicting prognosis of squamous cell and adenocarcinomas of the lung. *Cancer Res.* 2006;66:7466-7472.
5. Pisters KM, Evans WK, Azzoli CG, et al. Cancer Care Ontario and American Society of Clinical Oncology adjuvant chemotherapy and adjuvant radiation therapy for stages I-IIIA resectable non small-cell lung cancer guideline. *J Clin Oncol.* 2007;25:5506-5518.

4 Pleural, Interstitial Lung, and Pulmonary Vascular Disease

Introduction

There was a broad range of interesting and clinically relevant publications in pleural, interstitial, and pulmonary vascular disease in the past 12 months. We will start with a look at pulmonary hypertension (PH). A noninvasive algorithm to rule out pulmonary arterial hypertension (PAH) in echocardiographic PH is proposed that may reduce the need to perform right heart catheterizations. In scleroderma-associated PH, trend in NT-pro—brain natriuretic proteins and tricuspid annular plane systolic excursion in 2 separate articles were predictive of outcomes in this difficult to manage disease.

Two additional articles looked at the effect of endothelin receptor antagonists (ERAs) in different populations. The agents were found to be less efficacious in men and a trend toward less efficacy in blacks was noted. Additionally, ERAs were found to be efficacious and safe in the long term in children with PAH. Long-term safety and efficacy were also studied in both inhaled treprostinil and oral sildenafil. An intriguing article also prospectively evaluated the effect of sildenafil in left-sided heart failure with preserved ejection fraction. A practical approach to the critically ill PAH patient was also postulated.

In pleural disease, a battery of pro- and antiinflammatory cytokines was compared against gold-standard studies and the classics won out. Talc was found to be safe and effective in the treatment of primary spontaneous pneumothorax, but it was special talc.

In interstitial lung disease, an automated algorithm was designed and validated to evaluate severity of disease. Risk factors for mortality were also reviewed, and delayed referral to a specialty center was identified as an independent predictor of poor outcome. Finally, though effective therapy remains elusive, treatment of gastroesophageal reflux disease was found to correlate with improved outcomes in this devastating disease.

Christopher D. Spradley, MD, FCCP

Pulmonary Vascular Disease

A noninvasive algorithm to exclude pre-capillary pulmonary hypertension
Bonderman D, Wexberg P, Martischnig AM, et al (Med Univ of Vienna, Austria)
Eur Respir J 37:1096-1103, 2011

Current guidelines recommend right heart catheterisation (RHC) in symptomatic patients at risk of pre-capillary pulmonary hypertension (PH) with echocardiographic systolic pulmonary artery pressures ≥36 mmHg. Growing awareness for PH, a high prevalence of post-capillary PH and the inability to distinguish between pre- and post-capillary PH by echocardiography have led to unnecessary RHCs. The aim of our study was to assess whether standard noninvasive diagnostic procedures are able to safely exclude pre-capillary PH.

Data from 251 patients referred for suspicion of pre-capillary PH were used to develop a noninvasive diagnostic decision tree. A prospectively collected data set of 121 consecutive patients was utilised for temporal validation.

According to the decision tree, patients were stratified by the presence or absence of an electrocardiographic right ventricular strain pattern (RVS) and serum N-terminal brain natriuretic peptide (NT-proBNP) levels below and above 80 pg·mL^{-1}. In the absence of RVS and elevated NT-proBNP, none of the patients in the prospective validation cohort were diagnosed with pre-capillary PH by RHC. Combining echocardiography with the diagnostic algorithm increased specificity to 19.3% (p = 0.0009), while sensitivity remained at 100%.

Employing ECG and NT-proBNP on top of echocardiography helps recognise one false positive case per five patients referred with dyspnoea and echocardiographic suspicion of PH, while not missing true pre-capillary PH.

▶ The traditional teaching concerning right heart failure is that the most common cause is left heart failure. Awareness in the healthcare and the lay public has shifted the focus to pulmonary arterial hypertension (PAH). Indeed, current guidelines advocate the gold standard study, right heart catheterization, for all patients with echocardiographic evidence of pulmonary artery systolic pressure ≥36 mm Hg. In this setting, 55% of patients sent to pulmonary hypertension referral centers are found to have Dana Point group 2 disease (owing to left ventricular dysfunction.)

Right heart catheterization is a relatively benign test, but it is invasive. Procedural risks include, but are not limited to, infection, bleeding, pneumothorax (depending on the approach), dysrhythmia, and the dreaded and potentially deadly pulmonary artery rupture. Bonderman and colleagues devised a simple noninvasive approach to rule out precapillary pulmonary hypertension by analyzing data from 251 consecutive patients referred for suspicion of PAH. They then validated their findings using a prospective pool of 121 patients.

The algorithm presented identified a significant percentage of referred patients who could be ruled out for PAH without subjecting them to right heart catheterization. No patient with precapillary PAH was excluded. Interestingly, electrocardiogram is recommended in the initial evaluation of presumed PAH by current guidelines. In addition, N-terminal brain natriuretic peptide at baseline has prognostic implications for patients with PAH.

Application of this simple approach may reduce cost and exposure to a potentially harmful invasive test.

C. D. Spradley, MD

Usefulness of Serial N-Terminal Pro–B-Type Natriuretic Peptide Measurements for Determining Prognosis in Patients With Pulmonary Arterial Hypertension

Mauritz G-J, Rizopoulos D, Groepenhoff H, et al (Inst for Cardiovascular Res and VU Univ Med Ctr, Amsterdam, The Netherlands; Erasmus Univ Med Ctr, Rotterdam, The Netherlands)
Am J Cardiol 108:1645-1650, 2011

Previous studies have shown the prognostic benefit of N-terminal pro–brain natriuretic peptide (NT–pro-BNP) in pulmonary arterial hypertension (PAH) at time of diagnosis. However, there are only limited data on the clinical utility of serial measurements of the inactive peptide NT–pro-BNP in PAH. This study examined the value of serial NT–pro-BNP measurements in predicting prognosis PAH. We retrospectively analyzed all available NT–pro-BNP plasma samples in 198 patients who were diagnosed with World Health Organization group I PAH from January 2002 through January 2009. At time of diagnosis median NT–pro-BNP levels were significantly different between survivors (610 pg/ml, range 6 to 8,714) and nonsurvivors (2,609 pg/ml, range 28 to 9,828, p <0.001). In addition, NT–pro-BNP was significantly associated (p <0.001) with other parameters of disease severity (6-minute walking distance, functional class). Receiver operating curve analysis identified ≥1,256 pg/ml as the optimal NT–pro-BNP cutoff for predicting mortality at time of diagnosis. Serial measurements allowed calculation of baseline NT–pro-BNP (i.e., intercept obtained by back-extrapolation of concentration time graph), providing a better discrimination between survivors and nonsurvivors than NT–pro-BNP at time of diagnosis alone (p = 0.010). Furthermore, a decrease of NT–pro-BNP of >15%/year was associated with survival. In conclusion, a serum NT–pro-BNP level <1,256 pg/ml at time of diagnosis identifies poor outcome in patients with PAH. In addition, a decrease in NT–pro-BNP of >15%/year is associated with survival in PAH (Fig 5).

▶ Mauritz and colleagues have asked a compelling question. We know that N-terminal pro-brain natriuretic peptide (NT–pro-BNP) levels can be used to predict outcome in pulmonary arterial hypertension (PAH) at baseline based

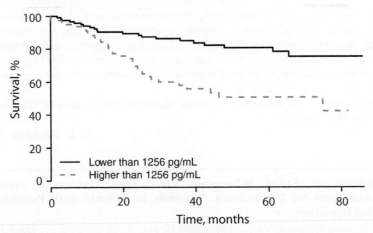

FIGURE 5.—Kaplan—Meier estimate for time to death for low (<1,256 pg/ml) and high (>1,256 pg/ml) values of baseline N-terminal pro—B-type natriuretic peptide. (Reprinted from the American Journal of Cardiology, Mauritz G-J, Rizopoulos D, Groepenhoff H, et al. Usefulness of serial N-terminal Pro—B-type natriuretic peptide measurements for determining prognosis in patients with pulmonary arterial hypertension. *Am J Cardiol.* 2011;108:1645-1650. Copyright 2011, with permission from Elsevier.)

on multiple studies. Can the marker be followed over time as well? The precedent does exist in the realm of left-sided heart failure.

The team identified a level of greater than 1256 pg/mL (Fig 5) as a predictor of mortality at baseline in close agreement with prior work. The team also found that a reduction of NT—pro-BNP of greater than 15% per year predicts long-term survival. This applied even in early diagnosis. In light of these findings, the authors conclude that simply maintaining a low threshold may not be an appropriate therapeutic goal.

Issues with the study centered around its retrospective design and wide biovariability between measurements. The latter necessitated linear regression for extrapolation. This will limit practical application. That said, the finding is compelling and may add a new tool to the pulmonary hypertension disease monitoring process. As is frequently the case in this field, a well-designed prospective study may shed more light on the applicability of these findings.

C. D. Spradley, MD

Tricuspid Annular Plane Systolic Excursion Is a Robust Outcome Measure in Systemic Sclerosis-associated Pulmonary Arterial Hypertension
Mathai SC, Sibley CT, Forfia PR, et al (Johns Hopkins Univ School of Medicine, Baltimore, MD; Univ of Pennsylvania School of Medicine, Philadelphia; Emory Univ School of Medicine, Atlanta, GA; et al)
J Rheumatol 38:2410-2418, 2011

Objective.—The tricuspid annular plane systolic excursion (TAPSE) strongly reflects right ventricular (RV) function and predicts survival in idiopathic pulmonary arterial hypertension (PAH). But its role in systemic sclerosis (SSc)-associated PAH has not been established. Our objective was to validate the TAPSE in the assessment of RV function and prediction of survival in SSc-PAH.

Methods.—Fifty consecutive patients with SSc-PAH who underwent echocardiography with TAPSE measurement within 1 h of clinically indicated right heart catheterization were followed prospectively. The relationship between TAPSE and measures of RV function and measures of survival was assessed.

Results.—The majority of the cohort were women in New York Heart Association class III/IV with severe PAH (mean cardiac index 2.4 ± 0.8 l/min/m^2). RV function was significantly impaired (mean cardiac index 2.1 ± 0.7 vs 2.9 ± 0.8 l/min/m^2; $p < 0.01$) and RV after load was significantly greater (mean pulmonary vascular resistance 11.1 ± 5.1 vs 5.8 ± 2.5 Wood units; $p < 0.01$) in subjects with a TAPSE ≤1.7 cm. The proportion surviving in the low TAPSE group was significantly lower [0.56 (95% CI 0.37—0.71) and 0.46 (95% CI 0.28—0.62) vs 0.87 (95% CI 0.55—0.96) and 0.79 (95% CI 0.49—0.93), 1- and 2-year survival, respectively]. TAPSE ≤1.7 cm conferred a nearly 4-fold increased risk of death (HR 3.81, 95% CI 1.31—11.1, $p < 0.01$).

Conclusion.—TAPSE is a robust measure of RV function and strongly predicts survival in patients with PAH-SSc. Future studies are needed to identify the responsiveness of TAPSE to PAH-specific therapy and to assess its diagnostic utility in PAH-SSc.

▶ Echocardiography is currently accepted as the screening test of choice for pulmonary arterial hypertension (PAH). Unfortunately, data derived from the study are notoriously inconsistent. This has now been proven in multiple studies comparing echocardiography with right heart catheterization, frequently performed within 1 hour in patients suspected of or carrying a diagnosis of PAH. Additionally, the geometry of the right ventricle (RV) makes measurements that are routine in the assessment of the conical left ventricle (specifically ejection fraction) extremely difficult.

Based on the finding that the right ventricle shortens during systole, the tricuspid annular plane systolic excursion (TAPSE) was identified as a possible marker of RV function. Subsequently, studies identified a TAPSE of less than 1.8 cm in a population of patients with various forms of PAH to be a strong predictor of mortality (7-fold risk).

PAH in association with systemic sclerosis (SSc-PAH) carries a notoriously poor prognosis. Unfortunately, echocardiographic studies and even well-established hemodynamic markers of PAH severity from right heart catheterization such as right atrial pressure, cardiac index, and pulmonary vascular resistance do not seem to correlate well with prognosis in systemic sclerosis (SSc)-PAH. Mathai and colleagues set out to determine weather TAPSE could be applied to this vulnerable population. Their findings were sound. In patients with SSc-PAH, the authors demonstrated that a TAPSE less than or equal to 1.7 cm conferred a 4-fold risk of death (Fig 2 in the original article).

As a noninvasive, easily reproducible measurement, the TAPSE provides robust information concerning patient prognosis in a difficult-to-manage population. Use of this type of data may assist in decision making when patients are faced with the complex and difficult treatment options that are currently available to them.

C. D. Spradley, MD

Race and Sex Differences in Response to Endothelin Receptor Antagonists for Pulmonary Arterial Hypertension
Gabler NB, French B, Strom BL, et al (Univ of Pennsylvania, Philadelphia; et al)
Chest 141:20-26, 2012

Background.—Recently studied therapies for pulmonary arterial hypertension (PAH) have improved outcomes among populations of patients, but little is known about which patients are most likely to respond to specific treatments. Differences in endothelin-1 biology between sexes and between whites and blacks may lead to differences in patients' responses to treatment with endothelin receptor antagonists (ERAs).

Methods.—We conducted pooled analyses of deidentified, patient-level data from six randomized placebo-controlled trials of ERAs submitted to the US Food and Drug Administration to elucidate heterogeneity in treatment response. We estimated the interaction between treatment assignment (ERA vs placebo) and sex and between treatment and white or black race in terms of the change in 6-min walk distance from baseline to 12 weeks.

Results.—Trials included 1,130 participants with a mean age of 49 years; 21% were men, 74% were white, and 6% were black. The placebo-adjusted response to ERAs was 29.7 m (95% CI, 3.7-55.7 m) greater in women than in men ($P = .03$). The placebo-adjusted response was 42.2 m for whites and -1.4 m for blacks, a difference of 43.6 m (95% CI, -3.5-90.7 m) ($P = .07$). Similar results were found in sensitivity analyses and in secondary analyses using the outcome of absolute distance walked.

Conclusions.—Women with PAH obtain greater responses to ERAs than do men, and whites may experience a greater treatment benefit than do blacks. This heterogeneity in treatment-response may reflect pathophysiologic differences between sexes and races or distinct disease phenotypes.

▶ The BREATH and ARIES trials[1,2] demonstrated the efficacy of endothelin receptor antagonist (ERA) therapy in the treatment of pulmonary arterial hypertension (PAH). The authors of this study ask the question, "Does race and sex difference impact response to specific therapy for PAH?" This is a worthy question given the known difference in response to therapy for systemic hypertension found in different ethnic groups. In PAH, this may be particularly important in light of the fact that most PAH patients are female.

Interestingly, men are known to have higher levels of circulating ET-1 than women, and black patients have higher circulating levels than whites.

The study retrospectively reviewed data from randomized placebo-controlled trials of ERAs in the treatment of PAH. Women in these studies demonstrated a 29.7 m greater improvement in 6-minute walk distance than men, and a 43.6 m greater response was noted in whites compared with blacks. The first observation was statistically significant. The second was hampered by small sample size.

This study dispels the myth of one-size-fits-all adherence to guidelines in PAH therapy. Unfortunately, given the small numbers of patients affected by this disease, the likelihood of efficacious targeted therapy for specific populations may be a fantasy. That said, in light of these findings, response to therapy in men and minorities may need to be monitored closely. Unfortunately, tailored alternatives have not been identified. Future studies are definitely needed.

C. D. Spradley, MD

References

1. Rubin LJ, Badesch DB, Barst RJ, et al. Bosentan therapy for pulmonary arterial hypertension. *N Engl J Med.* 2002;346:896-903.
2. Galiè N, Olschewski H, Oudiz RJ, et al; Ambrisentan in Pulmonary Arterial Hypertension, Randomized, Double-Blind, Placebo-Controlled, Multicenter, Efficacy Studies (ARIES) Group. Ambrisentan for the treatment of pulmonary arterial hypertension: results of the ambrisentan in pulmonary arterial hypertension, randomized, double-blind, placebo-controlled, multicenter, efficacy (ARIES) study 1 and 2. *Circulation.* 2008;117:3010-3019.

Long-term efficacy of bosentan in treatment of pulmonary arterial hypertension in children

Hislop AA, Moledina S, Foster H, et al (Univ College London, UK)
Eur Respir J 38:70-77, 2011

The aim of the present study was to evaluate a 5-yr experience of bosentan in children with pulmonary arterial hypertension (PAH). A retrospective, observational study was made of children in the UK Pulmonary Hypertension Service for Children (Great Ormond Street Hospital for Children, London, UK) who were given bosentan as monotherapy or in combination, from February 2002 to May 2008 and followed up for ≥6 months.

Detailed studies were made of 101 children with idiopathic PAH (IPAH) (n=42) and PAH associated with congenital heart disease (n=59). Before treatment, World Health Organization (WHO) functional class, 6-min walk distance (6MWD), height, weight and haemodynamic data were determined. Evaluations were analysed after 6 months and annually to a maximum of 5 yrs.

Median duration of treatment was 31.5 months. Initial improvement in WHO functional class and 6MWD was maintained for up to 3 yrs. Height and weight increased but the z-scores did not improve. After 3 yrs, bosentan was continued as monotherapy in only 21% of children with IPAH, but in 69% of repaired cases and 56% of those with Eisenmenger syndrome. The Kaplan—Meier survival estimates for the 101 patients were 96, 89, 83 and 60% at 1, 2, 3 and 5 yrs, respectively.

A treatment regime that includes bosentan is safe and appears to be effective in slowing disease progression in children with PAH.

▶ This British study of long-term efficacy and safety of bosentan in the treatment of idiopathic and associated pulmonary arterial hypertension in children demonstrated efficacy and safety of the compound that is comparable with what has been demonstrated in the adult population. Multiple compelling observations were made during this study.

The average exposure to bosentan was 31.5 months. Survival at 1, 2, 3, and 5 years was 96%, 89%, 83%, and 60%, respectively. Interestingly, only 3 subjects demonstrated liver function abnormalities, and only 1 of those required permanent discontinuation of therapy (0.99%). Twenty-one percent of patients with IPAH maintained monotherapy, and 69% of patients with repaired congenital disease and 56% with Eisenmenger's physiology remained on the single agent. Only 7 surviving patients discontinued drug: 1 for toxicity, 1 for hypotension, 1 was weaned off, and 4 refused liver function test monitoring.

The patients demonstrated improvement in height and weight but did not catch up to their peers. They also demonstrated improvement in functional class (Fig 2 in the original article) and walk distance (Fig 3 in the original article). Interestingly, a cohort of patients that was observed for an average of 5 months prior to initiation of therapy demonstrated rapid deterioration before therapy and never made up for it. Although bosentan was well tolerated in the study, survival benefit fell sharply after 3 years regardless of escalation of therapy (Fig 5 in the original article).

This study demonstrated efficacy and safety of bosentan in the pediatric population, mirroring findings of adult studies. Additional findings in the study led the authors to argue for early initiation of therapy and initial use of combination drugs. Although more work is needed to support the second recommendation, it is hard to argue with this initial study.

C. D. Spradley, MD

Long-term effects of inhaled treprostinil in patients with pulmonary arterial hypertension: The TReprostinil sodium Inhalation Used in the Management of Pulmonary arterial Hypertension (TRIUMPH) study open-label extension

Benza RL, Seeger W, McLaughlin VV, et al (Allegheny General Hosp, Pittsburgh, PA; Univ of Giessen Lung Ctr, Germany; Univ of Michigan Health System, Ann Arbor; et al)
J Heart Lung Transplant 30:1327-1333, 2011

Background.—Inhaled treprostinil improved functional capacity as add-on therapy in the short-term management of patients with pulmonary arterial hypertension (PAH). This study investigated the long-term effects of inhaled treprostinil in patients concurrently receiving oral background therapy.

Methods.—A total of 206 patients (81% women) completing the 12-week double-blind phase of the Treprostinil Sodium Inhalation Used in the Management of Pulmonary Arterial Hypertension (TRIUMPH) study transitioned into an open-label extension. Patients were assessed every 3 months for changes in 6-minute walk distance (6MWD), Borg dyspnea score, New York Heart Association (NYHA) functional class, quality of life (QOL) scores, and signs and symptoms of PAH.

Results.—Patients were primarily NYHA class III (86%), with a mean baseline 6MWD of 349 ± 81 meters. A median change in 6MWD of 28, 31, 32, and 18 meters in patients continuing therapy was observed at 6, 12, 18, and 24 months, respectively. This effect was more prominent in those patients originally allocated to active therapy in the double-blind phase. Survival rates for patients remaining on therapy were 97%, 94%, and 91% at 12, 18, and 24 months, respectively. In addition, 82%, 74%, and 69% of patients maintained treatment benefit as evidenced by lack of clinical worsening at 12, 18, and 24 months. The most common adverse events were known effects of prostanoid therapy (headache [34%], nausea [21%], and vomiting [10%]) or were due to the route of administration (cough [53%], pharyngolaryngeal pain [13%], and chest pain [13%]).

Conclusions.—Long-term therapy with inhaled treprostinil demonstrated persistent benefit for PAH patients who remained on therapy for up to 24 months.

▶ A total of 4 open-label extension studies in pharmacologic therapy for pulmonary arterial hypertension are reviewed in this text. This particular study is unique in that it evaluates the efficacy of add-on inhaled prostacyclin to established oral therapy.

The TRIUMPH study showed the efficacy of inhaled treprostinil in improving 6-minute walking distance in patients on stable background therapy with sildenafil or bosentan. The question of whether the median 20 M gained with the addition of the therapy would be maintained or improved upon was answered by this open-label extension study.

The study found statistically significant increase in 6-minute walk distance from baseline at all time points in the study. Additionally, survival of the cohort that began the study in New York Heart Association class III was 90% after 2 years.

The study suffers from the typical issues associated with open-label extension studies, in that it represents a population heavily influenced by the inclusion of a large cohort of responders. That said, inhaled treprostinil is an attractive option for additional therapy in patients who do not have robust response to monotherapy with oral agents, especially when there are contraindications or patient resistance to subcutaneous or intravenous therapy. Indeed, percentage of patients reporting improvement from baseline at 24 months was 36%. A total of 90% demonstrated improvement or no change in classification. When confronted with the dismal natural history of pulmonary hypertension, these findings should be viewed in a positive light.[1]

C. D. Spradley, MD

Reference

1. Channick RN, Olschewski H, Seeger W, Staub T, Voswinckel R, Rubin LJ. Safety and efficacy of inhaled treprostinil as add-on therapy to bosentan in pulmonary arterial hypertension. *J Am Coll Cardiol.* 2006;48:1433-1437.

Long-term Treatment With Sildenafil Citrate in Pulmonary Arterial Hypertension: The SUPER-2 Study

Rubin LJ, on behalf of the SUPER-2 Study Group (Univ of California at San Diego; et al)
Chest 140:1274-1283, 2011

Background.—The long-term safety and tolerability of sildenafil treatment of pulmonary arterial hypertension (PAH) were assessed.

Methods.—Two hundred fifty-nine of 277 randomized and treated patients completed a 12-week, double-blind, placebo-controlled trial (SUPER-1 [Sildenafil Use in Pulmonary Arterial Hypertension]) of oral sildenafil in treatment-naive patients with PAH (96% functional class II/III) and entered an open-label uncontrolled extension study (SUPER-2) that continued until the last patient completed 3 years of sildenafil treatment. Patients titrated to sildenafil 80 mg tid; one dose reduction for tolerability was allowed during the titration phase.

Results.—The median duration of sildenafil treatment across SUPER-1 and SUPER-2 was 1,242 days (range, 1-1,523 days); 170 patients (61%) completed both studies, and 89 patients discontinued from SUPER-2. After 3 years, 87% of 183 patients on treatment were receiving sildenafil 80 mg tid. Of patients remaining under follow-up, 3%, 10%, and 18% were receiving a second approved PAH therapy at 1, 2, and 3 years, respectively. At 3 years post-SUPER-1 baseline, 127 patients had an increased 6-min walk distance (6MWD); 81 improved and 86 maintained functional class. Most adverse events were of mild or moderate severity. At 3 years, 53 patients had died (censored, n = 37). Three-year estimated survival rate was 79%; if all censored patients were assumed to have died, 3-year survival rate was 68%. No deaths were considered to be treatment related.

Conclusions.—Long-term treatment of PAH initiated as sildenafil monotherapy was generally well tolerated. After 3 years, the majority of patients (60%) who entered the SUPER-1 trial improved or maintained their functional status, and 46% maintained or improved 6MWD.

Trial Registry.—ClinicalTrials.gov; No.: NCT00159887; URL: www. clinicaltrials.gov.

▶ The SUPER trial demonstrated the efficacy of sildenafil citrate for improvement in 6-minute walk distance and functional class at 12 weeks, thus establishing the drug as a treatment for PAH.[1] The SUPER 2 extension study aimed to demonstrate the long-term safety and tolerability of sildenafil citrate. Three-year survival was 79% for the study. If censored patients were assumed dead, the survival rate fell to 68%. At study end, 71% of patients were on monotherapy with sildenafil (add-on therapy was allowed). Forty-six percent of patients experienced sustained improvement in 6-minute walk distance, and 60% demonstrated maintenance or improvement in functional class. Lack of improvement at 12 weeks of active therapy for patients who walked less than 325 m (Fig 3 in the original article) was predictive of poor outcomes, and 19% of study subjects died.

The drug was well tolerated and safe, and thus in light of its goal, this was a positive study. This is impressive in light of the fact that the study pushed the dose of the medication in 87% of the subjects to 80 mg three times daily. Unfortunately, this makes comparison to real-world clinical scenarios in terms of outcomes quite difficult, because the current approved dosing in the United States is 20 mg three times daily. That said, open-label extension studies are generally not designed to evaluate efficacy, and only long-term prospective placebo-controlled trials can adequately answer this question.

On the basis of this study, one can conclude that sildenafil is a safe and well-tolerated long-term therapy for PAH. The additional finding concerning poor outcomes in nonresponders at 12 weeks of therapy may also prove helpful in making the decision to escalate or alter therapy.

C. D. Spradley, MD

Reference

1. Galiè N, Ghofrani HA, Torbicki A, et al; Sildenafil Use in Pulmonary Arterial Hypertension (SUPER) Study Group. Sildenafil citrate therapy for pulmonary arterial hypertension. *N Engl J Med.* 2005;353:2148-2157.

Pulmonary Hypertension in Heart Failure With Preserved Ejection Fraction: A Target of Phosphodiesterase-5 Inhibition in a 1-Year Study
Guazzi M, Vicenzi M, Arena R, et al (Univ of Milan, Italy; Virginia Commonwealth Univ, Richmond)
Circulation 124:164-174, 2011

Background.—The prevalence of heart failure with preserved ejection fraction is increasing. The prognosis worsens with pulmonary hypertension and right ventricular (RV) failure development. We targeted pulmonary hypertension and RV burden with the phosphodiesterase-5 inhibitor sildenafil.

Methods and Results.—Forty-four patients with heart failure with preserved ejection fraction (heart failure signs and symptoms, diastolic dysfunction, ejection fraction $\geq 50\%$, and pulmonary artery systolic pressure >40 mm Hg) were randomly assigned to placebo or sildenafil (50 mg thrice per day). At 6 months, there was no improvement with placebo, but sildenafil mediated significant improvements in mean pulmonary artery pressure $(-42.0 \pm 13.0\%)$ and RV function, as suggested by leftward shift of the RV Frank-Starling relationship, increased tricuspid annular systolic excursion $(+69.0 \pm 19.0\%)$ and ejection rate $(+17.0 \pm 8.3\%)$, and reduced right atrial pressure ($-54.0 \pm 7.2\%$). These effects may have resulted from changes within the lung (reduced lung water content and improved alveolar-capillary gas conductance, $+15.8 \pm 4.5\%$), the pulmonary vasculature (arteriolar resistance, $-71.0 \pm 8.2\%$), and left-sided cardiac function (wedge pulmonary pressure, $-15.7 \pm 3.1\%$; cardiac index, $+6.0 \pm 0.9\%$; deceleration time, $-13.0 \pm 1.9\%$; isovolumic relaxation time, $-14.0 \pm 1.7\%$; septal mitral annulus velocity, $-76.4 \pm 9.2\%$). Results were similar at 12 months.

Conclusions.—The multifaceted response to phosphodiesterase-5 inhibition in heart failure with preserved ejection fraction includes improvement in pulmonary pressure and vasomotility, RV function and dimension, left ventricular relaxation and distensibility (structural changes and/or ventricular interdependence), and lung interstitial water metabolism (wedge pulmonary pressure decrease improving hydrostatic balance and right atrial pressure reduction facilitating lung lymphatic drainage). These results enhance our understanding of heart failure with preserved ejection fraction and offer new directions for therapy.

Clinical Trial Registration.—URL: http://www.clinicaltrials.gov. Unique identifier: NCT01156636. (Fig 1)

▶ In this compelling study, the authors prospectively evaluated the effect of sildenafil citrate versus placebo on 44 patients with pulmonary hypertension in heart failure with preserved ejection fraction (HFpEF), Dana Point classification 2.2. Patients showed improvement in multiple hemodynamic parameters known to impact survival (Fig 1), as well as quality of life. The results of this study may point to possible medical therapy for a disease that currently has no established treatment. Follow-up large-scale studies with firm clinical endpoints will surely shed more light on these findings.

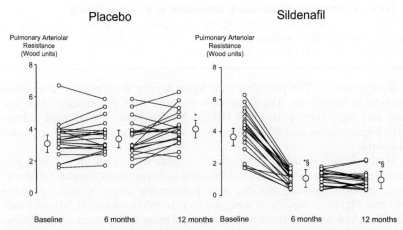

FIGURE 1.—Individual and mean ($\pm$ SD) values for pulmonary arteriolar resistance at baseline and after 6 and 12 months of placebo or sildenafil. *$P<0.01$ vs baseline; $^{\S}P<0.01$ vs corresponding placebo value. (Reprinted from Guazzi M, Vicenzi M, Arena R, et al. Pulmonary hypertension in heart failure with preserved ejection fraction: a target of phosphodiesterase-5 inhibition in a 1-year study. *Circulation.* 2011;124:164-174, with permission from American Heart Association, Inc.)

Caution, however, is warranted. Because of established safety, easy accessibility, and no requirement for toxicity monitoring, phosphodiesterase-5 therapy is already frequently prescribed on the basis of echocardiographic findings consistent with pulmonary hypertension without thorough workup. This occurs even though the agents have not been shown to delay clinical worsening in pulmonary arterial hypertension (PAH). Availability of a drug with efficacy in PAH and HFpEF may lead to inadequate or inappropriate treatment in patients who would benefit from more aggressive therapy, continuous positive airway pressure, or surgical thromboendarterectomy.

C. D. Spradley, MD

Intensive Care Unit Management of Patients with Severe Pulmonary Hypertension and Right Heart Failure
Hoeper MM, Granton J (Hannover Med School, Germany; Univ of Toronto, Ontario, Canada)
Am J Respir Crit Care Med 184:1114-1124, 2011

Despite advances in medical therapies, pulmonary arterial hypertension (PAH) continues to cause significant morbidity and mortality. Although the right ventricle (RV) can adapt to an increase in afterload, progression of the pulmonary vasculopathy that characterizes PAH causes many patients to develop progressive right ventricular failure. Furthermore, acute right ventricular decompensation may develop from disorders that lead to either an acute increase in cardiac demand, such as sepsis, or to an increase in ventricular afterload, including interruptions in medical therapy, arrhythmia, or pulmonary embolism. The poor reserve of the right ventricle, RV ischemia, and adverse right ventricular influence on left ventricular filling may lead to a global reduction in oxygen delivery and multiorgan failure. There is a paucity of data to guide clinicians caring for acute right heart failure in PAH. Treatment recommendations are frequently based on animal models of acute right heart failure or case series in humans with other causes of pulmonary hypertension. Successful treatment often requires that invasive hemodynamics be used to monitor the effect of strategies that are based primarily on biological plausibility. Herein we have developed an approach based on the current understanding of RV failure in PAH and have attempted to develop a treatment paradigm based on physiological principles and available evidence (Table 1).

▶ No solid evidence-based data exist to guide the management of critically ill patients with severe pulmonary hypertension (PH). The authors of this article have taken what is known from animal models, what is understood from human physiology, and what has been observed in this patient population and have created an elegant algorithm (Fig 1 in the original article).

The focus of this review is on critically ill patients with Dana Point Group 1 disease or pulmonary arterial hypertension (PAH) (Table 1). This population poses unique challenges. If the patient presents with prior diagnosis, he or she

---

TABLE 1.—Updated Clinical Classification of Pulmonary Hypertension

---

1. Pulmonary arterial hypertension (PAH)
   1.1. Idiopathic PAH
   1.2. Heritable
      1.2.1. BMPR2
      1.2.2. ALK1, endoglin (with or without hereditary hemorrhagic telangiectasia)
      1.2.3. Unknown
   1.3. Drugs and toxins induced
   1.4. Associated with
      1.4.1. Connective tissue diseases
      1.4.2. HIV infection
      1.4.3. Portal hypertension
      1.4.4. Congenital heart diseases
      1.4.5. Schistosomiasis
      1.4.6. Chronic hemolytic anemia
   1.5. Persistent pulmonary hypertension of the newborn
1'. Pulmonary venoocclusive disease and/or pulmonary capillary hemangiomatosis
2. Pulmonary hypertension due to left heart disease
   2.1. Systolic dysfunction
   2.2. Diastolic dysfunction
   2.3. Valvular disease
3. Pulmonary hypertension due to lung diseases and/or hypoxia
   3.1. Chronic obstructive pulmonary disease
   3.2. Interstitial lung disease
   3.3. Other pulmonary diseases with mixed restrictive and obstructive pattern
   3.4. Sleep-disordered breathing
   3.5. Alveolar hypoventilation disorders
   3.6. Chronic exposure to high altitude
   3.7. Developmental abnormalities
4. Chronic thromboembolic pulmonary hypertension
5. PH with unclear and/or multifactorial mechanisms
   5.1. Hematological disorders: myeloproliferative disorders, splenectomy.
   5.2. Systemic disorders: sarcoidosis, pulmonary Langerhans cell histiocytosis,
      lymphangioleiomyomatosis, neurofibromatosis, vasculitis
   5.3. Metabolic disorders: glycogen storage disease, Gaucher disease, thyroid disorders
   5.4. Others: tumoral obstruction, fibrosing mediastinitis, chronic renal failure on dialysis

Definition of Abbreviations: ALK1 = activin receptor-like kinase-1 gene; BMPR2 = bone morphogenetic protein receptor-2 gene; PH = pulmonary hypertension.
From Reference 2.

---

is frequently on maximized medical therapy, and thus the focus is on finding reversible causes of acute decompensation. When the patient presents with new diagnosis, this is frequently in the setting of severe right heart failure. Current strategies for management of the critically ill (intubation, aggressive fluid resuscitation) can prove fatal. Because of the physiologic paradoxes imposed by pulmonary vascular disease, invasive hemodynamic monitoring in the form of pulmonary artery catheterization is vital. Negative fluid balance, perhaps even in the setting of sepsis, may be a worthy goal.

Frequently, the outcome for patients with PH in the intensive care unit is dismal. The authors point out the obvious final common pathway. If the patient is a candidate for transplantation, application of extracorporeal life support may be indicated.

There is nothing like a PH patient in the medical intensive care unit to challenge the skills and confidence of the most seasoned intensivist. With the stepwise approach advocated here, one can be reassured that, in the absence of data, one can still proceed with logic as a weapon. A prospective application of this algorithm in multiple centers would be a logical next step; however, such a study would prove exceedingly difficult to implement. In the meantime, I will keep this review handy.

C. D. Spradley, MD

Interstitial Lung Disease

Proinflammatory and Antiinflammatory Cytokine Levels in Complicated and Noncomplicated Parapneumonic Pleural Effusions

Marchi E, Vargas FS, Acencio MM, et al (Univ of São Paulo Med School, Brazil; et al)
Chest 141:183-189, 2012

Objectives.—This study aimed to evaluate a panel of proinflammatory and antiinflammatory cytokines in noncomplicated and complicated parapneumonic pleural effusions and to correlate their levels with pleural fluid biochemical parameters.

Methods.—Serum and pleural effusion were collected from 60 patients with noncomplicated (n = 26) or complicated (n = 34) parapneumonic effusions and assayed for cytologic, biochemical, and proinflammatory and antiinflammatory cytokines. Student t test was used to compare serum and pleural fluid values, Spearman correlation to analyze the relationship between pleural fluid cytokines and biochemical parameters, and accuracy of pleural fluid cytokine levels to determine the optimal cutoff value for identification of complicated effusions. Corrections for multiple comparisons were applied and a P value $< .05$ was accepted as significant.

Results.—Serum and pleural fluid cytokine levels of IL-8, vascular endothelial growth factor (VEGF), IL-10, and tumor necrosis factor (TNF) soluble receptor (sR) II were similar between groups. In contrast, complicated effusions had higher levels of pleural fluid IL-1β, IL-1 receptor antagonist (ra), and TNF sRI. Negative correlations were found between pleural fluid glucose with IL-1β and TNF sRI and positive correlations between lactic dehydrogenate (LDH) with IL-1β, IL-8, and VEGF. Pleural fluid levels of IL-1β, IL-1ra, and TNF sRI were more accurate than IL-8, VEGF, IL-10, and TNF sRII in discriminating complicated effusions.

Conclusions.—Both proinflammatory and antiinflammatory cytokine levels in pleural fluid are elevated in complicated in comparison with noncomplicated parapneumonic pleural effusions, and they correlate with both pleural fluid glucose and LDH levels. IL-1β, IL-1ra, and TNF sRI had higher sensitivity and specificity than IL-8, VEGF, IL-10, and TNF sRII in discriminating complicated effusions.

▶ The goal of this study was to evaluate the levels of pro-inflammatory and anti-inflammatory cytokines in parapneumonic effusions. The key finding was that both classes of cytokines were elevated in pleural fluid samples obtained from complicated effusions. Interestingly, their levels were no more predictive of complicated parapneumonic effusion than the well-established pleural fluid lactate dehydrogenase and glucose.

The authors do remind us that the gold standard for making the decision between complicated and uncomplicated effusions is pH. They also point out that, unfortunately, proper handling of the sample (collection in a gas syringe and analysis through use of a blood gas machine) is rarely done, so results are unreliable. In our clinic, we actually use citrate lab tubes to ease collection and transport and have found results equivalent to gas syringe collection (presented in abstract form).

Of cytokines measured, interleukin (IL)-1β, IL-Ira, and tumor necrosis factor soluble receptor demonstrated the highest sensitivities. Although not necessarily ready for prime time in terms of fluid analysis and bedside decision making, these cellular signaling molecules may provide insight into the inflammatory process underlying the complicated parapneumonic effusion and may also provide us with future targets for novel directed therapies.

C. D. Spradley, MD

Automated Quantification of High-Resolution CT Scan Findings in Individuals at Risk for Pulmonary Fibrosis
Rosas IO, Yao J, Avila NA, et al (Natl Insts of Health, Bethesda, MD)
Chest 140:1590-1597, 2011

Background.—Automated methods to quantify interstitial lung disease (ILD) on high-resolution CT (HRCT) scans in people at risk for pulmonary fibrosis have not been developed and validated.

Methods.—Cohorts with familial pulmonary fibrosis (n = 126) or rheumatoid arthritis with and without ILD (n = 86) were used to develop and validate a computer program capable of quantifying ILD on HRCT scans, which imaged the lungs semicontinuously from the apices to the lung bases during end-inspiration in the prone position. This method uses segmentation, texture analysis, training, classification, and grading to score ILD.

Results.—Quantification of HRCT scan findings of ILD using an automated computer program correlated with radiologist readings and detected disease of varying severity in a derivation cohort with familial pulmonary fibrosis or their first-degree relatives. This algorithm was validated in an independent cohort of subjects with rheumatoid arthritis with and without ILD. Automated classification of HRCT scans as normal or ILD was significant in the derivation and validation cohorts ($P < .001$ and $P < .001$, respectively). Areas under receiver operating characteristic curves performed independently for each group were 0.888 for the derivation cohort and 0.885 for the validation cohort. Pulmonary function test results, including FVC and diffusion capacity, correlated with computer-generated HRCT scan scores for ILD($r = -0.483$ and $r = -0.532$, respectively).

Conclusions.—Automated computer scoring of HRCT scans can objectively identify ILD and potentially quantify radiographic severity of lung disease in populations at risk for pulmonary fibrosis.

▶ The authors of this study used a cohort of patients with familial interstitial lung disease (ILD) and their family members to develop an automated algorithm for the detection and quantification of ILD with high-resolution CT scan (HRCT) findings. They then validated the algorithm with a cohort of patients with rheumatoid arthritis both with and without ILD.

The program was successful at discriminating between normal and ILD in both cohorts (both *P*s < .001). The algorithm also correlated well with pulmonary function testing. There was also strong agreement between computer scoring and expert assessment by 2 independent radiologists (Fig 2 in the original article).

This is the first time a systematic approach has been used to design and validate an automated algorithm for quantification of ILD using HRCT. This technology may be a valuable tool for detecting early disease in vulnerable populations and tracking disease progression in the future. Can such a technique be designed to differentiate between different types of ILD? Research in this field may change the way we diagnose and monitor patients with ILD in the near future.

C. D. Spradley, MD

Ascertainment of Individual Risk of Mortality for Patients with Idiopathic Pulmonary Fibrosis

du Bois RM, Weycker D, Albera C, et al (Imperial College, London, UK; Policy Analysis Inc, Brookline, MA; Univ of Turin, Italy; et al)
Am J Respir Crit Care Med 184:459-466, 2011

Rationale.—Several predictors of mortality in patients with idiopathic pulmonary fibrosis have been described; however, there is a need for a practical and accurate method of quantifying the prognosis of individual patients.

Objectives.—Develop a practical mortality risk scoring system for patients with idiopathic pulmonary fibrosis.

Methods.—We used a Cox proportional hazards model and data from two clinical trials (n = 1,099) to identify independent predictors of 1-year mortality among patients with idiopathic pulmonary fibrosis. From the comprehensive model, an abbreviated clinical model comprised of only those predictors that are readily and reliably ascertained by clinicians was derived. Beta coefficients for each predictor were then used to develop a practical mortality risk scoring system.

Measurements and Main Results.—Independent predictors of mortality included age, respiratory hospitalization, percent predicted FVC, 24-week change in FVC, percent predicted carbon monoxide diffusing capacity, 24-week change in percent predicted carbon monoxide diffusing capacity, and 24-week change in health-related quality of life. An abbreviated clinical model comprising only four predictors (age, respiratory hospitalization, percent predicted FVC, and 24-wk change in FVC), and the corresponding risk scoring system produced estimates of 1-year mortality risk consistent with observed data (9.9% vs. 9.7%; C statistic = 0.75; 95% confidence interval, 0.71–0.79).

Conclusions.—The prognosis for patients with idiopathic pulmonary fibrosis may be accurately determined using four readily ascertainable predictors. Our simplified scoring system may be a valuable tool for determining prognosis and guiding clinical management. Additional research is needed to validate the applicability and accuracy of the scoring system (Table 4).

▶ Treatment options for patients with idiopathic pulmonary fibrosis (IPF) are severely limited. Multiple recent multicenter randomized placebo controlled trials have failed to demonstrate clinical benefit of pharmacotherapy. Given the progressive and fatal nature of the disease, mortality prediction tools would prove valuable in a clinical setting to assist in decision making. Participate in a clinical trial? Proceed with transplant evaluation and listing? Reevaluate code status?

The authors of this study applied multiple known independent predictors of mortality to data derived from 2 of the large clinical trials in IPF; 1099 subjects were included. The authors found that age, respiratory hospitalization, percentage predicted forced vital capacity (FVC), and 24-week change in FVC used in a scoring system (Table 4) were strongly predictive of mortality at 1 year. Impressively, change in FVC of only 5% in 24 weeks was associated with a greater than

TABLE 4.—Mortality Risk Scoring System for Patients With Idiopathic Pulmonary Fibrosis

(1) Sum Individual Scores Corresponding to Level of Each Risk Factor for a Given Patient*		(2) Find Expected 1-Year Probability of Death Corresponding to Total Risk Score	
Risk Factors	Score	Total Risk Score	Expected 1-Year Risk of Death
Age			
≥70	8		
60–69	4	0–4	<2%
<60	0	8–14	2–5%
History of respiratory hospitalization		16–21	5–10%
Yes	14	22–29	10–20%
No	0	30–33	20–30%
% Predicted FVC		34–37	30–40%
≤50	18	38–40	40–50%
51–65	13	41–43	50–60%
66–79	8	44–45	60–70%
≥80	0	47–49	70–80%
24-Week change in % predicted FVC		>50	>80%
≤ −10	21		
−5 to −9.9	10		
> −4.9	0		

*For example: total score for a patient aged 70 years, with no history of respiratory hospitalization, a % predicted FVC of 51–65, and a 24-week change in % predicted FVC of −5 to −9.9, is 31 (8 + 0 + 13 + 10) and predicted 1-year probability of death, 20–30%.

2-fold risk of death. Strikingly, this change in FVC is within the accepted variability of the test.

The study is limited by the fact that the patient pool consisted of primarily patients with mild and moderate disease at assumed low risk of death, and validation is needed; however, this prediction tool may prove valuable in the future when counseling patients with IPF concerning treatment options and goals of therapy.

C. D. Spradley, MD

Delayed Access and Survival in Idiopathic Pulmonary Fibrosis: A Cohort Study

Lamas DJ, Kawut SM, Bagiella E, et al (Columbia Univ, NY; Univ of Pennsylvania School of Medicine, Philadelphia)
Am J Respir Crit Care Med 184:842-847, 2011

Rationale.—Idiopathic pulmonary fibrosis is often initially misdiagnosed. Delays in accessing subspecialty care could lead to worse outcomes among those with idiopathic pulmonary fibrosis.

Objectives.—To examine the association between delayed access to subspecialty care and survival time in idiopathic pulmonary fibrosis.

Methods.—We performed a prospective cohort study of 129 adults who met American Thoracic Society criteria for idiopathic pulmonary fibrosis evaluated at a tertiary care center. Delay was defined as the time from the onset of dyspnea to the date of initial evaluation at a tertiary care center. We used competing risk survival methods to examine survival time and time to transplantation.

Measurements and Main Results.—The mean age was 63 years and 76% were men. The median delay was 2.2 years (interquartile range 1.0–3.8 yr), and the median follow-up time was 1.1 years. Age and lung function at the time of evaluation did not vary by delay. A longer delay was associated with an increased risk of death independent of age, sex, forced vital capacity, third-party payer, and educational attainment (adjusted hazard ratio per doubling of delay was 1.3, 95% confidence interval 1.03 to 1.6). Longer delay was not associated with a lower likelihood of undergoing lung transplantation.

Conclusions.—Delayed access to a tertiary care center is associated with a higher mortality rate in idiopathic pulmonary fibrosis independent of disease severity. Early referral to a specialty center should be considered for those with known or suspected interstitial lung disease.

▶ A common scenario in pulmonary clinic plays out as follows. A patient is referred for shortness of breath and carries a clinical diagnosis of chronic obstructive pulmonary disorder. The patient is on multiple bronchodilators as well as inhaled and systemic steroids. Examination reveals rales two-thirds of the way up the chest. The patient is hypoxic. Pulmonary function testing reveals severe restriction with reduction in the diffusion capacity. Chest imaging reveals severe interstitial lung disease. The patient presented with the initial complaint over 2 years before the referral.

Based on the findings in this study of a prospective cohort referred to a tertiary referral center, this delay alone is a strong predictor of mortality. Specifically, a doubling in the delay confers a hazard ratio of 1.3. Those in the last quartile (> 4 years) had a 3.4-fold increased risk of mortality (Fig 3 in the original article). This was independent of markers of disease severity. Interestingly, delay to referral did not impact likelihood of transplantation.

This is a troubling finding. The question is, how do we speed up the referral process and save lives? This study should be taken as a call to action to educate primary care providers and the public about the disease.

C. D. Spradley, MD

Gastroesophageal Reflux Therapy Is Associated with Longer Survival in Patients with Idiopathic Pulmonary Fibrosis
Lee JS, Ryu JH, Elicker BM, et al (Univ of California San Francisco; Mayo Clinic, Rochester, MN)
Am J Respir Crit Care Med 184:1390-1394, 2011

Rationale.—Gastroesophageal reflux (GER) is highly prevalent in patients with idiopathic pulmonary fibrosis (IPF). Chronic microaspiration secondary to GER may play a role in the pathogenesis and natural history of IPF.

Objectives.—To investigate the relationship between GER-related variables and survival time in patients with IPF.

Methods.—Regression analysis was used to investigate the relationship between GER-related variables and survival time in a retrospectively identified cohort of patients with well-characterized IPF from two academic medical centers.

Measurements and Main Results.—Two hundred four patients were identified for inclusion. GER-related variables were common in this cohort: reported symptoms of GER (34%), a history of GER disease (45%), reported use of GER medications (47%), and Nissen fundoplication (5%). These GER-related variables were significantly associated with longer survival time on unadjusted analysis. After adjustment, the use of GER medications was an independent predictor of longer survival time. In addition, the use of gastroesophageal reflux medications was associated with a lower radiologic fibrosis score. These findings were present regardless of center.

Conclusions.—The reported use of GER medications is associated with decreased radiologic fibrosis and is an independent predictor of longer survival time in patients with IPF. These findings further support the hypothesis that GER and chronic microaspiration may play important roles in the pathobiology of IPF.

▶ This retrospective study evaluated the relationship between report of gastroesophageal reflux (GER) treatment and survival in patients with interstitial pulmonary fibrosis (IPF) at 2 academic medical centers. The study found statistically significant survival advantage for report of GER symptoms versus no report, diagnosis of GER versus no diagnosis, GER medication use and no use, and history or not of Nissen fundoplication (Fig 1 in the original article). Use of GER medications was also associated with lower high-resolution CT fibrosis scores.

These findings are intriguing, especially in light of the extremely disheartening results of randomized placebo-controlled trials targeted at treatment of IPF. The retrospective nature and small sample size of this study prevent any firm conclusions from being drawn. Given the high prevalence of GER in patients with IPF, the patients on therapy may receive more aggressive therapy across the board. They may also seek therapy for GER symptoms early in the course of disease, resulting in lead-time bias.

It is clear that large-scale randomized prospective trials are needed to prove a strong causal association. That said, in light of these findings, one cannot be faulted for aggressively seeking symptoms of GER and initiating therapy in patients with IPF.

C. D. Spradley, MD

Pleural Disease

Short-term safety of thoracoscopic talc pleurodesis for recurrent primary spontaneous pneumothorax: a prospective European multicentre study
Bridevaux P-O, Tschopp J-M, Cardillo G, et al (Univ Hosps of Geneva, Switzerland; Réseau Santé Valais, Crans Montana, Switzerland; Carlo Forlanini Hosp, Rome, Italy; et al)
Eur Respir J 38:770-773, 2011

The safety of talc pleurodesis is under dispute following reports of talc-induced acute respiratory distress syndrome (ARDS) and death. We investigated the safety of large-particle talc for thoracoscopic pleurodesis to prevent recurrence of primary spontaneous pneumothorax (PSP).

418 patients with recurrent PSP were enrolled between 2002 and 2008 in nine centres in Europe and South Africa. The main exclusion criteria were infection, heart disease and coagulation disorders. Serious adverse events (ARDS, death or other) were recorded up to 30 days after the procedure. Oxygen saturation, supplemental oxygen use and temperature were recorded daily at baseline and after thoracoscopic pleurodesis (2 g graded talc).

During the 30-day observation period following talc poudrage, no ARDS (95% CI 0.0—0.9%), intensive care unit admission or death were recorded. Seven patients presented with minor complications (1.7%, 95% CI 0.7—3.4%). After pleurodesis, mean body temperature increased by 0.41°C (95%CI 0.33—0.48°C; p < 0.001) at day 1 and returned to baseline value at day 5. Pleural drains were removed after day 4 in 80% of patients.

Serious adverse events, including ARDS or death, did not occur in this large, multicentre cohort. Thoracoscopic talc poudrage using larger particle talc to prevent recurrence of PSPS can be considered safe.

▶ This prospective study of 481 patients treated with large-particle talc poudrage for recurrent primary spontaneous pneumothorax (PSP) aimed to evaluate the safety and efficacy of the technique. The study used a talc product with an average particle size of 31.5 microns. Motivation for the study was to address concerns surrounding talc-induced acute respiratory distress syndrome (ARDS). By using particles that were much larger than pleural stoma, the hope was that the risk of ARDS would be minimized. Indeed, there was not a single case of ARDS in the entire series.

Temperature rise, oxygen requirement, and duration of drain were also measured. Temperature rise was essentially universal but abated by day 4. Oxygen requirement peaked at baseline but dropped considerably by day 5. Drains were removed by day 4 in 80% of patients. Pleurodesis failed in 4 cases, resulting in need for surgical intervention for persistent air leak.

This study presents a strong case for the efficacy and safety of large particle talc pleurodesis for recurrent PSP, thus providing an alternative to surgical intervention. It also appears to be quite safe. Unfortunately, the talc used in the study is currently not available in the United States.

C. D. Spradley, MD

5 Community-Acquired Pneumonia

Introduction

The first section in this chapter is devoted to studies about prognostic tools and prognostic criteria. Severity/prognostic scoring systems have been well developed in community-acquired pneumonia and generally are useful in sicker patients. They tend to be less useful in patients who do not require higher levels of care or who may require that level of care but do not have classic characteristics. Many studies being published now focus on the less sick patients and on tools that are more useful for this group. One of the studies selected seeks to validate guideline-based minor criteria for intensive care unit (ICU) admission; another is a meta-analysis comparing all the current tools that seek to guide ICU admission. A third study evaluates the widely used CURB-65 prognostic tool and finds limited usefulness in less sick patients. The final study in this group has a different orientation as it reviews an important biomarker in terms of its prognostic value. It is a meta-analysis of the use of procalcitonin in determining antibiotic therapy and, based on the studies reviewed, proposes clinical algorithms.

The second section includes a group of studies focused on outcomes of patients with community-acquired pneumonia. The initial study in this section suggests that inflammatory responses can be used to predict outcomes: the better the inflammatory response, the better the outcome. Other studies address the role (or lack of role) of dexamethasone in treatment of acute pneumonia, whether or not timing of first antibiotic dose affects mortality (an important controversial area), and whether hospital-associated pneumonia is really a separate entity from other community-acquired pneumonias, particularly in terms of outcomes.

The final section includes a disparate group of articles addressing important topics in community-acquired pneumonia. These include articles about antibiotic use in nursing home patients, seasonal-influenza—associated pneumonias, and a summary of the British Thoracic Society audit of the appropriate use of the UK community-acquired pneumonia guidelines—a good approach, I think, in monitoring guideline implementation to improve guideline use. The final 2 articles are meta-analyses examining whether thiazolidinediones, widely used antidiabetic drugs, are associated with an increased risk of pneumonia and the spectrum of pneumococcal empyemas in the new era of changing serotypes of pneumococcal disease due to the introduction early in the century of pneumococcal conjugate vaccines.

Janet R. Maurer, MD, MBA

Validation of the Infectious Diseases Society of America/American Thoratic Society Minor Criteria for Intensive Care Unit Admission in Community-Acquired Pneumonia Patients Without Major Criteria or Contraindications to Intensive Care Unit Care

Chalmers JD, Taylor JK, Mandal P, et al (Univ of Edinburgh, UK; et al)
Clin Infect Dis 53:503-511, 2011

Background.—The 2007 Infectious Disease Society of America/American Thoracic Society (IDSA/ATS) guidelines for community-acquired pneumonia (CAP) recommended new criteria to guide admission to the intensive care unit (ICU) for patients with this condition. Although the major criteria (requirement for mechanical ventilation or septic shock requiring vasopressor support) are well established, the value of the minor criteria alone have not been fully validated.

Methods.—We performed a prospective observational study of consecutive adult patients with CAP admitted to NHS Lothian (Scotland, United Kingdom). Patients meeting the IDSA/ATS major criteria on admission were excluded, along with patients not suitable for ICU care owing to advanced directives or major comorbid illnesses. Performance characteristics for the IDSA/ATS minor criteria were calculated and compared with those for alternative scoring systems identified in the literature. Two definitions of severe CAP were used as primary end points: ICU admission, and subsequent requirement for mechanical ventilation or vasopressor support (MV/VS); 30-day mortality was a secondary outcome.

Results.—The study included 1062 patients with CAP potentially eligible for ICU admission. Each of the 9 minor criteria was associated with increased risk of MV/VS and 30-day mortality in univariate analysis. Two hundred seven patients had ≥3 minor criteria (19.5%). The IDSA/ATS 2007 criteria had an area under the receiver operating characteristic curve of 0.85 (0.82–0.88) for prediction of MV/VS, 0.85 (0.82–0.88) for prediction of ICU admission, and 0.78 (0.74–0.82) for prediction of 30-day mortality. The IDSA/ATS 2007 criteria were at least equivalent to more established scoring systems for prediction of MV/VS and ICU admission and equivalent to alternative scoring systems for predicting 30-day mortality in this patient population.

Conclusions.—In a population of patients with CAP without contraindications to ICU care, the IDSA/ATS minor criteria predict subsequent requirement for MV/VS, ICU admission, and 30-day mortality.

▶ In their 2007 jointly issued guidelines for management of community-acquired pneumonia (CAP), the American Thoracic Society and Infectious Diseases

Society of America not only recommended antibiotic regimens but also attempted to provide guidance on appropriate site of care.[1] For patients requiring hospitalization, the authors tried to determine clinical factors that would help clinicians determine if intensive care unit (ICU) care was indicated in any individual patient. Using existing validated risk-stratifying instruments and other evidence to guide them, they arrived at 2 types of criteria for ICU admission, major and minor. If patients with CAP had either of the 2 major criteria, septic shock requiring vasopressor support or acute respiratory failure requiring mechanical ventilation, they met criteria for ICU care. However, in addition to the major criteria, the guidelines also name 9 minor criteria, all identified in at least 1 major publication or in a prognostic index as a risk factor for mortality, and state that if a patient with CAP has at least 3 of the minor criteria, ICU admission is indicated. The problem is that this is an unvalidated recommendation; while few disagree that the major criteria are clear indications for ICU care, the minor criteria are much less compelling. In addition, no prospective studies have hitherto studied different combinations of the minor criteria, and it is not clear that any 3 of the minor criteria are equivalent to any other 3 in terms of assessing the likely need for ICU care or outcomes. The 9 minor criteria are respiratory rate > 30 per minute, alveolar partial pressure of oxygen/fraction of inspired oxygen (Pao_2/Fio_2) ratio < 250, multilobar infiltrates, confusion/disorientation, uremia, leukopenia, thrombocytopenia, hypothermia, and hypotension requiring aggressive fluid resuscitation.[1] Chalmers et al identified patients with CAP with at least 3 of the minor criteria (and no major criteria) and observed that the use of the minor criteria was able to predict the need for ICU care as well as outcomes. Their study did not determine if any specific combinations of minor criteria were better predictors than others. Guo et al[2] in a study of 1230 patients with CAP observed specifically combinations of minor factors and found that certain combinations were more predictive than others. For example, the combination of Pao_2/Fio_2 ratio < 250, uremia, and confusion was the best predictor of mortality, whereas leukopenia, hypothermia, and hypotension were not predictive of mortality. Although more studies on combinations of minor criteria in predicting ICU needs and outcome will certainly be helpful, another approach may be to add biomarker level measurements into the mix as a second layer of severity assessment once a patient with CAP fulfills minor criteria for severity. The usefulness of biomarkers in predicting pneumonia severity is an area that has been much more extensively clarified since the guidelines were published and may aid in better definition within the minor criteria. Ramírez et al[3] used this approach. They studied almost 700 patients with CAP with minor criteria only and measured a variety of biomarkers. A major finding was that patients with severe CAP by minor criteria, but low levels of procalcitonin (one of the most useful prognostic biomarkers identified to date), never required ICU admission. It is necessary to much better clarify the role of minor criteria in determining the level of care and prognosis and, additionally, the added definition that biomarkers will undoubtedly provide.

J. R. Maurer, MD, MBA

References

1. Mandell LA, Wunderink RG, Anzueto A, et al. Infectious Diseases Society of America/American Thoracic Society consensus guidelines on the management of community-acquired pneumonia in adults. *Clin Infect Dis.* 2007;44:S27-S72.
2. Guo Q, Li HY, Zhou YP, et al. Weight of the IDSA/ATS minor criteria for severe community-acquired pneumonia. *Respir Med.* 2011;105:1543-1549.
3. Ramírez P, Ferrer M, Martí V. Inflammatory biomarkers and prediction for intensive care unit admission in severe community-acquired pneumonia. *Crit Care Med.* 2011;39:2211-2217.

Severity assessment tools to guide ICU admission in community-acquired pneumonia: systematic review and meta-analysis
Chalmers JD, Mandal P, Singanayagam A, et al (Univ of Edinburgh, UK; Royal Infirmary of Edinburgh, UK; et al)
Intensive Care Med 37:1409-1420, 2011

Background.—The aim of this meta-analysis was to determine if severity assessment tools can be used to guide decisions regarding intensive care unit (ICU) admission of patients with community-acquired pneumonia.

Methods.—A search of PUBMED and EMBASE (1980—2009) was conducted to identify studies reporting pneumonia severity scores and prediction of ICU admission. Two reviewers independently collected data and assessed study quality. Performance characteristics were pooled using a random-effects model.

Results.—Sufficient data were collected to perform a meta-analysis on five current scoring systems: the Pneumonia Severity Index (PSI), the CURB65 score, the CRB65 score, the American Thoracic Society (ATS) 2001 criteria and the Infectious Disease Society of America/ATS (IDSA/ATS) 2007 criteria. The analysis was limited due to large variations in the ICU admission criteria, ICU admission rates and patient characteristics between different studies and different healthcare systems. In the pooled analysis, PSI, CURB65 and CRB65 performed similarly in terms of sensitivity and specificity across a range of cut-offs. Patients in CURB65 group 0 were at lowest risk of ICU admission (negative likelihood ratio 0.14; 95% confidence interval 0.06—0.34) while the ATS 2001 criteria had the highest positive likelihood ratio (7.05; 95% confidence interval 4.39—11.3).

Conclusion.—Large variations exist in the use of ICU resources between different studies and different healthcare systems. Scoring systems designed to predict 30-day mortality perform less well when ICU admission is taken into account. Further studies of dedicated ICU admission scores are required (Fig 2).

▶ Severity assessment tools for community-acquired pneumonia—primarily the CURB65, CRB65 and PSI—are now routinely used when patients present to the emergency department. They have been particularly useful in identifying patients who require admission and in predicting 30-day mortality. Less attention has

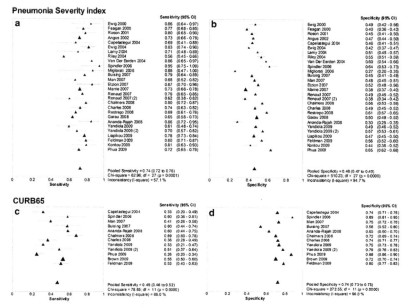

FIGURE 2.—Pooled sensitivity and specificity forest plots for the Pneumonia Severity Index (PSI; using PSI ≥IV as the selected cutpoint) and the CURB65 score (confusion, urea, respiratory rate, blood pressure and age ≥65 years; using CURB65 ≥3 as the selected high-risk cut-off point). a Sensitivity for PSI, b specificity for PSI, c sensitivity for CURB65, d specificity for CURB65. (With kind permission from Springer Science+Business Media: Chalmers JD, Mandal P, Singanayagam A, et al. Severity assessment tools to guide ICU admission in community-acquired pneumonia: systematic review and meta-analysis. *Intensive Care Med.* 2011;37:1409-1420.)

been paid to whether these tools are useful in predicting early the need for intensive care unit (ICU) admission. In addition, several other tools have been developed but not as well validated.[1-3] It is important to have a good predictor early for ICU admission, as recent data suggest that delayed ICU admission in those who need this level of care can result in higher mortality.[4] The American Thoracic Society/Infectious Disease Society of America guidelines[5] provide major and minor criteria for ICU admission: the major criteria describe critically ill patients by any standards, however, and the minor criteria have not been clearly validated.[6,7] In the end, this meta-analysis showed how difficult it is to try to identify a good predictor in this setting (Fig 2). The analysis was significantly compromised because of the heterogeneity of admission standards for different ICUs. If ICUs have widely varying admission requirements, it is next to impossible to design a predictor for admission, so all the tools studied had relatively poor sensitivity for ICU admission. But I think the message here is not about the usefulness of the severity assessment tools, but rather about heterogeneity around ICU admission criteria. ICUs consume a huge amount of resources and only those patients who truly need that level of care should be admitted to them. The focus should be on creating relatively homogeneous criteria around what clinical characteristics require that level of care.

J. R. Maurer, MD, MBA

References

1. Buising KL, Thursky KA, Black JF, et al. Identifying severe community-acquired pneumonia in the emergency department: a simple clinical prediction tool. *Emerg Med Australas.* 2007;19:418-426.
2. Renaud B, Labarère J, Coma E, et al. Risk stratification of early admission to the intensive care unit of patients with no major criteria of severe community-acquired pneumonia: development of an international prediction rule. *Crit Care.* 2009;13: R54.
3. Charles PG, Wolfe R, Whitby M, et al; Australian Community-Acquired Pneumonia Study Collaboration. SMART-COP: a tool for predicting the need for intensive respiratory or vasopressor support in community-acquired pneumonia. *Clin Infect Dis.* 2008;47:375-384.
4. Restrepo MI, Mortensen EM, Rello J, Brody J, Anzueto A. Late admission to the ICU in patients with community-acquired pneumonia is associated with higher mortality. *Chest.* 2010;137:552-557.
5. Mandell LA, Wunderink RG, Anzueto A, et al. Infectious Diseases Society of America/American Thoracic Society consensus guidelines on the management of community-acquired pneumonia in adults. *Clin Infect Dis.* 2007;44:S27-S72.
6. Chalmers JD, Taylor JK, Mandal P, et al. Validation of the Infectious Diseases Society of America/American Thoracic Society minor criteria for intensive care unit admission in community-acquired pneumonia patients without major criteria or contraindications to intensive care unit care. *Clin Infect Dis.* 2011;53:503-511.
7. Guo Q, Li HY, Zhou YP, et al. Weight of the IDSA/ATS minor criteria for severe community-acquired pneumonia. *Respir Med.* 2011;105:1543-1549.

Low CURB-65 is of limited value in deciding discharge of patients with community-acquired pneumonia

Aliberti S, Ramirez J, Cosentini R, et al (Univ of Milan-Bicocca, Monza, Italy; Univ of Louisville, KY; IRCCS Fondazione Cà Granda, Ospedale Maggiore Policlinico, Milan, Italy; et al)
Respir Med 105:1732-1738, 2011

Background.—The relationship between clinical judgment and indications of the CURB-65 score in deciding the site-of-care for patients with community-acquired pneumonia (CAP) has not been fully investigated. The aim of this study was to evaluate reasons for hospitalization of CAP patients with CURB-65 score of 0 and 1.

Methods.—An observational, retrospective study of consecutive CAP patients was performed at the Fondazione Cà Granda, Milan, Italy, between January 2005 and December 2006. The medical records of hospitalized patients with CAP having a CURB-65 score of 0 and 1 were identified and reviewed to determine whether there existed a clinical basis to justify hospitalization.

Results.—Among the 580 patients included in the study, 218 were classified with a CURB-65 score of 0 or 1. Among those, 127 were hospitalized, and reasons that justified hospitalization were found in 104 (83%) patients. Main reasons for hospitalization included the presence of hypoxemia on admission (35%), failure of outpatient therapy (14%) and the presence of cardiovascular events on admission (9.7%). Used as the sole indicator for inappropriate hospitalization, the CURB-65 score had a poor positive predictive value of 52%.

Conclusions.—Although the CURB-65 has been proposed as a tool to guide the site of care decision by international guidelines, this score is not ideal by itself, and should not be regarded as providing decision support information if a score of 0 and 1 is present. In CAP patients with CURB-65 scores of 0 or 1, further evaluations should be performed and completed by clinical judgment.

▶ One of the most useful predictor tools in community-acquired pneumonia is CURB-65 and its derivative CRB-65. This tool developed by the British Thoracic Society uses confusion, blood urea nitrogen (CURB-65 only), respiratory rate, blood pressure, and age on presentation to predict severity/mortality of the pneumonia.[1] Patients are stratified into low, intermediate, and high risk for mortality. Systematic reviews and meta-analyses have validated the usefulness of this simple tool in predicting mortality.[2,3] Thus, the BTS has also suggested that those patients with low mortality risk, that is, patients who meet 1 or none of the CURB-65 criteria, can likely be treated as outpatients. However, it is not clear that just using these 4 criteria is adequate to make that judgment. How important is clinical judgment in making decisions about admission? Fully 83% of those in this study admitted with CURB-65 scores of 0 or 1 had good reasons for admission. Choudhury et al[4] did a similar study and had similar findings: only 19.3% seemed to have no justification for admission. Reasons for admission in this low-risk group included other markers of severity, further management that could not be provided in the community, and unsafe social circumstances. It is clear that a scoring tool cannot supplant clinical judgment entirely just yet because at least 80% of the CURB-65 low-risk patients who were admitted in 2 different studies were appropriately admitted.

J. R. Maurer, MD, MBA

References

1. Lim WS, van der Eerden MM, Laing R, et al. Defining community acquired pneumonia severity on presentation to hospital: an international derivation and validation study. *Thorax*. 2003;58:377-382.
2. Chalmers JD, Singanayagam A, Akram AR, et al. Severity assessment tools for predicting mortality in hospitalised patients with community-acquired pneumonia. Systematic review and meta-analysis. *Thorax*. 2010;65:878-883.
3. Loke YK, Kwok CS, Niruban A, Myint PK. Value of severity scales in predicting mortality from community-acquired pneumonia: systematic review and meta-analysis. *Thorax*. 2010;65:884-890.
4. Choudhury G, Chalmers JD, Mandal P, et al. Physician judgement is a crucial adjunct to pneumonia severity scores in low-risk patients. *Eur Respir J*. 2011; 38:643-648.

Procalcitonin Algorithms for Antibiotic Therapy Decisions: A Systematic Review of Randomized Controlled Trials and Recommendations for Clinical Algorithms
Schuetz P, Chiappa V, Briel M, et al (Harvard School of Public Health, Boston, MA; Massachusetts General Hosp, Boston; McMaster Univ, Hamilton, Ontario, Canada)
Arch Intern Med 171:1322-1331, 2011

Previous randomized controlled trials suggest that using clinical algorithms based on procalcitonin levels, a marker of bacterial infections, results in reduced antibiotic use without a deleterious effect on clinical outcomes. However, algorithms differed among trials and were embedded primarily within the European health care setting. Herein, we summarize the design, efficacy, and safety of previous randomized controlled trials and propose adapted algorithms for US settings. We performed a systematic search and included all 14 randomized controlled trials (N=4467 patients) that investigated procalcitonin algorithms for antibiotic treatment decisions in adult patients with respiratory tract infections and sepsis from primary care, emergency department (ED), and intensive care unit settings. We found no significant difference in mortality between procalcitonin-treated and control patients overall (odds ratio, 0.91; 95% confidence interval, 0.73-1.14) or in primary care (0.13; 0-6.64), ED (0.95; 0.67-1.36), and intensive care unit (0.89; 0.66-1.20) settings individually. A consistent reduction was observed in antibiotic prescription and/or duration of therapy, mainly owing to lower prescribing rates in low-acuity primary care and ED patients, and shorter duration of therapy in moderate- and high-acuity ED and intensive care unit patients. Measurement of procalcitonin levels for antibiotic decisions in patients with respiratory tract infections and sepsis appears to reduce antibiotic exposure without worsening the mortality rate. We propose specific procalcitonin algorithms for low-, moderate-, and high-acuity patients as a basis for future trials aiming at reducing antibiotic overconsumption.

▶ Concern about overuse of antibiotics and their role in creating resistant organisms continues to be a major problem. Critical as antibiotics are to managing infections, there are many reasons other than their impact on drug resistance to prescribe them only in appropriate situations and to use them only as long as necessary—annoying to life-threatening side effects, cost, and drug-drug interactions. Until recently, the standard approach in antibiotic treatment was to prescribe the drugs for a set period, eg, 7 or 10 days, or to continue antibiotics for 24 to 48 hours after significant improvement in symptoms. This approach is not very scientific. The need to better monitor antibiotic therapy has resulted in many studies in recent years that concentrate on inflammatory and proinflammatory markers. Levels of some of these markers, particularly procalcitonin, have been shown in multiple reports to not only support diagnosis of pneumonia, but also to predict the severity/prognosis of the pneumonia.[1,2] Serial levels can also be used to determine when it is safe to discontinue antibiotics. Why is procalcitonin so useful? This is not entirely clear, but it is reliably released within a few hours in response to bacterial toxins and bacteria-specific mediators,[1] and it falls rapidly when the bacteria respond to treatment and the patient's immune system.[3] In addition, this biomarker does not appear to respond to viral-related proinflammatory cytokines or other confusing pictures, such as heart failure, so it is relatively specific.[4] The value of this review is that it brings together the data from all the highest quality studies on procalcitonin and pulls it together and interprets it into algorithms that are accessible to the practicing clinician (Figs 2 and 3 in the original article).

J. R. Maurer, MD, MBA

References

1. Becker KL, Nylén ES, White JC, Müller B, Snider RH Jr. Procalcitonin and the calcitonin gene family of peptides in inflammation, infection, and sepsis: a journey from calcitonin back to its precursors. *J Clin Endocrinol Metab.* 2004;89:1512-1525.
2. Müller F, Christ-Crain M, Bregenzer T, et al; ProHOSP Study Group. Procalcitonin levels predict bacteremia in patients with community-acquired pneumonia: a prospective cohort trial. *Chest.* 2010;138:121-129.
3. Karlsson S, Heikkinen M, Pettilä V, et al; Finnsepsis Study Group. Predictive value of procalcitonin decrease in patients with severe sepsis: a prospective observational study. *Crit Care.* 2010;14:R205.
4. Delerme S, Chenevier-Gobeaux C, Doumenc B, Ray P. Usefulness of B natriuretic peptides and procalcitonin in emergency medicine. *Biomark Insights.* 2008;3: 203-217.

Inflammatory responses predict long-term mortality risk in community-acquired pneumonia
Guertler C, Wirz B, Christ-Crain M, et al (Univ Hosp Basel, Switzerland; et al)
Eur Respir J 37:1439-1446, 2011

Long-term outcomes in patients surviving community-acquired pneumonia (CAP) are still incompletely understood. This study investigates the association of clinical parameters and blood markers with long-term mortality.

We prospectively followed 877 CAP patients from a previous multi-centre trial for 18 months follow-up and investigated all-cause mortality following hospital discharge.

Overall mortality was 17.3% (95% CI 14.8−19.8%) with a 12.8% (95% CI 10.9−15.0%) mortality incidence rate per year. Initial risk assignment using the Pneumonia Severity Index was accurate during the 18 month follow-up. Multivariable regression models (hazard ratio, 95% CI) designated the following as independent risk factors for long-term mortality: male sex (1.7, 1.2−2.5); chronic obstructive pulmonary disease (1.5, 1.1−2.1); neoplastic disease (2.5, 1.7−3.7); and highest quartile of peak pro-adrenomedullin level (3.3, 1.7−6.2). Initial presentation with temperature >38.7°C (0.4, 0.2−0.6), chills (0.6, 0.4−0.99) and highest quartile of the inflammatory marker C-reactive-protein (0.3, 0.2−0.5) were independent protective factors. A weighted risk score based on these variables showed good discrimination (area under receiver operating characteristic curve 0.78, 95% CI 0.74—0.82).

Pronounced clinical and laboratory signs of systemic inflammatory host response upon initial hospital stay were associated with favourable long-term prognosis. Further studies should address whether closer monitoring of high-risk CAP patients after hospital discharge favourably impacts long-term mortality.

▶ Risk stratification and prognostic tools for community-acquired pneumonia (CAP) have focused primarily on the acute illness because the mortality rate is around 10% and even higher in older patients and those with comorbidities. Nevertheless, most patients survive the acute illness. Several investigators have studied outcomes beyond the initial month after discharge and generally have concluded that an episode of CAP confers an increased risk of death over the ensuing year or so. However, beyond that, the few studies that have been reported have suggested comorbidities and age as risk factors but have not clearly consistently delineated other predictors.[1,2] Most of the studies on long-term outcomes were published several years ago when the severity and prognostic tools used today to help in the management of acute illness were not available. A recent Canadian study used one of these tools, the Pneumonia Severity Index, to assess long-term mortality based on the severity scores at admission and found a correlation between initial severity and long-term outcome.[3] The current study extends this approach by including some inflammatory markers measured at admission to determine if they are helpful in long-term prognosis. Future studies tracking initial inflammatory markers over time, for example, tracking how rapidly they fall or to what level they fall, may add even more understanding of the disease and may help design strategies to reduce long-term mortality.

J. R. Maurer, MD, MBA

References

1. Brancati FL, Chow JW, Wagener MM, Vacarello SJ, Yu VL. Is pneumonia really the old man's friend? Two-year prognosis after community-acquired pneumonia. *Lancet.* 1993;342:30-33.
2. Hedlund JU, Ortqvist AB, Kalin ME, Granath F. Factors of importance for the long term prognosis after hospital treated pneumonia. *Thorax.* 1993;48:785-789.
3. Johnstone J, Eurich DT, Majumdar SR, Jin Y, Marrie TJ. Long-term morbidity and mortality after hospitalization with community-acquired pneumonia: a population-based cohort study. *Medicine (Baltimore).* 2008;87:329-334.

Dexamethasone and length of hospital stay in patients with community-acquired pneumonia: a randomised, double-blind, placebo-controlled trial
Meijvis SCA, Hardeman H, Remmelts HHF, et al (St. Antonius Hosp, Nieuwegein, Netherlands; Gelderse Vallei Hosp, Ede, Netherlands; et al)
Lancet 377:2023-2030, 2011

Background.—Whether addition of corticosteroids to antibiotic treatment benefits patients with community-acquired pneumonia who are not in intensive care units is unclear. We aimed to assess effect of addition of dexamethasone on length of stay in this group, which might result in earlier resolution of pneumonia through dampening of systemic inflammation.

Methods.—In our double-blind, placebo-controlled trial, we randomly assigned adults aged 18 years or older with confirmed community-acquired pneumonia who presented to emergency departments of two teaching hospitals in the Netherlands to receive intravenous dexamethasone (5 mg once a day) or placebo for 4 days from admission. Patients were ineligible if they were immunocompromised, needed immediate transfer to an intensive-care unit, or were already receiving corticosteroids or immunosuppressive drugs. We randomly allocated patients on a one-to-one basis to treatment groups with a computerised randomisation allocation sequence in blocks of 20. The primary outcome was length of hospital stay in all enrolled patients. This study is registered with ClinicalTrials.gov, number NCT00471640.

Findings.—Between November, 2007, and September, 2010, we enrolled 304 patients and randomly allocated 153 to the placebo group and 151 to the dexamethasone group. 143 (47%) of 304 enrolled patients had pneumonia of pneumonia severity index class 4—5 (79 [52%] patients in the dexamethasone group and 64 [42%] controls). Median length of stay was 6·5 days (IQR 5·0—9·0) in the dexamethasone group compared with 7·5 days (5·3—11·5) in the placebo group (95% CI of difference in medians 0—2 days; p=0·0480). In-hospital mortality and severe adverse events were infrequent and rates did not differ between groups, although 67 (44%) of 151 patients in the dexamethasone group had hyperglycaemia compared with 35 (23%) of 153 controls (p<0·0001).

Interpretation.—Dexamethasone can reduce length of hospital stay when added to antibiotic treatment in non-immunocompromised patients with community-acquired pneumonia (Fig 2).

▶ Corticosteroid use in community-acquired pneumonia as an adjunctive treatment to antibiotics is controversial. The few small trials that have studied steroid use in community-acquired pneumonia have had varying results.[1-3] The rationale for steroid use is appealing. Steroids are anti-inflammatory in that they down regulate proinflammatory cytokine transcription that should attenuate the cytokine response/cascade and allow quicker resolution of the inflammation. The differences in this study compared with previous similar studies is that it used dexamethasone, which has a relatively long half-life, and the dexamethasone was given early after presentation and for 4 days (giving a biological effect for up to 11 days). However, the reduction in hospital stay that is reported barely reaches statistical significance (Fig 2). Of note, the authors also secondarily evaluated quality of life of patients after discharge and found more improvement in the steroid-treated group. On a related topic, Brun-Buisson et al[4] retrospectively reviewed the 2009 French Reseau d Rescherche in Ventilation Artificielle registry of critically ill patients looking for the use of corticosteroids in patients with Influenza A/H1N1 pneumonia and adult respiratory distress syndrome. About 40% of those patients had received steroids and among that group the death rate was significantly higher. I think it is safe to say that questions remain unanswered,

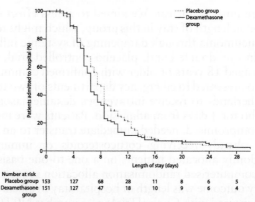

FIGURE 2.—Kaplan-Meier analysis of the effect of dexamethasone on length of hospital stay in all enrolled patients. Patients who died or were admitted to the intensive-care unit were censored on the day of death or the day of admission to the intensive-care unit. (Reprinted from The Lancet, Meijvis SCA, Hardeman H, Remmelts HHF, et al. Dexamethasone and length of hospital stay in patients with community-acquired pneumonia: a randomised, double-blind, placebo-controlled trial. *Lancet*. 2011;377:2023-2030. © 2011, with permission from Elsevier.)

and the final word is not yet in on the use of corticosteroids in community-acquired pneumonia.

J. R. Maurer, MD, MBA

References

1. Mikami K, Suzuki M, Kitagawa H, et al. Efficacy of corticosteroids in the treatment of community-acquired pneumonia requiring hospitalization. *Lung*. 2007; 185:249-255.
2. Confalonieri M, Urbino R, Potena A, et al. Hydrocortisone infusion for severe community-acquired pneumonia: a preliminary randomized study. *Am J Respir Crit Care Med*. 2005;171:242-248.
3. Marik P, Kraus P, Sribante J, Havlik I, Lipman J, Johnson DW. Hydrocortisone and tumor necrosis factor in severe community-acquired pneumonia. A randomized controlled study. *Chest*. 1993;104:389-392.
4. Brun-Buisson C, Richard JC, Mercat A, Thiébaut AC, Brochard L, REVA-SRLF A/H1N1v 2009 Registry Group. Early corticosteroids in severe Influenza A/H1N1 pneumonia and acute respiratory distress syndrome. *Am J Respir Crit Care Med*. 2011;183:1200-1206.

Hospital-reported Data on the Pneumonia Quality Measure "Time to First Antibiotic Dose" Are Not Associated With Inpatient Mortality: Results of a Nationwide Cross-sectional Analysis

Quattromani E, Powell ES, Khare RK, et al (Northwestern Univ, Chicago, IL)
Acad Emerg Med 18:496-503, 2011

Objectives.—Significant controversy exists regarding the Centers for Medicare & Medicaid Services (CMS) "time to first antibiotics dose" (TFAD) quality measure. The objective of this study was to determine whether hospital performance on the TFAD measure for patients admitted from the emergency department (ED) for pneumonia is associated with decreased mortality.

Methods.—This was a cross-sectional analysis of 95,704 adult ED admissions with a principal diagnosis of pneumonia from 530 hospitals in the 2007 Nationwide Inpatient Sample. The sample was merged with 2007 CMS Hospital Compare data, and hospitals were categorized into TFAD performance quartiles. Univariate association of TFAD performance with inpatient mortality was evaluated by chi-square test. A population-averaged logistic regression model was created with an exchangeable working correlation matrix of inpatient mortality adjusted for age, sex, comorbid conditions, weekend admission, payer status, income level, hospital size, hospital location, teaching status, and TFAD performance.

Results.—Patients had a mean age of 69.3 years. In the adjusted analysis, increasing age was associated with increased mortality with odds ratios (ORs) of >2.3. Unadjusted inpatient mortality was 4.1% (95% confidence interval [CI] = 3.9% to 4.2%). Median time to death was 5 days (25th–75th interquartile range = 2–11). Mean TFAD quality performance was 77.7% across all hospitals (95% CI = 77.6% to 77.8%). The risk-adjusted OR of mortality was 0.89 (95% CI = 0.77 to 1.02) in the highest performing TFAD quartile, compared to the lowest performing TFAD quartile. The second highest performing quartile OR was 0.94 (95% CI = 0.82 to 1.08), and third highest performing quartile was 0.91 (95% CI = 0.79 to 1.05).

Conclusions.—In this nationwide heterogeneous 2007 sample, there was no association between the publicly reported TFAD quality measure performance and pneumonia inpatient mortality.

▶ The excessive costs of medical care in the United States combined with unremarkable outcomes has led to a burgeoning focus on quality and, more specifically, on value, which is quality divided by price. The focus on improved quality has been led by the Centers for Medicare and Medicaid Services, followed by other payers and accrediting bodies, and has taken several forms. The quality of care delivered by individual providers is typically assessed by adherence to standard of care as hopefully defined by evidence-based guidelines or specific safety or preventive care measures. Surgeons also may be assessed by complication rates, for example. Hospitals are scored on, among other things, quality measures that may include length of stay, resource use, complications, safety, transitions in care, and readmissions. Unfortunately, because of the demand for quality performance measures, not all of them have been based on ideal clinical evidence because in many areas of medicine, high-quality prospective studies are not available. A good example of this is the measure referenced in the report by Quattromani et al. The "time to first antibiotic dose" quality measure originally required that antibiotics be administered within 4 hours (subsequently changed to 6 hours) of presentation in the emergency room for a hospital to be considered adherent. This measure was based on analysis of 2 retrospective databases of patients with pneumonia, not on a prospective study that typically would be considered most appropriate as high-quality clinical evidence.[1,2] (The Quattromani et al study is, in fact, another retrospective review that comes to a different conclusion.) Subsequent prospective studies have had difficulty confirming the benefits of very early antibiotic administration.[3,4] Indeed, it has been argued that the time frame requirement for adherence has led to significant overuse of antibiotics in patients who later turn out not to have pneumonia. The issue of performance measures based on poor-quality evidence can potentially result in more harm than good. This concern was addressed in a report by Wilson and Schünemann.[5] They assess the quality of the evidence supporting 6 pulmonary-related performance measures: pneumococcal vaccination, blood cultures, antibiotic administration within 6 hours, use of guideline-compliant antibiotic administration, 1-step smoking cessation counseling, and influenza vaccination. Only influenza vaccination had good evidence to support its use. Thus, the authors concluded that the evidence behind many performance measures is not of stellar quality. This is a concern in part because it implies that performance measures may foster care delivery that is not appropriate. The messages from these studies seem to be that we should be cautious about rushing to create performance measures without good supporting evidence, and most importantly, we should identify and focus prospective clinical trials on areas where good evidence for effective care is lacking.

J. R. Maurer, MD, MBA

References

1. Meehan TP, Fine MJ, Krumholz HM, et al. Quality of care, process, and outcomes in elderly patients with pneumonia. *JAMA*. 1997;278:2080-2084.
2. Houck PM, Bratzler DW, Nsa W, Ma A, Bartlett JG. Timing of antibiotic administration and outcomes for Medicare patients hospitalized with community-acquired pneumonia. *Arch Intern Med*. 2004;164:637-644.
3. Marrie TJ, Wu L. Factors influencing in-hospital mortality in community-acquired pneumonia: a prospective study of patients not initially admitted to the ICU. *Chest*. 2005;127:1260-1270.
4. Silber SH, Garrett C, Singh R, et al. Early administration of antibiotics does not shorten time to clinical stability in patients with moderate-to-severe community-acquired pneumonia. *Chest*. 2003;124:1798-1804.
5. Wilson KC, Schünemann HJ. An appraisal of the evidence underlying performance measures for community-acquired pneumonia. *Am J Respir Crit Care Med*. 2011; 183:1454-1462.

Epidemiology, Antibiotic Therapy, and Clinical Outcomes in Health Care—Associated Pneumonia: A UK Cohort Study
Chalmers JD, Taylor JK, Singanayagam A, et al (Univ of Edinburgh, UK; Royal Infirmary of Edinburgh, UK)
Clin Infect Dis 53:107-113, 2011

Background.—The recently introduced concept of health care—associated pneumonia (HCAP), referring to patients with frequent healthcare contacts and at higher risk of contracting resistant pathogens, is controversial.

Methods.—This prospective observational study recorded the clinical features, microbiology, and outcomes in a UK cohort of hospitalized patients with pneumonia. The primary outcome was 30-day mortality. Logistic regression was used to adjust for confounders when determining the impact of HCAP on clinical outcomes.

Results.—A total of 20.5% of patients met the HCAP criteria. HCAP patients were older than patients with community-acquired pneumonia (CAP) (median 76 y, IQR 65−83 vs 65 y, IQR 48−77; *P* < .0001) and more frequently had major comorbidities (62.1% vs 45.2%; *P* < .0001). Patients with HCAP had higher initial severity compared to CAP patients (Pneumonia Severity Index, mean 3.7 [SD 1.1] vs mean 3.1 [SD 1.3]; *P* < .0001) but also worse functional status using the Eastern Cooperative Oncology Group scale (mean 2.4 [SD 1.44] vs mean 1.4 [SD 1.13]; *P* < .0001) and more frequently had treatment restrictions such as do not resuscitate orders (59.9% vs 29.8%; *P* < .0001). Consequently mortality was increased (odds ratio [OR] 2.15 [1.44−3.22]; *P* =.002) in HCAP patients on univariate analysis. Multivariate analysis suggested this relationship was primarily due to confounders rather than a higher frequency of treatment failure due to resistant organisms (adjusted OR .97 [.61−1.55]; *P* =.9). The frequencies of *Pseudomonas aeruginosa*, methicillin-resistant *Staphylococcus aureus*, and Gram-negative Enterobacteriaceae were low in both cohorts.

Conclusions.—HCAP is common in the United Kingdom and is associated with a high mortality. This increased mortality was primarily related to underlying patient-related factors rather than the presence of antibiotic-resistant pathogens. This study did not establish a clear indication to change prescribing practices in a UK cohort (Table 3).

▶ Traditionally, pneumonia caused by infectious organisms had been designated either as community acquired or hospital acquired. In 2005, however, the unified guidelines for management of pneumonia published by the American Thoracic Society and the Infectious Diseases Society of America added an

TABLE 3.—Demographic Comparison of Patients With CAP and Those With HCAP

	CAP Patients	HCAP Patients	*P* Value
N	1071	277	
Demographics			
Age, median (IQR)	65 (48−77)	76 (65−83)	<.0001
Gender, % male	48.9%	53.8%	.2
Comorbidities			
Congestive cardiac failure	15.8%	29.6%	<.0001
Liver disease	4.9%	4.3%	.8
Renal failure	6.3%	8.3%	.3
Cerebrovascular disease	10.1%	18.8%	.0001
COPD	18.3%	30.0%	<.0001
Diabetes	9.3%	13.4%	.06
Risk factors for aspiration	11.6%	22.4%	<.0001
Functional status, mean (SD)	1.4 (1.13)	2.4 (1.44)	<.0001

NOTE. CAP, community-acquired pneumonia; COPD, chronic obstructive pulmonary disease; HCAP, health care−associated pneumonia; IQR, interquartile range.

additional designation: health care—acquired pneumonia.[1] The justification for this is that a group of patients exists that is prone to developing pneumonia, who are not in hospital, but theoretically have risks for organisms that resemble those seen in hospital-acquired episodes. In particular, these guidelines singled out patients hospitalized within the last 90 days, nursing home residents, dialysis patients, home infusion or other home care patients, and family members known to carry drug-resistant organisms.[1] This new pneumonia designation did not come, however, from carefully done prospective studies but rather from the results of a single retrospective review, which suggested that the subgroup of the population in frequent contact with health care facilities or long-term care facilities tended to be infected with organisms similar to hospital-acquired pneumonia.[2] The health care—associated designation has been controversial, and investigators have struggled to better define the universe of this entity or even if it exists as distinct from either community-acquired or hospital-acquired infection. Most studies supporting the designation have come from the United States, whereas European studies have been less supportive.[3]

This study provides a new insight. The initial rational in creating the health care—associated pneumonia designation was to call out the need to use a different antibiotic approach to address the more hospital-acquired pneumonialike organisms thought to be involved and responsible for higher mortalities. Chalmers et al did find higher mortality in these patients, but it was due to the characteristics of the patients—older age and comorbidities—not to the organisms involved (Table 3). Studies from the United States have not yet defined how much of the increased mortality in the United States is due to demographic and comorbid factors rather than the organisms involved. However, there have been suggestions to better define these roles. This should be an important focus of prospective studies since excessive use of broad-spectrum drugs is not only harmful—especially to elderly patients—but also of course is the cause of our large number of multidrug-resistant bacteria. It may be that the most useful aspect of the health care—associated designation is for prognostic purposes.

J. R. Maurer, MD, MBA

References

1. American Thoracic Society, Infectious Diseases Society of America. Guidelines for the management of adults with hospital-acquired, ventilator-associated, and healthcare-associated pneumonia. *Am J Respir Crit Care Med.* 2005;171:388-416.
2. Kollef MH, Shorr A, Tabak YP, Gupta V, Liu LZ, Johannes RS. Epidemiology and outcomes of health-care-associated pneumonia: results from a large US database of culture-positive pneumonia. *Chest.* 2005;128:3854-3862.
3. Shorr AF, Zilberberg MD, Micek ST, Kollef MH. Prediction of infection due to antibiotic-resistant bacteria by select risk factors for health care-associated pneumonia. *Arch Intern Med.* 2008;168:2205-2210.

Patterns of Antimicrobial Use for Respiratory Tract Infections in Older Residents of Long-Term Care Facilities

Vergidis P, Hamer DH, Meydani SN, et al (Boston Univ, MA; et al)
J Am Geriatr Soc 59:1093-1098, 2011

Objectives.—To describe patterns of antimicrobial use for respiratory tract infections (RTIs) in older residents of long-term care facilities (LTCFs).

Design.—Data from a prospective, randomized, controlled study of the effect of vitamin E supplementation on RTIs conducted from April 1998 through August 2001 were analyzed.

Setting.—Thirty-three LTCFs in the greater Boston area.

Participants.—Six hundred seventeen subjects aged 65 and older residing in LTCFs.

Measurements.—RTIs, categorized as acute bronchitis, pneumonia, common cold, influenza-like illness, pharyngitis, and sinusitis, were studied for appropriateness of antimicrobial use, type of antibiotics used, and factors associated with their use. For cases in which drug treatment was administered, antibiotic use was rated as appropriate (when an effective drug was used), inappropriate (when a more-effective drug was indicated), or unjustified (when use of any antimicrobial was not indicated).

Results.—Of 752 documented episodes of RTI, overall treatment was appropriate in 79% of episodes, inappropriate in 2%, and unjustified in 19%. For acute bronchitis, treatment was appropriate in 35% and unjustified in 65% of cases. For pneumonia, treatment was appropriate in 87% of episodes. Of the most commonly used antimicrobials, macrolide use was unjustified in 43% of cases. No statistically significant differences in the patterns of antibiotic use were observed when stratified according to age, sex, race, or comorbid conditions, including diabetes mellitus, dementia, and chronic kidney disease.

Conclusion.—Antimicrobials were unjustifiably used for one-fifth of RTIs and more than two-thirds of cases of acute bronchitis, suggesting a need for programs to improve antibiotic prescribing at LTCFs.

▶ Residents of long-term care facilities are prone to respiratory tract infections likely because of their close proximity to each other, their chronic comorbidities, and their overall frailty. There are many concerns, however, about overuse of antibiotics in these facilities because of the potential to create populations of multiresistant bacteria[1] and because of serious side effects such as colitis caused by *Clostridium difficile*. In fact, *C difficile* colitis is reported to be the most common cause of infectious diarrhea in nursing home settings.[2] In their 2007 guidelines on the management of community-acquired pneumonia, the American Thoracic Society and Infectious Disease Society of America identified long-term care facility residents who develop pneumonia as having healthcare-associated pneumonia, a new designation of out-of-hospital—acquired pneumonia, considered to be more likely caused by hospital-acquired types of organisms.[3] While controversy about this designation and how well it applies to residents of long-term care facilities exists, it is nevertheless important to better understand the use of antibiotics in long-term care residents. The data in this study are almost a decade old, but it is not likely that patterns of care have changed much. These data come from a large prospective study and show unjustified use of antibiotics in all types of respiratory tract infections, but particularly in acute bronchitis. Because national guidelines for management of both pneumonia and bronchitis exist, as do performance measures to assess adherence to the guidelines (standards of care), it is appropriate to make quality measurement and quality improvement an integral part of the infection protocols in these facilities.

J. R. Maurer, MD, MBA

References

1. O'Fallon E, Kandel R, Schreiber R, D'Agata EM. Acquisition of multidrug-resistant gram-negative bacteria: incidence and risk factors within a long-term care population. *Infect Control Hosp Epidemiol.* 2010;31:1148-1153.
2. Simor AE, Bradley SF, Strausbaugh LJ, Crossley K, Nicolle LE, SHEA Long-Term-Care Committee. Clostridium difficile in long-term-care facilities for the elderly. *Infect Control Hosp Epidemiol.* 2002;23:696-703.
3. Mandell LA, Wunderink RG, Anzueto A, et al. Infectious diseases society of America/American thoracic society consensus guidelines on the management of community-acquired pneumonia in adults. *Clin Infect Dis.* 2007;44:S27-S72.

How deadly is seasonal influenza-associated pneumonia? The German Competence Network for Community-Acquired Pneumonia
von Baum H, the CAPNETZ Study Group (Ulm Univ Hosp, Germany; et al)
Eur Respir J 37:1151-1157, 2011

The emergence of new influenza virus subtypes has rekindled the interest in the clinical course and outcome of patients with influenza-associated pneumonia.

Based on prospective data from 5,032 patients with community-acquired pneumonia (CAP) included in the German Competence Network for Community-Acquired Pneumonia (CAPNETZ), we studied the incidence, clinical characteristics and outcome of patients with influenza-associated CAP and compared these findings with patients without influenza. Diagnosis relied on a positive PCR for influenza in throat washings.

160 patients with influenza-associated CAP were identified (3.2% of total population, 12% of those with defined aetiology). 34 (21%) patients with seasonal influenza had a concomitant pathogen (mostly *Streptococcus pneumoniae*). Patients with influenza-associated CAP were significantly older, had been vaccinated less often and had preceding antibacterial treatment less often. 30-day mortality was low (4.4%) and not different to that of patients with pneumonia caused by bacterial (6.2%) or viral (other than influenza) pathogens (4%). Patients with influenza plus a bacterial pathogen (mixed influenza-associated pneumonia) had a higher mortality than those with pure influenza-associated pneumonia (9% *versus* 3.2%).

Mortality was higher in patients with mixed compared with pure influenza-associated pneumonia. However, we could not observe any excess mortality in patients with influenza-associated pneumonia.

▶ The German Competence Network for Community Acquired Pneumonia (CAPNETZ) published 2 reports focused on seasonal influenza. Understandably, the interest in morbidity and mortality of influenza infections has risen significantly both in the health care community and in the general public in the wake of the publicity around the H1N1 pandemic of 2009. In that pandemic, the death rate was somewhat lower than many anticipated, but it was substantial, particularly in young, healthier people. In influenza pandemics, susceptibility to bacterial pneumonia is generally thought to be increased, and this results in increased morbidity and mortality.[1,2] Bacterial pneumonia was reported in more than 18% of those hospitalized with H1N1 disease in the 2009 pandemic.[3] Outside of pandemics, however, the association of usual seasonal influenza and bacterial pneumonia and the impact on mortality has been less clear. In this report from the Competence Network for Community-Acquired Pneumonia (CATNETZ), seasonal influenza had a relatively small rate of associated bacterial pneumonia, and it occurred in the more typical risk group of older, unvaccinated patients. Overall the excess mortality was low in contrast to the H1N1 pandemic. In a related CATNETZ report, Tessemer et al[4] were able to show that influenza vaccinations appear to decrease the severity of community-acquired pneumonia (CAP) during influenza season. The authors compared the severity of community-acquired pneumonia cases during influenza season and during the off-season. Influenza-vaccinated patients with CAP had less severe pneumonias than unvaccinated patients during the flu season, but in the off-season, vaccination status made no difference. Another good reason to get your annual flu shot!

J. R. Maurer, MD, MBA

References

1. Louria DB, Blumenfeld HL, Ellis JT, Kilbourne ED, Rogers DE. Studies on influenza in the pandemic of 1957–1958. II. Pulmonary complications of influenza. *J Clin Invest.* 1959;38:213-265.
2. Morens DM, Taubenberger JK, Fauci AS. Predominant role of bacterial pneumonia as a cause of death in pandemic influenza: implications for pandemic influenza preparedness. *J Infect Dis.* 2008;198:962-970.
3. Viasus D, Paño-Pardo JR, Pachon J, et al; Novel Influenza A(H1N1) Study Group of the Spanish Network for Research in Infectious Diseases (REIPI). Pneumonia complicating pandemic (H1N1) 2009: risk factors, clinical features, and outcomes. *Medicine.* 2011;90:328-336.
4. Tessmer A, Welte T, Schmidt-Ott R, et al; CAPNETZ Study Group. Influenza vaccination is associated with reduced severity of community-acquired pneumonia. *Eur Respir J.* 2011;38:147-153.

British Thoracic Society adult community acquired pneumonia audit 2009/10

Lim WS, On behalf of the British Thoracic Society (Nottingham City Hosp, UK; et al)
Thorax 66:548-549, 2011

Background.—The updated British Thoracic Society (BTS) Guidelines for the management of Community Acquired Pneumonia (CAP) in adults was published in October 2009. In conjunction with the Guidelines, the first national BTS audit of adult CAP was conducted.

Methods.—An audit tool was developed as part of the Guidelines. Members of the BTS were invited to participate in the audit capturing data relating to acutely ill adults admitted to hospitals in the UK and treated for CAP within the period 1 December 2009 and 31 January 2010. Data entry using the web-based audit tool closed in May 2010.

Results.—Of 2749 submissions from 64 institutions; 8 were excluded due to inconsistent data. The mean age of patients was 71 years (range 16–105 years). The CURB65 score was 0 to 1 in 40% of patients, 2 in 30% and 3 to 5 in 30%. Five hundred and three (18.3%) patients died in hospital within 30 days, 101 (20.1%) within 1 day of admission. Initial empirical antibiotics were in accordance with local CAP guidelines in 1478 (55.5%) patients and were administered intravenously in 712 (65%), 603 (74%) and 743 (90%) patients with CURB65 scores 0 to 1, 2 and 3 to 5 respectively. Within 4 hours of admission, a chest x-ray was obtained in 83% of patients and the first dose of antibiotics was administered in 58%.

Conclusions.—The burden of CAP is high. Efforts should be directed at improving adherence to local CAP guidelines and specific processes of care.

▶ The British Thoracic Society (BTS) has a series of audit tools for different respiratory conditions that are published on their website. These tools are typically published in conjunction with their guidelines and cover such topics as bronchiectasis, adult and pediatric asthma, and pleural procedures. When the adult community-acquired pneumonia (CAP) guidelines were updated in 2009, an audit tool was created for them, and this report is the first report of that audit. As stated in the guidelines, "the management of CAP is a sufficiently common and important issue to warrant the development of audit measures of the process of care and outcome to evaluate the quality of care for CAP, using guidelines as a standard of management."[1] Individual physicians can register at the BTS to access the audit tool and report their data, which they can then compare with the national data compiled from them and their peers. There are many good reasons to collect these data: they can be used as an individual quality improvement tool; they can be used to evaluate the overall care of pneumonia in the country or in specific regions; and, possibly most important of all, as a large database, they can be used to learn a great deal about the epidemiology of CAP.

J. R. Maurer, MD, MBA

Reference

1. Lim WS, Baudouin SV, George RC, et al; Pneumonia Guidelines Committee of the BTS Standards of Care Committee. BTS guidelines for the management of community acquired pneumonia in adults: update 2009. *Thorax.* 2009;64:iii1-iii55.

Long-term use of thiazolidinediones and the associated risk of pneumonia or lower respiratory tract infection: systematic review and meta-analysis
Singh S, Loke YK, Furberg CD (Johns Hopkins Univ School of Medicine, Baltimore, MD; Univ of East Anglia, Norwich, UK; Wake Forest Univ School of Medicine, Winston-Salem, NC)
Thorax 66:383-388, 2011

Introduction.—The peroxisome proliferator-activated receptor-γ agonists rosiglitazone and pioglitazone activate glucocorticoid receptors and have an immunomodulatory effect. The authors aimed to systematically determine the risk of pneumonia or lower respiratory tract infections associated with thiazolidinediones.

Methods.—Systematic searches of MEDLINE, EMBASE, regulatory documents and trial registries were carried out for randomised controlled trials of thiazolidinediones with no date restrictions through March 2010. The authors selected long-term (≥ 1 year) randomised controlled trials of thiazolidinediones versus a placebo, metformin or sulfonylurea control for prevention or treatment of type 2 diabetes that reported on pneumonia or lower respiratory tract infection adverse events or serious adverse events (hospitalisation, disability or death). Relative risks (RRs) were estimated using a fixed-effects meta-analysis, and statistical heterogeneity was assessed using the I^2 statistic.

Results.—Thirteen trials (n=17 627, including 8163 patients receiving thiazolidinediones and 9464 patients receiving control therapy) with a duration of follow-up of 1–5.5 years were included after a detailed screening of 58 studies. Thiazolidinediones were associated with a statistically significantly increased risk for any pneumonia or lower respiratory tract infection (n=130/8163 vs 100/9464; RR 1.40; 95% CI 1.08 to 1.82; p=0.01; I^2=0%) and serious pneumonia or lower respiratory tract infection (n=111/7391 vs 87/8692; RR 1.39; 95% CI 1.05 to 1.83; p=0.02; I^2=0%).

Interpretation.—Long-term thiazolidinedione use is associated with a modestly increased risk of any pneumonia or lower respiratory tract infection and serious pneumonia or lower respiratory tract infection in patients with type 2 diabetes.

▶ Thiazolidinediones are relatively new agents whose primary indication is to treat type II diabetes. They improve insulin sensitivity by increasing activity of the nuclear receptor peroxisome proliferator-activated receptor gamma (PPARγ). These drugs have also been studied in asthma patients because PPARγ activation has anti-inflammatory and immunomodulary effects in the lung. Rosiglitazone has been shown to be effective in asthmatics in at least 1 prospective, randomized controlled trial, and pioglitazone has shown activity in animals.[1,2] However, these drugs have been shown to have some bothersome long-term use toxicities, including myocardial infarction, heart failure, potential macular edema, and fractures.[3-6] Another important consideration in asthmatics is pneumonia. This is of concern with these drugs because they have a similar effect to that of glucocorticoids in the lung, and even inhaled steroids have been shown to increase pneumonia in chronic obstructive pulmonary disease patients.[7] Prior smaller studies with the thiazolidinediones have been inconsistent, so this meta-analysis is useful in putting some perspective around the risk of these drugs. In a risk-benefit analysis, it seems likely that the relative risks of these drugs is relatively great when compared with the benefits, especially since there are a number of effective drugs for asthma that have fewer risks.

J. R. Maurer, MD, MBA

References

1. Spears M, Donnelly I, Jolly L, et al. Bronchodilatory effect of the PPAR-gamma agonist rosiglitazone in smokers with asthma. *Clin Pharmacol Ther.* 2009;86:49-53.
2. Narala VR, Ranga R, Smith MR, et al. Pioglitazone is as effective as dexamethasone in a cockroach allergen-induced murine model of asthma. *Respir Res.* 2007;8:90.
3. Singh S, Loke YK, Furberg CD. Long-term risk of cardiovascular events with rosiglitazone: a meta-analysis. *JAMA.* 2007;298:1189-1195.
4. Singh S, Loke YK, Furberg CD. Thiazolidinediones and heart failure: a teleo-analysis. *Diabetes Care.* 2007;30:2148-2153.
5. Merante D, Menchini F, Truitt KE, Bandello FM. Diabetic macular edema: correlations with available diabetes therapies—evidence across a qualitative review of published literature from MEDLINE and EMBASE. *Drug Saf.* 2010;33:643-652.
6. Loke YK, Singh S, Furberg CD. Long-term use of thiazolidinediones and fractures in type 2 diabetes: a meta-analysis. *CMAJ.* 2009;180:32-39.
7. Singh S, Amin AV, Loke YK. Long-term use of inhaled corticosteroids and the risk of pneumonia in chronic obstructive pulmonary disease: a meta-analysis. *Arch Intern Med.* 2009;169:219-229.

The Spectrum of Pneumococcal Empyema in Adults in the Early 21st Century

Burgos J, Lujan M, Falcó V, et al (Universitat Autònoma de Barcelona, Spain; Corporacio Sanitaria Parc Tauli, Sabadell, Spain; et al)
Clin Infect Dis 53:254-261, 2011

Background.—Increased rates of empyema have been reported in children after the introduction of the pneumococcal conjugate vaccine (PCV7). Our objective was to describe the risk factors for pneumococcal empyema in adults and to analyze the differences in the incidence, disease characteristics, and serotype distribution between the pre- and post-PCV7 eras.

Methods.—An observational study of all adults hospitalized with invasive pneumococcal disease (IPD) who presented with empyema in 2 Spanish hospitals was conducted during the periods 1996—2001 (prevaccine period) and 2005—2009 (postvaccine period). Incidences of empyema were calculated. A multivariate analysis was performed to identify variables associated with pneumococcal empyema.

Results.—Empyema was diagnosed in 128 of 1080 patients with invasive pneumococcal disease. Among patients aged 18–50 years, the rates of pneumococcal pneumonia with empyema increased from 7.6% to 14.9% ($P = .04$) and the incidence of pneumococcal empyema increased from 0.5 to 1.6 cases per 100,000 person-years (198% [95% confidence interval {CI}, 49%–494%]). The incidence of empyema due to serotype 1 increased significantly from 0.2 to 0.8 cases per 100,000 person-years (253% [95% CI, 67%–646%]). Serotype 1 caused 43.3% of cases of empyema during the postvaccine period. Serotypes 1 (odds ratio [OR], 5.88; [95% CI, 2.66–13]) and 3 (OR, 5.49 [95% CI, 1.93–15.62]) were independently associated with development of empyema.

Conclusions.—The incidence of pneumococcal empyema in young adults has increased during the postvaccine period, mainly as a result of the emergence of serotype 1. Serotypes 1 and 3 are the main determinants of development of this suppurative complication.

▶ The introduction of 7-valent conjugated pneumococcal vaccine in young children in 2001 changed the face of invasive pneumococcal disease by both greatly reducing infections with the serotypes included in the vaccine and resulting in some unintended consequences. In some countries like the United States, where there was immediate uniform and high uptake of the vaccine, a rapid drop-off of invasive pneumococcal disease was seen not only in the vaccinated children but also in older members of the households.[1] This reduction in overall invasive disease has been sustained; however, there has been an increase in invasive infections with some serotypes such as 19A and others not covered by the 7-valent vaccine.[2] In countries like Spain, where introduction of the vaccine was more gradual and less uniform, there was also a fall-off of invasive disease in children and adults of the serotypes contained in the 7-valent vaccine but a rapid increase in nonvaccine serotypes that caused invasive disease, and overall there was a relatively small reduction in invasive disease.[3] The primary nonvaccine serotypes now isolated in Europe are 1, 19A, 3, 6A, and 7F.[4] Changes in serotype distribution have now been described essentially wherever the conjugated vaccines have been used, and along with those changes has come a changing face of the disease. One such change is reported here by Burgos et al. They note a surprising rise in empyema rates in both children and adults, particularly in young adults less than 50 years old. What is not reported, but should be further studied, is the morbidity associated with these empyemas, something that could be significant and an unfortunate result of the 7-valent vaccine. With the changing face of invasive disease and the emergence of invasive disease from other serotypes, however, the vaccine makers are happily creating new vaccines directed against an ever-increasing number of serotypes.

J. R. Maurer, MD, MBA

References

1. Whitney CG, Farley MM, Hadler J, et al; Active Bacterial Core Surveillance of the Emerging Infections Program Network. Decline in invasive pneumococcal disease after the introduction of protein-polysaccharide conjugate vaccine. *N Engl J Med.* 2003;348:1737-1746.
2. Pilishvili T, Lexau C, Farley MM, et al; Active Bacterial Core Surveillance/Emerging Infections Program Network. Sustained reductions in invasive pneumococcal disease in the era of conjugate vaccine. *J Infect Dis.* 2010;201:32-41.
3. Guevara M, Barricarte A, Gil-Setas A, et al. Changing epidemiology of invasive pneumococcal disease following increased coverage with the heptavalent conjugate vaccine in Navarre, Spain. *Clin Microbiol Infect.* 2009;15:1013-1019.
4. Isaacman DJ, McIntosh ED, Reinert RR. Burden of invasive pneumococcal disease and serotype distribution among Streptococcus pneumoniae isolates in young children in Europe: impact of the 7-valent pneumococcal conjugate vaccine and considerations for future conjugate vaccines. *Int J Infect Dis.* 2010;14:e197-e209.

6 Lung Transplantation

Predictors of Acute Rejection After Lung Transplantation
Mangi AA, Mason DP, Nowicki ER, et al (Cleveland Clinic, OH)
Ann Thorac Surg 91:1754-1762, 2011

Background.—Acute rejection (AR) after lung transplantation (LTx) impacts survival and quality of life. The objective of this study, therefore, was to identify risk factors for AR after LTx, focusing on donor- and recipient-specific factors, operative variables, and immunologic issues, including pretransplant panel-reactive antibody (PRA) levels, and donor—recipient human leukocyte antigen (HLA) mismatch.

Methods.—From March 1996 to November 2007, 481 adults undergoing LTx had 3237 serial transbronchial biopsy specimens that were evaluated for perivascular rejection (grade A0 to A4). Longitudinal analysis was used to characterize the prevalence of rejection grade and influence of donor, recipient, technical, and immunologic variables.

Results.—AR was highest ($54\% \geq A1$) in the first 2 months after LTx, decreased at 6 months ($16\% \geq A1$), then remained steady. Prevalence of AR at any time was dominated by donor-specific factors of young age ($p < 0.0001$), blunt trauma ($p = 0.008$), and nonblack race ($p = 0.012$) and by recipient class II PRA exceeding 10% ($p = 0.005$). AR within 2 months was associated with HLA mismatch at the DR locus ($p = 0.0006$) and use of non-O blood-group donors ($p = 0.008$). AR at 4 years and longer after LTx was associated with HLA mismatch at the B locus ($p = 0.01$).

Conclusions.—Only a few recipient and operative factors were identified for AR after LTx. Moderately sensitized recipients identified by class II PRA exceeding 10% and those with HLA mismatches at the B and DR loci appear to be more susceptible to AR; however, such immunologic variations appear to be well controlled with current donor selection and immunosuppression protocols. The impact of donor-specific variables on AR is surprisingly strong and warrants closer inspection.

▶ Acute rejection following lung transplantation occurs in up to half of patients and results in significant morbidity. In addition, it is recognized as an important risk factor for the development of chronic lung allograft dysfunction. It is a little surprising, then, that risk factors for acute rejection have not been better defined than they are. This study, designed to identify both donor and recipient risk factors for rejection, found few statistically significant recipient risk factors—for example, donor-positive/recipient-negative cytomegalovirus status was not a significant risk factor. This study has limitations, the most significant of which is that it is from a single center and is retrospective. Nevertheless, it should serve to focus more research on the donor factors that have been identified here to determine whether they can be modified. If it is not possible to modify donor risk factors, another approach is to try to predict which at-risk patients will actually develop it. This information could potentially lead to strategies to prevent episodes. Miyoshi et al have reported that rises in immunoglobulin M in the donor organ and directed against the grafts can occur days before the clinical onset of acute rejection.[1] Early detection using this or other biomarkers might at least allow early and more successful treatment.

J. R. Maurer, MD, MBA

Reference

1. Miyoshi K, Sano Y, Yamane M, Toyooka S, Oto T, Miyoshi S. Elevation of anti-donor immunoglobulin M levels precedes acute lung transplant rejection. *Ann Thorac Surg.* 2011;92:1233-1238.

Timing of basiliximab induction and development of acute rejection in lung transplant patients

Swarup R, Allenspach LL, Nemeh HW, et al (Henry Ford Hosp, Detroit, MI)
J Heart Lung Transplant 30:1228-1235, 2011

Background.—Acute rejection affects more than 36% of recipients within the first year post-transplantation. The interleukin-2 (IL-2) receptor antagonist basiliximab has been associated with decreased frequency and severity of acute rejection. We investigated whether the timing of induction administration would impact the frequency and severity of acute rejection in the first year after transplantation.

Methods.—In this study we reviewed 119 patients who underwent lung transplantation at Henry Ford Hospital from October 1994 to January 2009. Prior to January 2000 no patients received induction. From January 2000 to March 2006 the initial dose was given after implantation, and from March 2006 to 2009 basiliximab was given prior to implantation. The primary outcome was cumulative acute rejection score (CAR) in the first post-operative year comparing post- vs pre-implant induction.

Results.—The CAR score for pre-implant basiliximab was 2.5 ± 2.3. This was significantly lower than CAR score of 4.6 ± 3.9 in the post-implant group ($p = 0.025$). The no-induction group had the highest CAR score at 6.3 ± 3.8 ($p = 0.077$ compared with the post group). The mean follow-up times in the post and pre group were 5.9 ± 2.3 and 2.3 ± 0.7 years, respectively ($p < 0.001$). There was no difference in freedom from bronchiolitis obliterans syndrome (BOS), survival or invasive infections between pre- and post-implant induction groups.

Conclusions.—Basiliximab prior to implant is associated with a lower cumulative acute rejection score over 1 year compared with induction

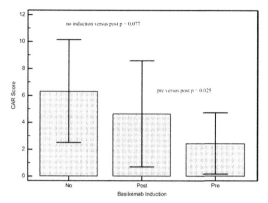

FIGURE 1.—Cumulative acute rejection (CAR) score (mean ± SD) at 1 year post-transplantation for the no-induction, post-implant induction and pre-implant induction groups with survival of ≥1 year. The pre group shows the lowest overall CAR score compared with the no- and post-induction groups. (Reprinted from The journal of Heart and Lung Transplantation, Swarup R, Allenspach LL, Nemeh HW, et al. Timing of basiliximab induction and development of acute rejection in lung transplant patients. *J Heart Lung Transplant.* 2011;30:1228-1235. Copyright 2011, with permission from International Society for Heart and Lung Transplantation.)

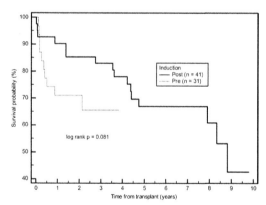

FIGURE 4.—Survival comparison in the post- and pre-induction groups. The post group had a 90% survival rate at 1 year, which was higher than expected. The survival difference between the two groups did not reach significance over the time period of study. (Reprinted from The journal of Heart and Lung Transplantation, Swarup R, Allenspach LL, Nemeh HW, et al. Timing of basiliximab induction and development of acute rejection in lung transplant patients. *J Heart Lung Transplant.* 2011;30:1228-1235. Copyright 2011, with permission from International Society for Heart and Lung Transplantation.)

post-implantation. Despite a lower cumulative acute rejection score, there was no significant difference in freedom from BOS or survival (Figs 1 and 4).

▶ Induction immunosuppression in lung transplant recipients has been controversial primarily because of the susceptibility of the lung graft to different types of infectious complications in the early time period during which induction is used and the risk of development of posttransplant lymphoproliferative disorders is greatest. According to the most recent International Society for Heart and Lung

Transplant registry report, the percent of new transplants receiving any induction has gradually risen from around 40% to between 50% and 60%. Of those receiving induction, the type varies. Between 2000 and 2010, the use of polyclonal antilymphocyte/antithymocyte globulin fell from 20% to 10%; the use of alemtuzumab rose to approximately 8%, and the use of interleukin (IL)-2 receptor antagonists rose from approximately 20% to more than 40%.[1] The popularity of IL-2 receptor antagonists is based on their relative ease of use, relative lack of side effects, and general effectiveness in preventing acute rejection episodes. Nevertheless, as many as a third of posttransplants have acute rejection episodes, even with induction therapy. This ongoing incidence of acute rejection has led to centers trying newer, very aggressive monoclonal antibody approaches such as alemtuzumab (anti-CD25), about which outcomes are just starting to appear.[2] The timing of induction has been little studied and that was the point of the current paper. Using an IL-2 receptor antagonist, a much more selective and benign antilymphocyte approach than drugs such as alemtuzumab, the authors showed a lower cumulative rate of acute rejection when the induction agent was given before the graft was implanted (Figs 1 and 4). Studies looking at the detail of induction approaches, as this study did, are needed to better refine appropriate early treatment and hopefully avoid the need for more aggressive approaches with higher risks.

J. R. Maurer, MD, MBA

References

1. Christie JD, Edwards LB, Kucheryavaya AY, et al. The registry of the international society for heart and lung transplantation: twenty-eighth adult lung and heart-lung transplant report—2011. *J Heart Lung Transplant*. 2011;30:1104-1122.
2. Shyu S, Dew MA, Pilewski JM, et al. Five-year outcomes with alemtuzumab induction after lung transplantation. *J Heart Lung Transplant*. 2011;30:743-754.

The protective role of laparoscopic antireflux surgery against aspiration of pepsin after lung transplantation

Fisichella PM, Davis CS, Lundberg PW, et al (Loyola Univ Med Ctr, Maywood, IL; et al)
Surgery 150:598-606, 2011

Background.—The goal of this study was to determine, in lung transplant patients, if laparoscopic antireflux surgery (LARS) is an effective means to prevent aspiration as defined by the presence of pepsin in the bronchoalveolar lavage fluid (BALF).

Methods.—Between September 2009 and November 2010, we collected BALF from 64 lung transplant patients at multiple routine surveillance assessments for acute cellular rejection, or when clinically indicated for diagnostic purposes. The BALF was tested for pepsin by enzyme-linked immunosorbent assay (ELISA). We then compared pepsin concentrations in the BALF of healthy controls ($n = 11$) and lung transplant patients with and without gastroesophageal reflux disease (GERD) on pH-monitoring ($n = 8$

and $n = 12$, respectively), and after treatment of GERD by LARS ($n = 19$). Time to the development of bronchiolitis obliterans syndrome was contrasted between groups based on GERD status or the presence of pepsin in the BALF.

Results.—We found that lung transplant patients with GERD had more pepsin in their BALF than lung transplant patients who underwent LARS ($P = .029$), and that pepsin was undetectable in the BALF of controls. Moreover, those with more pepsin had quicker progression to BOS and more acute rejection episodes.

Conclusion.—This study compared pepsin in the BALF from lung transplant patients with and without LARS. Our data show that: (1) the detection of pepsin in the BALF proves aspiration because it is not present in healthy volunteers, and (2) LARS appears effective as a measure to prevent the aspiration of gastroesophageal refluxate in the lung transplant population. We believe that these findings provide a mechanism for those studies suggesting that LARS may prevent nonallogenic injury to the transplanted lungs from aspiration of gastroesophageal contents.

▶ Several studies have addressed the issue of aspiration of refluxed stomach contents in transplant recipients with gastroesophageal reflux (GERD) and the possible impact on development of bronchiolitis obliterans syndrome (BOS).[1,2] In some centers, laparoscopic antireflux surgery (LARS) is applied almost routinely to patients found to have reflux either before or after transplantation. The studies of GERD are provocative but have raised several questions: If patients are aspirating, is there a direct causative relationship with BOS? Does surgery (LARS procedure) really prevent aspiration? Is surgery necessary to treat patients? The authors addressed the second question and were able to show that a surgical approach significantly reduced the amount of pepsin found in bronchoalveolar lavage fluid in patients known to have GERD. Thus, presumably, reflux is significantly reduced in refluxing patients. However, the remaining 2 questions that may delineate an actual causal relationship for BOS and the identification of nonsurgical treatment approaches remain unanswered. The authors correctly note that a long-term prospective, randomized study is necessary to better define the role of GERD in the outcomes of lung transplant recipients and to identify best practices of management when it is important.

J. R. Maurer, MD, MBA

References

1. Young LR, Hadjiliadis D, Davis RD, Palmer SM. Lung transplantation exacerbates gastroesophageal reflux disease. *Chest.* 2003;124:1689-1693.
2. Davis CS, Shankaran V, Kovacs EJ, et al. Gastroesophageal reflux disease after lung transplantation: pathophysiology and implications for treatment. *Surgery.* 2010; 148:737-744.

High Levels of Mannose-Binding Lectin Are Associated With Poor Outcomes After Lung Transplantation

Carroll KE, Dean MM, Heatley SL, et al (Dept of Respiratory Medicine St Vincent's Hosp, Victoria, Australia; Australian Red Cross Blood Service, Queensland, Australia; Australian Red Cross Blood Service, Adelaide, South Australia. Australia; et al)
Transplantation 91:1044-1049, 2011

Background.—Mannose-binding lectin (MBL) is a key molecule of the innate immune system and, in addition to the classical and alternative pathways, a principle driver of complement activation. Genetic mutations of MBL are common, result in low serum levels of MBL, and are associated with increased infection risk in solid-organ transplant recipients.

Methods.—We performed a retrospective study of *MBL2* genotype and plasma and bronchoalveolar lavage (BAL) MBL levels in 37 lung transplant recipients (LTR). Plasma MBL levels were measured pretransplant and both plasma and BAL MBL levels were measured at 3, 6, and 12 months after lung transplantation. *MBL2* genotyping was performed on recipient and donor peripheral blood mononuclear cells. Clinical variables analyzed included primary graft dysfunction, intensive care unit stay, acute allograft rejection, infection, bronchiolitis obliterans syndrome (BOS), and mortality.

Results.—Plasma MBL levels posttransplant were predicted by recipient, and not donor *MBL2* genotype. Compared with pretransplant levels, plasma MBL was significantly increased at 3, 6, and 12 months posttransplant ($P<0.05$). LTR who developed BOS or died during the study period had higher plasma MBL levels at 6 and 12 months posttransplant ($P \leq 0.05$) compared with LTR with stable graft function. MBL was not routinely detected in the lung allograft; however if present in the BAL at 3 and 6 months posttransplant, it was associated with the later development of BOS ($P<0.05$).

Conclusions.—Plasma MBL levels increase after lung transplantation and persistently increased MBL levels are associated with poor long-term outcomes.

▶ In recent years, several researchers investigating the pathogenesis of chronic lung allograft rejection have focused on the innate immune system looking for specific markers that might denote risk for poor outcomes. The innate immune system is a fundamental part of the body's first defense against microbial and other invaders until adaptive immunity develops. A critical part of innate immunity is the complement system that functions through the classical or alternative pathway or the mannose-binding lectin pathway (MBL). MBL levels have been studied in a variety of solid organ transplants, and abnormal levels have been associated with less-than-ideal outcomes. For example, in liver transplants, lower-than-normal levels have been associated with infection[1] whereas in kidney transplants, higher-than-normal levels have been associated with rejection-associated graft loss.[2] The most influential genotype appears to be MBL2, the genotype addressed in this study. As in reports of kidney transplants, the authors found that persistently high levels of MBL, possibly through its influence on complement activation, were associated with bronchiolitis obliterans syndrome and poor long-term outcomes. The importance of this provocative finding is unknown; future prospective studies are needed to further flesh out the role of the innate immune system in long-term graft outcomes.

J. R. Maurer, MD, MBA

References

1. Worthley DL, Johnson DF, Eisen DP, et al. Donor mannose-binding lectin deficiency increases the likelihood of clinically significant infection after liver transplantation. *Clin Infect Dis.* 2009;48:410-417.
2. Berger SP, Roos A, Mallat MJ, Fujita T, de Fijter JW, Daha MR. Association between mannose-binding lectin levels and graft survival in kidney transplantation. *Am J Transplant.* 2005;5:1361-1366.

Circulating Fibrocytes Correlate With Bronchiolitis Obliterans Syndrome Development After Lung Transplantation: A Novel Clinical Biomarker
LaPar DJ, Burdick MD, Emaminia A, et al (Univ of Virginia School of Medicine, Charlottesville)
Ann Thorac Surg 92:470-477, 2011

Background.—Development of bronchiolitis obliterans syndrome (BOS) after lung transplantation confers increased patient morbidity and mortality. Fibrocytes are circulating bone marrow—derived mesenchymal cell progenitors that influence tissue repair and fibrosis. Fibrocytes have been implicated in chronic pulmonary inflammatory processes. We investigated the correlation of circulating fibrocyte number with BOS development in lung transplant patients.

Methods.—We prospectively quantified circulating fibrocyte levels among lung transplant patients. Patients were stratified according to the development of BOS as indicated by predicted forced expiratory volume in 1 second. Fibrocyte activity was analyzed by flow cytometry (cluster of differentiation 45^+, collagen 1^+) in a blinded manner related to clinical presentation.

Results.—Thirty-nine patients (61.5% men) underwent double (33.3%), left (25.6%), or right (41.0%) lung transplantation. Average patient age was similar between BOS and non-BOS patients (58.3 ± 3.9 vs 60.3 ± 2.0 years, $p = 0.67$). Chronic obstructive lung disease was the most common indication for lung transplantation (41.0%). Median forced expiratory volume in 1 second was lower among BOS patients compared with non-BOS patients (1.08 vs. 2.18 L/s, $p = 0.001$). Importantly, circulating fibrocyte numbers were increased in BOS patients compared with non-BOS patients (8.91 vs 2.96×10^5 cells/mL, $p = 0.03$) by flow cytometry and were incrementally increased with advancing BOS stage ($p = 0.02$).

Conclusions.—Increased circulating fibrocyte levels correlate with the development of BOS after lung transplantation and positively correlate with advancing BOS stage. Quantification of circulating fibrocytes could serve as a novel biomarker and possible therapeutic target for BOS development in lung transplant patients.

▶ A number of biomarkers have been identified as being in increased quantities in patients who have chronic lung allograft dysfunction, especially bronchiolitis obliterans (BO). The difficulty with existing biomarkers is that they cannot be reliably used to predict the future development of BO, as elevated levels typically do not distinguish from other inflammatory conditions like infection. The appeal of fibrocytes is that they fit with the pathology seen in BO. In particular, the initial abnormal finding usually observed is a lymphocytic infiltration followed by fibroproliferation, increased extracellular matrix, and finally, fibrotic proliferation occluding the airway. The findings of increased circulating fibrocytes in this study are very interesting when viewed in the context of a second study published by Andersson-Sjöland et al.[1] That group studied fibroblasts in lung transplant patients 6 and 12 months following transplant. They found that, in general, fibroblasts in these patients were changed phenotypically to produce more proteoglycans, likely in response to wound healing. However, they found that in the subset of patients who were later destined to have BO, their fibroblasts were different—more inclined to produce versican in response to tumor growth factor—beta stimulation. Thus, patients who have increased levels of fibrocytes that are precursors to fibroblasts (under the right stimuli) might also be those patients who have the fibroblasts that produce versican, which has been associated with pathologic wound healing. This is clearly a promising finding that deserves much further investigation.

J. R. Maurer, MD, MBA

Reference

1. Andersson-Sjöland A, Thiman L, Nihlberg K, et al. Fibroblast phenotypes and their activity are changed in the wound healing process after lung transplantation. *J Heart Lung Transplant*. 2011;30:945-954.

Cytomegalovirus Replication Within the Lung Allograft Is Associated With Bronchiolitis Obliterans Syndrome

Paraskeva M, Bailey M, Levvey BJ, et al (Alfred Hosp Melbourne Vic 3181, Australia; Monash Univ, Melbourne, Victoria, Australia)
Am J Transplant 11:2190-2196, 2011

Early studies reported cytomegalovirus (CMV) pneumonitis as a risk factor for development of bronchiolitis obliterans syndrome (BOS) following lung transplantation. While improvements in antiviral prophylaxis have resulted in a decreased incidence of CMV pneumonitis, molecular diagnostic techniques allow diagnosis of subclinical CMV replication in the allograft. We hypothesized that this subclinical CMV replication was associated with development of BOS. We retrospectively evaluated 192 lung transplant recipients (LTR) from a single center between 2001 and

2009. Quantitative (PCR) analysis of CMV viral load and histological evidence of CMV pneumonitis and acute cellular rejection was determined on 1749 bronchoalveolar lavage (BAL) specimens and 1536 transbronchial biopsies. CMV was detected in the BAL of 41% of LTR and was significantly associated with the development of BOS (HR 1.8 [1.1—2.8], p = 0.02). This association persisted when CMV was considered more accurately as a time-dependent variable (HR 2.1 [1.3—3.3], p = 0.003) and after adjustment for significant covariates in a multivariate model. CMV replication in the lung allograft is common following lung transplantation and is associated with increased risk of BOS. As antiviral prophylaxis adequately suppresses CMV longer prophylactic strategies may improve long-term outcome in lung transplantation.

▶ Cytomegalovirus (CMV) infection and disease have always been major concerns in lung transplant recipients. Clinical CMV pneumonitis and asymptomatic, but active, CMV infection defined by presence of positive cultures or tissue inclusion bodies have been associated by some with accelerated or increased risk of bronchiolitis obliterans allograft dysfunction. The approach to preventing or reducing the negative impact of CMV has been to use antiviral prophylaxis. This is very effective during the time the prophylaxis is used, but routinely after prophylaxis is discontinued, CMV replication can again be detected. The impact of late CMV infection that occurs after prophylaxis is stopped is less clear. Recently, it has become possible by sophisticated polymerase chain reaction testing to identify CMV DNA very early in the replication process. In this study, the authors were able to identify even minimal levels of CMV replication after cessation of prophylaxis and were able to demonstrate that longer prophylaxis results in lower peak levels of CMV replication when the prophylaxis is stopped. This has been previously demonstrated; however, what the authors were also able to show using PCR is that even relatively minor CMV replication after prophylaxis cessation appeared to be associated significantly with bronchiolitis obliterans. The authors suggest this argues for longer CMV prophylaxis. This needs to be studied prospectively because this, as are most lung transplant studies, was retrospective. How long prophylaxis should be continued is still an unanswered question. That is an important parameter of future studies because while CMV is clearly risky, prophylaxis is both expensive and has its own side effects and other risks.

J. R. Maurer, MD, MBA

Survival Determinants in Lung Transplant Patients With Chronic Allograft Dysfunction
Verleden GM, Vos R, Verleden SE, et al (Katholieke Universiteit Leuven, Belgium)
Transplantation 92:703-708, 2011

Background.—Chronic lung allograft dysfunction (CLAD) remains the leading cause of mortality after lung transplantation.

Methods.—In this retrospective single-center study, we aimed to identify different phenotypes of and risk factors for mortality after CLAD diagnosis using univariate and multivariate Cox proportional hazard survival regression analysis.

Results.—CLAD was diagnosed in 71 of 294 patients (24.2%) at 30.9 ± 22.8 months after transplantation. Pulmonary function was obstructive in 51 (71.8%) of the CLAD patients, restrictive in 20 (28.2%) patients, of whom 17 had persistent parenchymal infiltrates on pulmonary computer tomography (CAT) scan. In univariate analysis, previous development of neutrophilic reversible allograft dysfunction (NRAD, $P=0.012$) and a restrictive pulmonary function ($P=0.0024$) were associated with a worse survival, whereas there was a strong trend for early development of CLAD and persistent parenchymal infiltrates on CAT scan ($P=0.067$ and 0.056, respectively). In multivariate analysis, early development of CLAD ($P=0.0067$), previous development of NRAD ($P=0.0016$), and a restrictive pulmonary function pattern ($P=0.0005$) or persistent parenchymal infiltrates on CAT scan ($P=0.0043$) remained significant.

Conclusion.—Although most CLAD patients develop an obstructive pulmonary function, 28% develop a restrictive pulmonary function, compatible with the recently defined restrictive allograft syndrome phenotype. Early-onset CLAD, previous development of NRAD, and the development of restrictive allograft syndrome are associated with worse survival after CLAD has been diagnosed.

▶ For many years, bronchiolitis obliterans has been considered the primary manifestation of chronic lung allograft rejection. To be sure, the bronchial lesions have been described in conjunction with obliterative vascular changes in several pathologic studies. However, with increasing experience and numbers of survivors, it has become clear that loss of allograft function with time probably has multiple manifestations other than obliterative bronchiolar changes. In a study that appeared prior to the article by Verleden et al, Sato et al[1] described a restrictive allograft syndrome (RAS) that accounted for 30% of their patients who developed chronic allograft dysfunction. The RAS form of chronic allograft dysfunction is an interstitial pattern on computed tomography and had a worse survival after onset than that of bronchiolitis obliterans. Verleden et al further evaluated the impact of a restrictive physiology on survival and found several early factors, ultimately leading to RAS similar to that identified by Sato et al.[1] Interestingly Verleden's group found about the same percentage of patients with chronic allograft dysfunction developed this restrictive picture and also confirmed the worse prognosis. These are important studies because they further clarify the complex course of lung allografts and identify important areas for further studies, eg, whether different early biomarkers point to the development of specific types of allograft dysfunction. In addition, this new information is important prognostically and may lead to different treatment approaches in different patients.

J. R. Maurer, MD, MBA

Reference

1. Sato M, Waddell TK, Wagnetz U, et al. Restrictive allograft syndrome (RAS): a novel form of chronic lung allograft dysfunction. *J Heart Lung Transplant.* 2011;30: 735-742.

Comparison of Hospitalized Solid Organ Transplant Recipients and Nonimmunocompromised Patients With Pandemic H1N1 Infection: A Retrospective Cohort Study

Minnema BJ, Patel M, Rotstein C, et al (Univ of Toronto, Ontario, Canada; et al)

Transplantation 92:230-234, 2011

Background.—Pandemic H1N1 influenza has been associated with a worldwide outbreak of febrile respiratory illness. Although impaired cell mediated immunity, such as that caused by transplant immunosuppression, has been identified as a risk factor for severe infection with this virus, the course of this infection has not been adequately characterized in solid organ transplant (SOT) recipients in comparison with nontransplanted controls. We report our experience with severe pH1N1 infection in transplant recipients and compare this group with nonimmunosuppressed patients.

Methods.—Data were retrospectively collected on all patients admitted to our institution with proven pH1N1 infection. Clinical characteristics, treatments, and outcomes were compared between SOT recipients and nonimmunocompromised controls.

Results.—Seventeen SOT recipients and 49 controls were identified. The control group had higher baseline rates of asthma ($P=0.02$) and smoking ($P=0.05$) at baseline. No difference in clinical features of H1N1 infection was detected except for a greater prevalence of wheeze in the non-SOT group ($P=0.02$). No statistical differences in outcomes could be detected between the groups. Several markers of severity, including use of high frequency oscillatory ventilation, extracorporeal membrane oxygenation, and death were slightly more frequent in the control group.

Conclusion.—SOT recipients admitted to hospital with pH1N1 infection did not have significantly more severe outcomes of their infection compared with their nonimmunocompromised counterparts, despite their immune suppressed status.

▶ In this study assessing the severity of H1N1 disease and outcomes in solid organ transplant recipients (SOT) compared with nonimmunocompromised patients, it may seem counterintuitive that SOT patients did not do worse than the controls. However, a closer look may help us understand these outcomes. Some of the sickest patients reported with H1N1 infection were younger patients with intact immune systems. Severe illness has been associated with what has been termed an early hyperinflammatory response to H1N1 involving Th1 and Th17 subsets of CD4$^+$ T lymphocyte helper cells. Thus, paradoxically, the immunosuppression of SOT might be protective in that SOT patients would not be able to mount this type of hyperimmune response.[1] In other types of influenza infections, SOT patients have more severe disease and worse outcomes compared with patients with normal immunity.[2] This finding supports the conjecture that the hyperimmune response in H1N1 is an important factor in the pathogenesis of severe disease.[2] More study of this phenomenon is necessary to determine if management aimed at targeting this immune response can improve outcomes.

J. R. Maurer, MD, MBA

References

1. Low CY, Kee T, Chan KP, et al. Pandemic (H1N1) 2009 infection in adult solid organ transplant recipients in Singapore. *Transplantation.* 2010;90:1016-1021.
2. Vilchez RA, McCurry K, Dauber J, et al. Influenza virus infection in adult solid organ transplant recipients. *Am J Transplant.* 2002;2:287-291.

Pneumonia Complicating Pandemic (H1N1) 2009: Risk Factors, Clinical Features, and Outcomes

Viasus D, for the Novel Influenza A(H1N1) Study Group of the Spanish Network for Research in Infectious Diseases (REIPI) (Hospital Universitari de Bellvitge-IDIBELL, Spain; et al)
Medicine 90:328-336, 2011

We performed an observational analysis of a prospective cohort of adults hospitalized for pandemic (H1N1) 2009 at 13 Spanish hospitals, from June to November 2009, to determine the risk factors, clinical features, and outcomes of pneumonia. Of 585 patients requiring hospitalization, chest radiography was obtained in 542. A total of 234 (43.1%) patients had pneumonia, of whom 210 underwent bacterial microbiologic studies. Of these patients, 174 (82.8%) had primary viral pneumonia and 36 (17.2%) had concomitant/secondary bacterial pneumonia. Bilateral pneumonia occurred in 48.3% of patients. *Streptococcus pneumoniae* was the most frequent pathogen among patients with bacterial pneumonia (26 of 36 patients). None of them had received pneumococcal vaccine. Compared with patients without pneumonia, those with pneumonia more frequently had shock during hospitalization (9.8% vs. 1%; p < 0.001), required intensive care unit admission (22.6% vs. 5.8%; p < 0.001), underwent mechanical ventilation (17.9% vs. 3.2%; p < 0.001), and had longer length of hospital stay (median, 7 d vs. 5 d; p < 0.001). In-hospital mortality was higher in patients with pneumonia than in the others (5.2% vs. 0%; p < 0.001). Absence of comorbid conditions (odds ratio [OR], 2.07; 95% confidence interval [CI], 1.32–3.24) was found to be an independent risk factor for pneumonia, whereas early (≤48 h) oseltamivir therapy (OR, 0.29; 95% CI, 0.19–0.46) was a protective factor. In conclusion, pneumonia is a frequent complication among adults hospitalized for pandemic (H1N1) 2009 and causes significant morbidity. Mortality in

TABLE 6.—Risk Factors for Pneumonia in Patients With Pandemic (H1N1) 2009: Multivariate Analysis

	OR (95% CI)	P
Age (16–49 yr)	1.35 (0.83–2.19)	0.22
Male sex	0.96 (0.63–1.47)	0.87
Current smoker	1.31 (0.83–2.08)	0.24
Alcohol abuse	2.17 (0.85–5.57)	0.10
Absence of comorbid conditions	2.07 (1.32–3.24)	0.001
Morbid obesity	0.92 (0.34–2.46)	0.87
Seasonal influenza vaccine	1.18 (0.62–2.22)	0.60
Early oseltamivir therapy (≤48 h)	0.29 (0.19–0.46)	<0.001

pandemic (H1N1) 2009 is low, but occurs mainly in patients with pneumonia. Early oseltamivir therapy is a protective factor for this complication (Table 6).

▶ Influenza infection typically has a relatively low rate of complications (predominantly pneumonia and especially bacterial pneumonia) except in particularly susceptible populations, but when complications occur, the morbidity and mortality escalates. With the emergence of pandemic H1N1 in 2009, there was great fear that—as in previous influenza pandemics—the rate of complications would be high. In fact, depending on the series that has been published from the H1N1 pandemic, as many as 66% of hospitalized patients had pneumonia.[1] The Viasus report categorizes risks factors for pneumonia in the 2009 pandemic and confirms that most deaths were in the subgroup of patients with pneumonia (Table 6). This is a large study (585 patients hospitalized in 13 different hospitals in Spain) with extensive demographic, clinical, and diagnostic information about patients with and without pneumonia. It should be a valuable reference to help clinicians caring for H1N1-infected patients recognize and treat early signs of pneumonia.

J. R. Maurer, MD, MBA

Reference

1. Louie JK, Acosta M, Winter K, et al; California Pandemic (H1N1) Working Group. Factors associated with death or hospitalization due to pandemic 2009 influenza A (H1N1) infection in California. *JAMA.* 2009;302:1896-1902.

Invasive Fungal Infections in Lung Transplant Recipients Not Receiving Routine Systemic Antifungal Prophylaxis: 12-Year Experience at a University Lung Transplant Center

Pinney MF, Rosenberg AF, Hampp C, et al (Orlando Regional Med Ctr, FL; Univ of Florida, Gainesville)
Pharmacotherapy 31:537-545, 2011

Study Objective.—To determine the rate of invasive fungal infection among the lung transplant population at a center that does not provide routine systemic antifungal prophylaxis, and to compare that rate with rates currently reported in the literature.

Design.—Retrospective medical record review.

Setting.—University-affiliated lung transplant center.

Patients.—Two hundred forty-two adults without cystic fibrosis who underwent lung transplantation between March 1, 1994, and June 30, 2006.

Measurements and Main Results.—Patients were followed by the adult lung transplant service. Twenty-three cases of invasive fungal infections were identified in 22 patients, resulting in a 9.1% overall invasive fungal infection rate in our study population. *Aspergillus* infections were the most common type of fungal infection identified, occurring in 11 (47.8%) of the 23 cases, with an overall rate of 4.5% (11/242 patients). Invasive fungal infections in lung transplant recipients have been reported in the literature at a rate 15–35%, with rates of *Aspergillus* infections reported as 3–15%.

Conclusion.—Despite the absence of routine systemic antifungal prophylaxis, the overall invasive fungal infection rate and the *Aspergillus* infection rate in these lung transplant recipients do not appear to be higher than the rates reported in the literature.

▶ A study published in 2004 reporting results of a survey of lung transplant centers and their antifungal posttransplant prophylaxis policies stated that of the 37 centers answering the survey, 28 routinely offered this type of antibiotic prophylaxis to recipients.[1] There was, however, no standard prophylactic agent, nor was there a standard timeframe for prophylaxis. Interestingly, inhaled amphotericin B was used by more than half the respondents, but systemic agents including azoles and intravenous amphotericin B were also used. A number of centers used more than 1 agent, and the average time of administration of prophylaxis was 3 months. The current article calls into question these practices. In this article, the authors report no higher rate of invasive fungal disease than that observed in institutions that routinely use prophylaxis. Of particular concern for lung transplants are infections with *Aspergillus* sp, which, when invasive, are often fatal. The investigators do note most of their invasive fungal infections were due to *Aspergillus* sp; however, that rate was no higher than reports in the literature. Antifungal prophylaxis is not benign. Some of the drugs can be nephrotoxic, which is a particular issue in posttransplant patients who are already taking the universally nephrotoxic calcineurin inhibitors. In addition to renal and other side effects, these drugs can also influence the levels of a number of other drugs commonly used in the posttransplant period, resulting in toxicity or inadequate drug levels. Not only would a more judicious "careful monitoring" approach be less expensive and onerous to patients, it might also result in better outcomes.

J. R. Maurer, MD, MBA

Reference

1. Dummer JS, Lazariashvilli N, Barnes J, Ninan M, Milstone AP. A survey of antifungal management in lung transplantation. *J Heart Lung Transplant.* 2004;23:1376-1381.

Increased Serum Vitamin A and E Levels After Lung Transplantation
Ho T, Gupta S, Brotherwood M, et al (St Michael's Hosp, Toronto, Ontario, Canada; et al)
Transplantation 92:601-606, 2011

Background.—Adult cystic fibrosis (CF) patients experience significant increases in serum vitamin A and E levels after lung transplantation. It is unclear whether this finding is specific to the CF population or inherent to the lung transplantation process.

Methods.—The objectives of this study were to assess pre- and postlung transplantation serum vitamin A and E levels in subjects with end-stage lung disease secondary to all causes. The study population consisted of adults who received a lung transplant at the Toronto Lung Transplant Program between 2004 and 2009. The mean change in serum vitamin A and E levels pre- and postlung transplant was evaluated using a paired t test, while differences in vitamin A and E levels between CF and non-CF subjects were determined using a Student's t test.

Results.—Thirty-two CF and 21 non-CF subjects who underwent lung transplantation were included in the study. Mean serum vitamin A and vitamin E levels increased significantly after transplant, from 1.2 to 3.5 μmol/L ($P<0.0001$) and from 21.9 to 33.2 μmol/L ($P<0.0001$), respectively. The proportion of individuals with serum levels above the upper limit of normal increased from 7.6% to 88.7% ($P<0.0001$) and from 11.3% to 24.5% ($P=0.02$) for vitamin A and vitamin E, respectively. The dosage of vitamin supplementation did not increase after transplant.

Conclusions.—Significant increases in serum vitamin A and E levels were seen in both CF and non-CF subjects after lung transplantation. Further research is needed to understand the cause and clinical implications of these findings.

▶ In this interesting study of oil-soluble vitamin A and E levels in pre- and post-lung transplant patients, the authors document a posttransplant increase in these vitamin levels to super-physiologic levels. The reason for the increase in vitamin A most likely is related in part to changes in intestinal absorption of vitamin A and a significant decrease in glomerular filtration rate caused by calcineurin inhibitors after transplant; however, the authors could not show a consistent correlation between pre- and posttransplant vitamin A levels and the changes in renal function. Vitamin E level changes are even more difficult to explain because this vitamin is primarily metabolized in the liver and excreted in the bile. The calcineurin inhibitors do impact the function of the liver's cytochrome P450 system, which may influence levels of both vitamins A and E. Causes of these changes deserve further investigation because hypervitaminosis has detrimental health effects. Hypervitaminosis A, in particular, is associated with increased risk of fracture, increased intracranial pressure, and liver toxicity. It seems prudent to monitor levels of these vitamins in long-term survivors and regularly assess medication regimens to avoid inappropriate vitamin supplementation.

J. R. Maurer, MD, MBA

Ocular complications in patients with lung transplants

Tarabishy AB, Khatib OF, Nocero JR, et al (Cleveland Clinic, OH)
Br J Ophthalmol 95:1295-1298, 2011

Aim.—To describe infectious and non-infectious ocular complications found in patients with lung transplants.

Methods.—545 patients underwent lung transplantation from January 1998 to September 2008 at the Cleveland Clinic. Patients who underwent ophthalmic examination at the Cole Eye Institute after lung transplantation were included in the study.

Outcomes.—Diagnoses, treatments, surgeries, laboratory parameters of immune status and patient survival were examined.

Results.—Of the 545 patients who received a lung transplant during the study period at the Cleveland Clinic, 46 (8.4%) patients underwent ophthalmology examination after a lung transplant. The most common ocular finding was posterior subcapsular cataract, found in 13/46 (28.3%) patients. Infectious ocular complications were present in 6/46 patients (13.0%) including fungal infections (rhino-orbital mucormycosis (n=1), disseminated *Pseudallescheria boydii* infection (n=2)), cytomegalovirus retinitis (n=1), varicella-zoster virus keratouveitis (n=1) and herpes zoster ophthalmicus (n=1). Five of six patients with infectious ocular complications died within 6 months of evaluation. Decreased absolute lymphocyte count was associated with infectious ocular complications (p=0.014).

Conclusions.—Many ocular conditions can occur in patients with lung transplants. Ocular infectious complications were uncommon but may be associated with increased mortality.

▶ Because of the systemic effects of immunosuppression, complications are seen in virtually all organ systems in lung transplant recipients, particularly infections and direct side effects of the drugs. That is the case in this series as well. However, the number of complications involving the eyes reported here is surprisingly few. In this series, the authors did not report any ocular neurotoxicity related to calcineurin inhibitors as has been reported previously in the literature.[1,2] The ocular neurotoxicity previously reported was caused by cyclosporine-related changes in the occipital lobe, some of which were reversible and some of which were permanent. The authors note that their patients are treated with tacrolimus (not cyclosporine), and that may be the reason they did not see this devastating complication. Tacrolimus has been associated with central pontine myelinolysis, but not directly with occipital lesions, causing blindness in this population, and generally has fewer central nervous system complications than cyclosporine. Fortunately, most of the complications reported here are treatable.

J. R. Maurer, MD, MBA

References

1. Knower MT, Pethke SD, Valentine VG. Reversible cortical blindness after lung transplantation. *South Med J.* 2003;96:606-612.

2. Drachman BM, DeNofrio D, Acker MA, Galetta S, Loh E. Cortical blindness secondary to cyclosporine after orthotopic heart transplantation: a case report and review of the literature. *J Heart Lung Transplant.* 1996;15:1158-1164.

Outcomes After Lung Transplantation and Practices of Lung Transplant Programs in the United States Regarding Hepatitis C Seropositive Recipients
Fong T-L, Cho YW, Hou L, et al (Univ of Southern California, Los Angeles, CA; et al)
Transplantation 91:1293-1296, 2011

Background.—The estimated prevalence of hepatitis C virus (HCV) infection among lung transplant (LT) recipients is 1.9%. Many thoracic transplant programs are reluctant to transplant HCV-seropositive patients due to concerns of hepatic dysfunction caused by immunosuppression. The aims of this study are to survey current practices of US LT programs regarding HCV-seropositive patients and using the Organ Procurement and Transplantation Network/United Network for Organ Sharing database and to assess the clinical outcomes of HCV-positive compared with HCV-negative LT recipients.

Methods.—A survey of US transplant centers that have performed more than 100 LTs was conducted. In addition, 170 HCV-seropositive and 9259 HCV-seronegative recipients who received HCV-seronegative donor organs between January 1, 2000, to December 31, 2007, were identified from the Organ Procurement and Transplantation Network/United Network for Organ Sharing database. Outcome variables including patient survival were compared between the two groups.

Results.—A total of 64.4% centers responded to the survey. Ten of 29 (34.5%) programs would not consider HCV-seropositive patients for LT. Among the 19 programs that will consider HCV-seropositive patients, only five centers would transplant actively viremic patients. Overall patient survival rates of HCV-seropositive patients were similar to HCV-seronegative patients (84.7% at 1 year, 63.9% at 3 years, 49.4% at 5 years for HCV-seropositive group vs. 82.0% at 1 year, 65.0% at 3 years, 51.4% at 5 years for HCV-seronegative group, $P=0.712$). Relative risk of recipients for death remained statistically insignificant after adjusting for recipient age, donor age, obesity, sensitization, serum creatinine, and medical condition at time of transplant (relative risk [RR] = 1.07 [0.84−1.38], $P=0.581$).

Conclusions.—Since 2000, patient survival rates of HCV-positive patients are identical to those who are HCV-negative. However, most of these HCV-seropositive patients were probably nonviremic.

▶ This study is important because it is the first comprehensive survey of practices regarding hepatitis C seropositive transplant recipients at large lung transplant centers as well as the outcomes from those centers. It is encouraging to see that the survival rates of the seropositive recipients were similar to those of seronegative recipients; however, it is also important to note—as the authors do—that most of these patients were likely nonviremic. A parallel study of heart transplant recipients, based on the US Scientific Registry of Transplant Recipients, evaluated the outcomes of 443 seropositive heart recipients after a mean of 5.6 years and found a significantly higher mortality rate in the seropositive patients compared with seronegative patients.[1] This was essentially an update of a study published in 2009 that had reached the same conclusion.[2] The difference in outcomes in the heart recipient studies versus the current study in lung transplant recipients is not clear, but it could be related to recipient selection. It would be prudent to look more carefully at the parameters used to select appropriate seropositive patients for transplant to ensure that those chosen have a reasonable chance of survival and that available grafts are appropriately distributed.

J. R. Maurer, MD, MBA

References

1. Lee I, Localio R, Brensinger CM, et al. Decreased post-transplant survival among heart transplant recipients with pre-transplant hepatitis C virus positivity. *J Heart Lung Transplant*. 2011;30:1266-1274.
2. Fong TL, Hou L, Hutchinson IV, Cicciarelli JC, Cho YW. Impact of hepatitis C infection on outcomes after heart transplantation. *Transplantation*. 2009;88:1137-1141.

Impact of Anastomotic Techniques on Airway Complications After Lung Transplant
van Berkel V, Guthrie TJ, Puri V, et al (Univ of Louisville School of Medicine, KY; Washington Univ School of Medicine, St Louis, MO)
Ann Thorac Surg 92:316-321, 2011

Background.—Airway complications are a source of morbidity and expense after lung transplant. Posttransplant stenosis can occur when the donor bronchus is rendered ischemic and is dependent upon collateral flow from the pulmonary capillary system. By shortening the donor bronchus, the tissue at risk for ischemia is reduced. In an effort to reduce airway complications, one surgeon at our institution began dividing the donor bronchus at the lobar carina.

Methods.—This is a retrospective analysis of all transplanted patients over the 2-year period before and after the institution of the technique change. To adjust for covariates, we performed a propensity score analysis. Outcome endpoints were postoperative airway complications, specifically, the need for therapeutic bronchoscopy, dilation, stenting, or retransplant.

Results.—After instituting the practice of dividing the bronchus at the lobar carina, the incidence of airway complication for the principle surgeon decreased from 13.2% (7 of 53) to 2.1% (1 of 48), resulting in an improved freedom from airway complication for that surgeon. Compared with all transplants performed during this period, the modified anastomosis resulted in fewer airway complications: 2.1% (1 of 48) versus 8.2% (19 of 231). The propensity analysis matched the 48 patients who received the modified anastomosis with 48 patients who received the standard two ring length anastomosis by surgical colleagues. The modified anastomosis group had fewer required interventions for airway complications and had significantly better freedom from airway complication when followed over time.

Conclusions.—Decreasing the amount of potentially ischemic tissue implanted from the donor bronchus can reduce posttransplant airway complications.

▶ Ischemia-reperfusion injury, acute rejection, infection, and airway anastomotic complications are the most common early complications encountered by lung transplant patients. The anastomotic complications arise because it is difficult to reattach small bronchial arteries to provide a blood supply to the donor bronchus or bronchi of the graft. Thus, there is a risk of ischemic injury and necrosis with dehiscence that typically first manifests between 1 week and 1 month after transplant, with ongoing stenosis developing and requiring management for many months. Multiple technical revisions have been tried to prevent this complication, which, at its worst, can result in death but often requires multiple bronchoscopic dilations or at least temporary stenting. Previous technique changes have included such approaches as bronchial artery revascularization[1] and telescoping anastomosis (the end of the donor and recipient bronchi overlap by at least 1 ring).[2] Neither has been particularly successful in significantly reducing airway issues (rates typically range between 10% and 20%) although surgical experience seems to make a difference. The use of shorter donor bronchi described in the current study has the advantage of exposing a minimal amount of ischemic tissue. The most compelling part of this study is that the airway complication rate of the same surgeon is compared before and after the change in technique, thereby removing the huge factor of individual surgical approach. The impressive drop in complications has the great advantage of improving quality of life for the graft recipient and greatly simplifying management while reducing the cost. This technique should be further studied over multiple surgeons and institutions to better establish the true complication rate.

J. R. Maurer, MD, MBA

References

1. Pettersson GB, Yun JJ, Nørgaard MA. Bronchial artery revascularization in lung transplantation: techniques, experience, and outcomes. *Curr Opin Organ Transplant.* 2010;15:572-577.
2. Garfein ES, McGregor CC, Galantowicz ME, Schulman LL. Deleterious effects of telescoped bronchial anastomosis in single and bilateral lung transplantation. *Ann Transplant.* 2000;5:5-11.

Lung transplantation in children with idiopathic pulmonary arterial hypertension: An 18-year experience
Goldstein BS, Sweet SC, Mao J, et al (Washington Univ School of Medicine, St Louis, MO)
J Heart Lung Transplant 30:1148-1152, 2011

Background.—The natural history of idiopathic pulmonary arterial hypertension (IPAH) in patients of all ages is one of relentless progression.

For those who fail medical therapy, lung transplantation remains the ultimate palliation. In the USA, IPAH is the second leading indication for lung transplantation in children and first for children 1 to 5 years of age. In this study, we report our 18-year experience with lung transplantation in children with IPAH.

Methods.—We performed a retrospective chart review of children with IPAH listed for lung transplant at our center between 1991 and 2009. Our data reflect a total of 26 children ranging in age from 1.6 to 18.9 years. Nineteen were transplanted and 7 died while waiting (27%). The impact of a number of pre-transplant variables on survival was evaluated.

Results.—Median survival for those transplanted was 5.8 years, with 1- and 5-year survival rates of 95% and 61%, respectively. Survival was independent of pre-transplant considerations such as age, weight, need for intravenous (IV) inotropes, use of IV pulmonary vasodilators, year of transplant and severity of right-sided cardiac pressures. There was 1 hospital death. Compared with the transplanted group, children who died waiting had a significantly higher incidence of supra-systemic right heart pressures ($p = 0.02$) and hemoptysis ($p = 0.01$).

Conclusions.—Our study is the largest to date to look at outcomes for lung transplantation in children with IPAH. Their median survival compares favorably with that of all pediatric lung transplant recipients, 5.8 years vs 4.5 years, respectively. We did not identify any pre-transplant variables that presaged a poorer outcome. Thus, survival seemed more related to factors that influence long-term outcomes in all transplant recipients such as rejection and infection. Lung transplantation remains a viable option for children with IPAH, especially for those with supra-systemic right heart pressures despite maximal medical therapy.

▶ Treatment with a variety of vasodilators has greatly improved the treatment and survival of patients with idiopathic pulmonary arterial hypertension in the last 10 to 15 years. More than 70% of children with this rare disease now live at least 5 years using these new treatments. However, for those patients who do not respond to the vasodilators, lung transplant remains an option. Although few lung transplants are performed in children, pulmonary hypertension remains the second most common indication. The authors note that one of the difficulties that have arisen in the successful vasodilator period is deciding when a child has truly failed this therapy and needs to be referred for transplant. To illustrate this, the authors note that 25% of the children on their transplant list died waiting, suggesting that they were placed on the list too late. The lesson here might be to consider referral of children for transplant who demonstrate suprasystemic right-sided cardiac pressures, even if their functional status appears to improve somewhat.

J. R. Maurer, MD, MBA

7 Sleep Disorders

Introduction

In my opinion, one of the most fascinating aspects of sleep medicine is its influence across a lifespan. Young and old alike, we all sleep. Sleep is a necessary part of life, yet its problems are distinctly different. In this YEAR BOOK's selection, I have included articles that involve sleep problems across a lifespan. We need to be aware of the expansion of recommendations for a safe sleeping environment for infants. Familiarity with this article is a must for healthcare providers caring for infants. As for adolescence and sleep, I encourage you also to read the selection on Sleep Duration or Bedtime? Exploring the Relationship between Sleep Habits and Weight Status and Activity Patterns. While much of the research focuses on sleep duration and weight change, this article examines sleep timing and patterns of weight and activity, which may be just as important. Additional research in this area may have significant public health impact, specifically delaying school start times. I have included a nice article about the link between sleep deprivation and metabolism for those of you who want to read more about this field. I have included articles this year on insomnia in older patients, particularly in very difficult-to-treat groups: Alzheimer dementia and residents in skilled nursing facilities. Insomnia is frequently encountered, particularly for the elderly, and pharmacologic treatment with hypnotics can be problematic for this population. Articles on cognitive behavioral therapy, activity and bright light, melatonin, magnesium, and zinc are included.

As usual, there were a lot of great articles this year about sleep disordered breathing. Portable monitoring is here—like it or not. While many have been in favor of the cost savings that portable monitoring brings in comparison with full polysomnography, the selection entitled An Integrated Health-Economic Analysis of Diagnostic and Therapeutic Strategies in the Treatment of Moderate to Severe Obstructive Sleep Apnea is a must-read. Further research in obstructive sleep apnea has expanded our knowledge about the consequences of sleep disordered breathing. Newer evidence by Chou et al supports a link between obstructive sleep apnea and chronic kidney disease. This study was conducted in a population without concomitant hypertension or diabetes. This year's selections also include a very interesting article that describes the risk of cognitive impairment and dementia in a group of women with obstructive sleep apnea who were followed longitudinally over nearly 5 years. I expect that we will hear more about the relationship between obstructive sleep apnea and cognitive impairment in the years to come and examine outcomes associated with use of continuous positive airway pressure. Be sure to read the selection by Parra et al, which describes the feasibility of using continuous positive airway pressure early in stroke. The effects of early continuous positive airway pressure on functional outcomes, quality of life, appearance of new cardiovascular events and mortality are very interesting.

Finally, I have included selections about sleep, safety and public impact. Our 24/7 lives generates problems including those associated with shift work and sleep deprivation. Interesting is the number of errors related to fatigue. While many groups, eg, truck drivers and pilots, have restrictions and emphasis on sleep, particularly obtaining adequate hours and management of obstructive sleep apnea, other groups are still examining fatigue and its risk. I recommend you read the selections entitled Prospective Evaluation of Consultant Surgeon Sleep Deprivation and Outcomes in More Than 4000 Consecutive Cardiac Surgical Procedures and Sleep Disorders, Health, and Safety in Police Officers.

In conclusion, I hope you find this YEAR BOOK's selection of articles intriguing and worthy of discussion. I certainly did.

Shirley F. Jones, MD, FCCP, DABSM

Diagnosis of Sleep-Disordered Breathing

An Integrated Health-Economic Analysis of Diagnostic and Therapeutic Strategies in the Treatment of Moderate-to-Severe Obstructive Sleep Apnea
Pietzsch JB, Garner A, Cipriano LE, et al (Wing Tech Inc, CA; Stanford Univ, CA)
Sleep 34:695-709, 2011

Study Objectives.—Obstructive sleep apnea (OSA) is a common disorder associated with substantially increased cardiovascular risks, reduced quality of life, and increased risk of motor vehicle collisions due to daytime sleepiness. This study evaluates the cost-effectiveness of three commonly used diagnostic strategies (full-night polysomnography, split-night polysomnography, unattended portable home-monitoring) in conjunction with continuous positive airway pressure (CPAP) therapy in patients with moderate-to-severe OSA.

Design.—A Markov model was created to compare costs and effectiveness of different diagnostic and therapeutic strategies over a 10-year interval and the expected lifetime of the patient. The primary measure of cost-effectiveness was incremental cost per quality-adjusted life year (QALY) gained.

Patients or Participants.—Baseline computations were performed for a hypothetical average cohort of 50-year-old males with a 50% pretest probability of having moderate-to-severe OSA (apnea-hypopnea index [AHI] $\geq$15 events per hour).

Measurements and Results.—For a patient with moderate-to-severe OSA, CPAP therapy has an incremental cost-effectiveness ratio (ICER) of $15,915 per QALY gained for the lifetime horizon. Over the lifetime horizon in a population with 50% prevalence of OSA, full-night polysomnography in conjunction with CPAP therapy is the most economically efficient strategy at any willingness-to-pay greater than $17,131 per-QALY gained because it dominates all other strategies in comparative analysis.

Conclusions.—Full-night polysomnography (PSG) is cost-effective and is the preferred diagnostic strategy for adults suspected to have moderate-to-severe OSA when all diagnostic options are available. Split-night PSG and unattended home monitoring can be considered cost-effective alternatives when full-night PSG is not available.

▶ The cost of health care is climbing. Management of chronic medical diseases such as obstructive sleep apnea (OSA) and its related comorbidities of cardiovascular disease, hypertension, and stoke will consume a significant portion of health care dollars. So studies examining both the cost-effectiveness and the comparative effectiveness of therapies are important. This study evaluated the cost-effectiveness of full-night polysomnogram, split-night polysomnogram, and unattended portable home monitoring plus continuous positive airway pressure (CPAP) therapy in patients with moderate to severe OSA. A variety of scenarios were considered and accounted for in a Markov model. This is a detailed and comprehensive study for which the investigators should receive accolades.

Pietzsch reports that use of CPAP has an incremental cost-effective ratio (ICER) of $15 915 per quality-adjusted life years (QALY), which falls well below $100 000 per QALY and thus is good value.[1] Estimates include that use of CPAP would result in an overall per-person risk of a fatal motor vehicle collision by approximately 48% and that nearly 670 motor vehicle collisions could be prevented per 100 000 persons.

I was very surprised by the results of this cost-effective effectiveness analysis between full-night polysomnogram, split-night polysomnogram, and unattended portable home monitoring (Fig 4 in the original article). Full-night polysomnography was determined to be the most cost-effective and preferred diagnostic strategy. How could this be, you ask? As with any economic model, certain assumptions need to be made, accurate or not. Although these assumptions are supported by the medical literature (ie, impact of OSA and treatment on quality of life), the literature itself is limited. A number of other assumptions are made, including the number of no-shows for in-laboratory studies, for example. In the end, it is the high number of false diagnoses in the unattended portable home monitoring that accounts for its higher ICER. False diagnosis leads to cost of therapy when it is not needed or, in contrast, cost of health care when OSA is not treated.

Am I going to stop using unattended portable home monitoring? No, I am not, but I have realized that it is not just the cost of the technology itself that makes something cost-effective. It is important to note that the cost-effectiveness analysis is modeled based on a population cohort of 50-year-old male patients with a prevalence of moderate to severe OSA of 50%. In situations in which the pretest probability of OSA is high, unattended portable home monitoring and split-night polysomnogram are both cost-effective. Furthermore, the authors do say that unattended portable home monitoring is cost-effective in situations where a full polysomnogram is not possible (limited availability, patient refusal to attend). I believe this a good article to facilitate discussion within your own practice settings.

S. F. Jones, MD, FCCP, DABSM

Reference

1. Weinstein MC, Skinner JA. Comparative effectiveness and heath care spending—implications for reform. *N Engl J Med.* 2010;362:460-465.

Therapeutic Decision-making for Sleep Apnea and Hypopnea Syndrome Using Home Respiratory Polygraphy: A Large Multicentric Study
Masa JF, the Spanish Sleep Network (San Pedro de Alcántara Hosp, Cáceres, Spain; et al)
Am J Respir Crit Care Med 184:964-971, 2011

Rationale.—Home respiratory polygraphy (HRP) is an alternative to polysomnography (PSG) for sleep apnea–hypopnea syndrome (SAHS) diagnosis. However, therapeutic decision-making is a different process than diagnosis.

Objectives.—This study aimed to determine the agreement between HRP and in-hospital PSG for therapeutic decision-making in a large-sample.

Methods.—Patients with an intermediate or high SAHS suspicion were included in a multicenter study (eight sleep centers) and assigned to home and hospital protocols in a random order. Therapeutic decisions (continuous positive airway pressure, no continuous positive airway pressure, or impossible decision) were made by an investigator in each center, based on using either HRP or PSG and a single set of auxiliary clinical variables. Patients and diagnostic methods (HRP and PSG) were assessed in random order using an electronic database. After a month the same therapeutic decision-making procedure was repeated with the same method.

Measurements and Main Results.—Of 366 randomized patients, 348 completed the protocol. The "impossible decision" case was not observed with either PSG or HRP. Therapeutic decisions using HRP had a sensitivity of 73%, a specificity of 77%, and an agreement level (sum of true positives and negatives) of 76%. Patients with higher HRP apnea–hypopnea index (AHI) scores ($\geq$30; 41% of the total sample) had a sensitivity of 94%, a specificity of 44%, and the agreement level was 91%.

Conclusions.—The HRP-based therapeutic decision was adequate when AHI was high, but deficient in the large population of patients with mild to moderate AHI. Therefore, both selecting patients with a high suspicion and severity of SAHS and future prospective cost-effectiveness studies are necessary.

▶ Advances in technologies in the diagnosis of obstructive sleep apnea have made testing more available and less costly. Furthermore, the Centers for Medicaid and Medicare Services and many insurance providers have accepted this as an alternative to the gold standard in laboratory polysomnogram. I have been seeing a growing number of type III devices being used by primary care providers and dentists. The diagnostic accuracy of some of the particular devices are good; however, type III monitors may underestimate the severity of disease simply because the apnea–hypopnea index (AHI) is determined using the recording time as the denominator. These inaccuracies are included in the decision of which patients to treat for obstructive sleep apnea (therapeutic decision making) and require clinical context. This article aimed to determine the agreement between home respiratory polygraphy (type III monitor) and in-hospital polysomnogram for therapeutic decision making in patients with an intermediate or high suspicion for obstructive sleep apnea. The investigators noted higher agreement between the in laboratory polysomnogram and home respiratory polygraphy at lower values of the apnea hypopnea index. However, the sensitivity of therapeutic decision making using home respiratory polygraphy was very much dependent on the pretest probability of disease severity. Where the pretest probability is lower— that is, when AHI is between 5 and 30 events per hour—the sensitivity, specificity, and agreement levels were much lower. When using home respiratory polygraphy in a population with mild to moderate degrees of obstructive sleep apnea, the probability of recommending continuous positive airway pressure that is in agreement with the in-laboratory polysomnogram is low. This is because of the disagreement between the apnea hypopnea indices of the in-laboratory and home tests. This study's findings dampen the use of the home respiratory polygraph in therapeutic decision making for patients with mild to moderate degrees of obstructive sleep apnea. I believe that studies examining cost effectiveness need to be explored further.

S. F. Jones, MD, FCCP, DABSM

Epidemiology of Sleep-Disordered Breathing

A prospective polysomnographic study on the evolution of complex sleep apnoea
Cassel W, Canisius S, Becker HF, et al (Philipps Univ Marburg, Germany; Asklepios Clinic Barmbek, Hamburg, Germany)
Eur Respir J 38:329-337, 2011

Complex sleep apnoea (CompSA) may be observed following continuous positive airway pressure (CPAP) treatment.

In a prospective study, 675 obstructive sleep apnoea patients (mean age 55.9 yrs; 13.9% female) participated. Full-night polysomnography was performed at diagnosis, during the first night with stable CPAP and after 3 months of CPAP.

12.2% (82 out of 675 patients) had initial CompSA. 28 of those were lost to follow-up. Only 14 out of the remaining 54 patients continued to satisfy criteria for CompSA at follow-up. 16 out of 382 patients not initially diagnosed with CompSA exhibited novel CompSA after 3 months. 30 (6.9%) out of 436 patients had follow-up CompSA. Individuals with CompSA were 5 yrs older and 40% had coronary artery disease. At diagnosis, they had similar sleep quality but more central and mixed apnoeas. On the first CPAP night and at follow-up, sleep quality was impaired (more wakefulness after sleep onset) for patients with CompSA. Sleepiness was improved with CPAP, and was similar for patients with or without CompSA at diagnosis and follow-up.

CompSA is not stable over time and is mainly observed in predisposed patients on nights with impaired sleep quality. It remains unclear to what extent sleep impairment is cause or effect of CompSA.

▶ Many of us who devote a significant portion of our time to seeing sleep medicine patients will encounter complex sleep apnea. I agree with the authors that this diagnosis is overapplied in clinical practice. The existing literature supports that complex sleep apnea can resolve over time,[1] and this article is in keeping with this. In this study, Cassel reports that 12.2% of subjects had complex apnea initially, but only 6.9% had it at 3-month follow-up. What makes this study interesting is the finding that patients without initial complex apnea had complex apnea by 3 months (Fig 2 in the original article). Comparisons between groups indicate that cardiovascular disease and hypertension are more common in those who have complex apnea at follow-up. There was more wake after sleep onset, arousals, poor sleep efficiency, and of course, central events noted on polysomnogram performed at 3 months between groups. A couple of things should be noted with these findings: (1) the evolution of complex apnea is fluid, and (2) continuous positive airway pressure (CPAP) does not resolve complex apnea over time in all individuals, and these individuals have more cardiovascular comorbidities and poorer quality sleep. It is possible that the 2 conditions are linked. This study argues that we should continue to follow up with patients clinically and with CPAP downloads, particularly those with cardiovascular disease for the development complex apnea.

S. F. Jones, MD, FCCP, DABSM

Reference

1. Javaher S, Smith J, Chung E. The prevalence and natural history of complex sleep apnea. *J Clin Sleep Med.* 2009;5:205-211.

Consequences of Sleep-Disordered Breathing

Cheyne–Stokes respiration and obstructive sleep apnoea are independent risk factors for malignant ventricular arrhythmias requiring appropriate cardioverter-defibrillator therapies in patients with congestive heart failure
Bitter T, Westerheide N, Prinz C, et al (Ruhr Univ Bochum, Georgstasse, Bad Oeynhausen, Germany; Univ of Bielefeld, Germany)
Eur Heart J 32:61-74, 2011

Aims.—The aim of this first large-scale long-term study was to investigate whether obstructive sleep apnoea (OSA) and/or central sleep apnoea

(CSA) are associated with an increased risk of malignant cardiac arrhythmias in patients with congestive heart failure (CHF).

Methods and Results.—Of 472 CHF patients who were screened for sleep disordered breathing (SDB) 6 months after implantation of a cardiac resynchronization device with cardioverter-defibrillator, 283 remained untreated [170 with mild or no sleep disordered breathing (mnSDB) and 113 patients declined ventilation therapy] and were included into this study. During follow-up (48 months), data on appropriately monitored ventricular arrhythmias as well as appropriate cardioverter-defibrillator therapies were obtained from 255 of these patients (90.1%). Time period to first monitored ventricular arrhythmias and to first appropriate cardioverter-defibrillator therapy were significantly shorter in patients with either CSA or OSA. Forward stepwise Cox models revealed an independent correlation for CSA and OSA regarding monitored ventricular arrhythmias [apnoea—hypopnoea index (AHI) ≥ 5 h^{-1}: CSA HR 2.15, 95% CI 1.40–3.30, $P < 0.001$; OSA HR 1.69, 95% CI 1.64–1.75, $P = 0.001$; AHI ≥ 15 h^{-1}: CSA HR 2.06, 95% CI 1.40–3.05, $P < 0.001$; OSA HR 1.69, 95% CI 1.14–2.51, $P = 0.02$] and appropriate cardioverter-defibrillator therapies (AHI ≥ 5 h^{-1}: CSA HR 3.24, 95% CI 1.86–5.64, $P < 0.001$; OSA HR 2.07, 95% CI 1.14–3.77, $P = 0.02$; AHI ≥ 15 h^{-1}: CSA HR 3.41, 95% CI 2.10–5.54, $P < 0.001$; OSA HR 2.10, 95% CI 1.17–3.78, $P = 0.01$).

Conclusion.—In patients with CHF, CSA and OSA are independently associated with an increased risk for ventricular arrhythmias and appropriate cardioverter-defibrillator therapies.

▶ Sleep disordered breathing is common in patients with congestive heart failure. It is important to recognize the significance of this comorbidity, particularly its associated negative outcomes. In patients with congestive heart failure, sleep disordered breathing is an independent predictor for life-threatening arrhythmias.[1] This study reveals patients with both central and obstructive sleep apnea were more likely to need pacing or defibrillation to treat ventricular arrhythmia than patients with no or minimal sleep disordered breathing. Both central and obstructive sleep apnea are independently associated with ventricular arrhythmias and appropriated therapies delivered by the device. This study is different in that the author examined the association of central and obstructive sleep apnea, separately, on arrhythmias and need for device therapy. Although the study does not explore causation, the authors hypothesized that hypoxemia and recurrent arousals from sleep may incite sympathetic activation. Future studies examining the effect of continuous positive airway pressure on mitigating the degree of arrhythmogenic potential are needed.

S. F. Jones, MD, FCCP, DABSM

Reference

1. Serizawa N, Yumino D, Kajimoto K, et al. Impact of sleep-disordered breathing on life-threatening ventricular arrhythmia in heart failure patients with implantable cardioverter-defibrillator. *Am J Cardiol.* 2008;102:1064-1068.

Obstructive sleep apnoea: a stand-alone risk factor for chronic kidney disease

Chou Y-T, Lee P-H, Yang C-T, et al (Chang Gung Memorial Hosp, Chiayi, Taiwan; Chang Gung Inst of Technology, Taoyuan, Taiwan; et al)
Nephrol Dial Transplant 26:2244-2250, 2011

Background.—Previous studies have found an association between obstructive sleep apnea (OSA) and chronic kidney disease (CKD). However, subjects with confounding factors such as diabetes and hypertension were not excluded. The purpose of the present study was to determine whether patients with OSA without meeting criteria for diabetes or hypertension would also show increased likelihood of CKD.

Methods.—We prospectively enrolled adult patients with a chief complaint of habitual snoring. Overnight polysomnography, fasting blood triglyceride, cholesterol, glucose, insulin, creatinine, albumin and hemoglobin A1c, and first voiding urine albumin and creatinine were examined. Estimated glomerular filtration rate (eGFR), urine albumin-to-creatinine ratio (UACR), homeostatic model assessment—insulin resistance and percentage of CKD were calculated.

Results.—The final analyses involved 40 patients who were middle-aged [44.8 (8.6) years] predominantly male (83%), obese [body mass index, 28.2 (5.1) kg/m^2] and more severe OSA, with an apnea–hypopnea index (AHI) of 51.6 (39.2)/h. The mean eGFR and UACR were 85.4 (18.3) mL/min/1.73m^2 and 13.4 (23.4) mg/g, respectively. The prevalence of CKD in severe OSA subjects is 18%. With stepwise multivariate linear regression analysis, AHI and desaturation index were the only independent predictor of UACR ($\beta = 0.26$, $P = 0.01$, $R^2 = 0.17$) and eGFR ($\beta = 0.32$, $P < 0.01$, $R^2 = 0.32$), respectively.

Conclusions.—High prevalence of CKD is present in severe OSA patients without hypertension or diabetes. Significantly positive correlations were found between severity of OSA and renal function impairment.

▶ Previous literature supporting an association between chronic kidney disease and obstructive sleep apnea included patients with diabetes and hypertension, both confounders. In this prospective study of 40 snorers conducted in a Taiwanese population, subjects were free of diabetes and hypertension. Apnea and hypopnea index and desaturation index were the only independent predictors of kidney urine albumin to creatinine ratio and estimated glomerular filtration rate. Of the patients in the sample, 14% to 18% had evidence of chronic kidney disease, with higher rates in those with severe obstructive sleep apnea. A possible mechanism for the finding is hyperfiltration induced by obstructive sleep apnea. Furthermore, the degree of microalbuminuria may be reversible.[1]

The study population is Southeast Asian, so the study should be replicated in other populations with different ethnicities. Assessment of estimated glomerular filtration rate should be considered in those with severe obstructive sleep apnea.

S. F. Jones, MD, FCCP, DABSM

Reference

1. Mauer M, Fioretto P, Woredekal Y, et al. Diabetic nephropathy. In: Schrier RW, ed. *Diseases of the Kidney and Urinary Tract.* 7th ed. Philadelphia, PA: Lippincott Williams and Wilkins; 2001:2083-2127.

Obstructive Sleep Apnea: Brain Structural Changes and Neurocognitive Function before and after Treatment
Canessa N, Castronovo V, Cappa SF, et al (Vita-Salute San Raffaele Univ, Milan, Italy; Vita-Salute San Raffaele Univ and San Raffaele Scientific Inst, Milan, Italy; et al)
Am J Respir Crit Care Med 183:1419-1426, 2011

Rationale.—Obstructive sleep apnea (OSA) is commonly associated with neurocognitive impairments that have not been consistently related to specific brain structure abnormalities. Knowledge of the brain structures involved in OSA and the corresponding functional implications could provide clues to the pathogenesis of cognitive impairment and its reversibility in this disorder.

Objectives.—To investigate the cognitive deficits and the corresponding brain morphology changes in OSA, and the modifications after treatment, using combined neuropsychologic testing and voxel-based morphometry.

Methods.—A total of 17 patients treatment-naive to sleep apnea and 15 age-matched healthy control subjects underwent a sleep study, cognitive tests, and magnetic resonance imaging. After 3 months of treatment, cognitive and imaging data were collected to assess therapy efficacy.

Measurements and Main Results.—Neuropsychologic results in pretreatment OSA showed impairments in most cognitive areas, and in mood and sleepiness. These impairments were associated with focal reductions of gray-matter volume in the left hippocampus (entorhinal cortex), left posterior parietal cortex, and right superior frontal gyrus. After treatment, we observed significant improvements involving memory, attention, and executive-functioning that paralleled gray-matter volume increases in hippocampal and frontal structures.

Conclusions.—The cognitive and structural deficits in OSA may be secondary to sleep deprivation and repetitive nocturnal intermittent hypoxemia. These negative effects may be recovered by consistent and thorough treatment. Our findings highlight the importance of early diagnosis and successful treatment of this disorder.

▶ In this article, the link between neuropsychological impairments and structural brain integrity is explored. The authors nicely described reduction of gray matter in certain regions of the brain along with poorer scores on all neurocognitive measures in patients with obstructive sleep apnea compared with controls. The structural and neurocognitive impairments both reversed following 3 months of treatment with Continuous Positive Airway Pressure (CPAP). The strengths of this article lie in the comparison between groups (OSA vs controls and pre-CPAP vs Post-CPAP). However, one of the limitations to the study is that the controls were not reevaluated in 3 months.

The authors make an argument about the pathophysiology of cognitive impairment in obstructive sleep apnea, linking references showing that hypoxia and hypercapnic-mediated damages cause structural changes, particularly in the hippocampal regions. Additional references support the ability of the hippocampus to regenerate neurons. The authors' research supports this further by their results showing that gray matter increases in the areas of the hippocampus and frontal regions following treatment with CPAP.

The implications of these findings could be used to educate patients and providers on the importance of early diagnosis and treatment for obstructive sleep apnea. This could serve as a motivational tool for patients to adhere to CPAP therapy.

S. F. Jones, MD, FCCP, DABSM

Sleep-Disordered Breathing, Hypoxia, and Risk of Mild Cognitive Impairment and Dementia in Older Women

Yaffe K, Laffan AM, Harrison SL, et al (Univ of California, San Francisco; California Pacific Med Ctr, San Francisco; et al)
JAMA 306:613-619, 2011

Context.—Sleep-disordered breathing (characterized by recurrent arousals from sleep and intermittent hypoxemia) is common among older adults. Cross-sectional studies have linked sleep-disordered breathing to poor cognition; however, it remains unclear whether sleep-disordered breathing precedes cognitive impairment in older adults.

Objectives.—To determine the prospective relationship between sleep-disordered breathing and cognitive impairment and to investigate potential mechanisms of this association.

Design, Setting, and Participants.—Prospective sleep and cognition study of 298 women without dementia (mean [SD] age: 82.3 [3.2] years) who had overnight polysomnography measured between January 2002 and April 2004 in a substudy of the Study of Osteoporotic Fractures. Sleep-disordered breathing was defined as an apnea-hypopnea index of 15 or more events per hour of sleep. Multivariate logistic regression was used to determine the independent association of sleep-disordered breathing with risk of mild cognitive impairment or dementia, adjusting for age, race, body mass index, education level, smoking status, presence of diabetes, presence of hypertension, medication use (antidepressants, benzodiazepines, or nonbenzodiazepine anxiolytics), and baseline cognitive scores. Measures of hypoxia, sleep fragmentation, and sleep duration were investigated as underlying mechanisms for this relationship.

Main Outcome Measures.—Adjudicated cognitive status (normal, dementia, or mild cognitive impairment) based on data collected between November 2006 and September 2008.

Results.—Compared with the 193 women without sleep-disordered breathing, the 105 women (35.2%) with sleep-disordered breathing were more likely to develop mild cognitive impairment or dementia (31.1% [n=60] vs 44.8% [n=47]; adjusted odds ratio [AOR], 1.85; 95% confidence interval [CI], 1.11-3.08). Elevated oxygen desaturation index (≥ 15 events/hour) and high percentage of sleep time (>7%) in apnea or hypopnea (both measures of disordered breathing) were associated with risk of developing mild cognitive impairment or dementia (AOR, 1.71 [95% CI, 1.04-2.83] and AOR, 2.04 [95% CI, 1.10-3.78], respectively). Measures of sleep fragmentation (arousal index and wake after sleep onset) or sleep duration (total sleep time) were not associated with risk of cognitive impairment.

Conclusion.—Among older women, those with sleep-disordered breathing compared with those without sleep-disordered breathing had an increased risk of developing cognitive impairment.

▶ This is a prospective longitudinal study of women without dementia. Polysomnography was performed, and after a mean of 4.7 years, nearly 45% of women with obstructive sleep apnea had developed mild cognitive impairment or dementia compared with 31% of women without obstructive sleep apnea. The oxygen desaturation index and a high percentage of total sleep time greater than 7% in apnea or hypopnea were associated with a higher incidence of mild cognitive impairment or dementia. It is interesting that sleep time with an oxygen saturation of less than 90% was not significantly associated with mild cognitive impairment or dementia. This suggests that intermittent hypoxemia poses a greater danger to the development of cognitive impairment than continuous hypoxemia. Interestingly, there is a lack of association between sleep fragmentation or duration and cognitive impairment, suggesting that the mechanism of cognitive impairment is more hypoxia mediated.

Further research should investigate whether continuous positive airway pressure (CPAP) may attenuate cognitive impairment. I have selected an article that highlights improvements in neurocognitive measures and recovery of structural losses with use of CPAP.[1] I encourage you to read that selection as well.

S. F. Jones, MD, FCCP, DABSM

Reference

1. Canessa N, Castronovo V, Cappa SF, et al. Obstructive sleep apnea: brain structural changes and neurocognitive function before and after treatment. *Am J Respir Crit Care Med.* 2011;183:1419-1426.

CPAP Treatment and Benefits

Continuous Positive Airway Pressure in Severe Obstructive Sleep Apnea Reduces Pain Sensitivity
Khalid I, Roehrs TA, Hudgel DW, et al (King Faisal Specialist Hosp & Res Ctr, Jeddah, Saudi Arabia; Sleep Disorders & Res Ctr, Detroit, MI; Univ of Manitoba, Winnipeg, CA)
Sleep 34:1687-1691, 2011

Study Objective.—To evaluate effects of CPAP on pain sensitivity in severe OSA patients.

Design.—Within-subject treatment study.

Setting.—Hospital-based sleep disorders center.

Patients.—Twelve severe OSA patients (7 men, 5 women), 50.2 ± 12.5 years, with no pain.

Interventions.—The morning after a diagnostic nocturnal polysomnogram (NPSG), patients underwent a training session of finger withdrawal latency (FWL) testing to a radiant heat stimulus, a validated human behavioral model of thermal nociception. Baseline FWL in seconds was obtained after the training session. CPAP pressure was titrated on a second night in the laboratory. Two nights after titration, patients returned to sleep in the laboratory on CPAP. FWL was tested in the morning after awakening, after 6-8 wks of CPAP use, and finally (within 6-8 weeks) after 2 nights of discontinuation of CPAP. Mean FWL in seconds (sec) was compared using MANOVAs with nights as the within subject variable.

Results.—Apnea-hypopnea index (AHI) decreased from 50.9 ± 14.5 to 1.4 ± 1.0 with CPAP, and sleep continuity improved. In parallel, FWL increased significantly from a mean baseline of 9.8 ± 1.3 sec to 13.7 ± 5.1 sec ($P = 0.01$) and with continued CPAP use (5.1 ± 2.3 h nightly) for 6-8 weeks FWL remained elevated (21.1 ± 16.2 sec). After the 2-night CPAP discontinuation, apnea/hypopneas returned and sleep was fragmented (AHI = 32.6 ± 19.8). FWL decreased to 11.6 ± 5.9 sec relative to intermediate-term CPAP use ($P = 0.03$).

Conclusion.—CPAP treatment reduces pain sensitivity in OSA patients. Future studies will focus on patients with OSA and chronic pain and identify mediating mechanisms.

▶ Pain seen in chronic conditions is associated with poor sleep quality. Poor sleep quality, such as arousals, is seen in patients with severe obstructive sleep apnea (OSA). The hypothesis that OSA patients are hyperalgesic because of fragmented sleep caused by the disorder is tested in this within-subject treatment study. The effects of continuous positive airway pressure (CPAP) on pain sensitivity in patients with severe obstructive sleep apnea are measured. Although the study size is small, I think the results are interesting and thought-provoking. Use of CPAP after just 2 days was associated with reductions in pain sensitivity. Longer durations of CPAP at 6 to 8 weeks were associated with more improvements, but these changes quickly dissipated just 2 days after withdrawal of CPAP (Fig 2 in the original article). Although the study did not explore causation, future studies should examine potential mechanisms. Are effects similar in patients with less severe OSA? Could use of CPAP reduce the amount of analgesics required to manage pain?

S. F. Jones, MD, FCCP, DABSM

Early treatment of obstructive apnoea and stroke outcome: a randomised controlled trial

Parra O, Sánchez-Armengol Á, Bonnin M, et al (Universitat de Barcelona, Spain; Unidad de Trastornos Respiratorios del Sueño, Barcelona, Spain; et al)
Eur Respir J 37:1128-1136, 2011

The aim of the present study was to assess the impact of nasal continuous positive airway pressure (nCPAP) in ischaemic stroke patients followed for 2 yrs.

Stroke patients with an apnoea-hypopnoea index ≥ 20 events$\cdot$h^{-1} were randomised to early nCPAP (n = 71; 3—6 days after stroke onset) or conventional treatment (n = 69). The Barthel Index, Canadian Scale, Rankin Scale and Short Form-36 were measured at baseline, and at 1, 3, 12 and 24 months.

The percentage of patients with neurological improvement 1 month after stroke was significantly higher in the nCPAP group (Rankin scale 90.9 *versus* 56.3% (p<0.01); Canadian scale 88.2 *versus* 72.7% (p<0.05)). The mean time until the appearance of cardiovascular events was longer in the nCPAP group (14.9 *versus* 7.9 months; p=0.044), although cardiovascular event-free survival after 24 months was similar in both groups. The cardiovascular mortality rate was 0% in the nCPAP group and 4.3% in the control group (p=0.161).

Early use of nCPAP seems to accelerate neurological recovery and to delay the appearance of cardiovascular events, although an improvement in patients' survival or quality of life was not shown.

▶ Obstructive sleep apnea (OSA) is a risk factor for stroke and other cardiovascular events. The literature examining effects of continuous positive airway pressure (CPAP) on outcomes is growing with a recent study showing that long-term CPAP treatment in moderate to severe OSA and ischemic stroke is associated with a reduction in excess risk of mortality.[1] In selection, Parra assesses the benefits of 2 years of early CPAP treatment on functional outcomes, quality of life, appearance of new cardiovascular events, and mortality and assesses the feasibility of using CPAP in the early phase of stroke.

The study is a prospective, randomized, controlled multicenter study. Patients had baseline and 1-, 3-, 12-, and 24-month follow-up. Patients who received CPAP within 6 days of an ischemic stroke had evidence of improved neurologic recovery at 1 month. There were no significant differences in the time points thereafter between groups. Furthermore, there were no cardiovascular-related deaths in the CPAP group during the study period compared with 3 in the control group, but this finding was not statistically significant. The time to first cardiovascular event was much longer in the CPAP group.

Although I think that the study will need to be repeated in a larger sample powered for cardiovascular mortality difference between groups, the findings are still very interesting. Patients and health care personnel both desire significant or complete and swift (if possible) neurologic recovery in patients with stroke. Could this be another tool to do so?

S. F. Jones, MD, FCCP, DABSM

Reference

1. Martínez-García MA, Soler-Cataluña JJ, Ejarque-Martínez L, et al. Continuous positive airway pressure treatment reduces mortality in patients with ischemic stroke and obstructive sleep apnea: a 5-year follow-up study. *Am J Respir Crit Care Med.* 2009;180:36-41.

Effects of Continuous Positive Airway Pressure Therapy Withdrawal in Patients with Obstructive Sleep Apnea: A Randomized Controlled Trial

Kohler M, Stoewhas A-C, Ayers L, et al (Univ of Zurich, Switzerland; Churchill Hosp, Oxford, UK)
Am J Respir Crit Care Med 184:1192-1199, 2011

Rationale.—To establish a new approach to investigate the physiological effects of obstructive sleep apnea (OSA), and to evaluate novel treatments, during a period of continuous positive airway pressure (CPAP) withdrawal.

Objectives.—To determine the effects of CPAP withdrawal.

Methods.—Forty-one patients with OSA and receiving CPAP were randomized to either CPAP withdrawal (subtherapeutic CPAP), or continued CPAP, for 2 weeks. Polysomnography, sleepiness, psychomotor performance, endothelial function, blood pressure (BP), heart rate (HR), urinary catecholamines, blood markers of systemic inflammation, and metabolism were assessed.

Measurements and Main Results.—CPAP withdrawal led to a recurrence of OSA within a few days and a return of subjective sleepiness, but was not associated with significant deterioration of psychomotor performance within 2 weeks. Endothelial function, assessed by flow-mediated dilatation, decreased significantly in the CPAP withdrawal group compared with therapeutic CPAP (mean difference in change, -3.2%; 95% confidence interval [CI], -4.5, -1.9%; $P < 0.001$). Compared with continuing CPAP, 2 weeks of CPAP withdrawal was associated with a significant increase in morning systolic BP (mean difference in change, $+8.5$ mm Hg; 95% CI, $+1.7$, $+15.3$ mm Hg; $P = 0.016$), morning diastolic BP (mean difference in change, $+6.9$ mm Hg; 95% CI, $+1.9$, $+11.9$ mm Hg; $P = 0.008$), and morning HR (mean difference in change, $+6.3$ bpm, 95% CI, $+0.4$, $+12.2$ bpm; $P = 0.035$). CPAP withdrawal was associated with an increase in urinary catecholamines but did not lead to an increase in markers of systemic inflammation, insulin resistance, or blood lipids.

Conclusions.—CPAP withdrawal usually leads to a rapid recurrence of OSA, a return of subjective sleepiness, and is associated with impaired endothelial function, increased urinary catecholamines, blood pressure, and heart rate. Thus the proposed study model appears to be suitable to evaluate physiological and therapeutic effects in OSA. Clinical trial registered with www.controlled-trials.com (ISRCTN93153804).

▶ In my practice, patients ask "what will happen to me if I don't wear continuous positive airway pressure (CPAP) for 1 night? What will happen to me if I don't take my CPAP machine with me on my 2-week vacation?" I think this study is interesting in that physiologic parameters were measured in patients who had discontinued CPAP for 2 weeks and were compared with controls (patients who continued to wear CPAP). There are both research-related and patient care implications to this study. The protocol implemented by the investigators has created a new model of the effects of untreated obstructive sleep apnea (OSA) that could be used in future studies to examine effects of new interventions. Withdrawal of CPAP led to an increase in number of apneas and hypopneas on as early as the first night with no further increase in apnea hypopnea index after a week of withdrawal (Fig 2 in the original article). Increases in Epworth sleepiness score were significant following withdrawal. The most impressive finding is the increase in morning systolic and diastolic blood pressure and morning heart rate (Fig 4 in the original article). This is something that I have observed in the laboratory, but these investigators have quantified these observations. Furthermore, with the observation of increase in urinary catecholamines, a surge in sympathetic activity is a possible etiology to these findings.

S. F. Jones, MD, FCCP, DABSM

Non-CPAP Treatment of Sleep-Disordered Breathing

Attenuation of Obstructive Sleep Apnea by Compression Stockings in Subjects with Venous Insufficiency

Redolfi S, Arnulf I, Pottier M, et al (Groupe Hospitalier Pitié-Salpêtrière, Paris, France; et al)
Am J Respir Crit Care Med 184:1062-1066, 2011

Rationale.—Fluid accumulation in the legs and its overnight redistribution into the neck appears to play a causative role in obstructive sleep apnea (OSA) in sedentary men. Chronic venous insufficiency (CVI) promotes fluid accumulation in the legs that can be counteracted by compression stockings.

Objectives.—To test the hypotheses that, in nonobese subjects with CVI and OSA, wearing compression stockings during the day will attenuate OSA by reducing the amount of fluid displaced into the neck overnight.

Methods.—Nonobese subjects with CVI and OSA were randomly assigned to 1 week of wearing compression stockings or to a 1-week control period without compression stockings, after which they crossed over to the other arm. Polysomnography and measurement of overnight changes in leg fluid volume and neck circumference were performed at baseline and at the end of compression stockings and control periods.

Measurements and Main Results.—Twelve subjects participated. Compared with the end of the control period, at the end of the compression stockings period there was a 62% reduction in the overnight leg fluid volume change ($P = 0.001$) and a 60% reduction in the overnight neck circumference increase ($P = 0.001$) in association with a 36% reduction in the number of apneas and hypopneas per hour of sleep (from 48.4 ± 26.9 to 31.3 ± 20.2, $P = 0.002$).

Conclusions.—Redistribution of fluid from the legs into the neck at night contributes to the pathogenesis of OSA in subjects with CVI. Prevention of fluid accumulation in the legs during the day, and its nocturnal displacement into the neck, attenuates OSA in such subjects.

▶ This is a very interesting article. Previously Redolfi[1,2] reported movements of fluid from the legs into the neck during sleep generates an increase in the neck circumference and also increases the number of apneas and hypopneas per hour (AHI). They take this further in this randomized double crossover study aimed to examine the effects of using standard thigh-high compression stockings during daytime hours in patients with chronic venous insufficiency and known obstructive sleep apnea (OSA). Use of stockings resulted in less body fluid, leg fluid volume, and bilateral ankle circumferences and less urine volume overnight. For nearly all subjects, there was a decrease in the neck circumference and a reduction in the AHI. On average, there was a 36% reduction in the AHI. The population represented those with severe OSA, as the average AHI was 48.4. While there was a significant reduction in the AHI with the compression stockings, the subjects still had severe OSA after treatment. It would be interesting to know if the same results would apply to those patients with mild to moderate degrees of OSA with and without chronic venous insufficiency.

This study is important in that it links rostral fluid displacement from the legs into the neck as a pathophysiologic mechanism for OSA. I think we will be seeing more mechanistic studies examining rostral fluid shift and its implication in other forms of sleep apnea. Perhaps this may be a form of adjunctive therapy in addition to continuous positive airway pressure?

S. F. Jones, MD, FCCP, DABSM

References

1. Redolfi S, Yumino D, Ruttanaumpawan P, et al. Relationship between overnight rostral fluid shift and obstructive sleep apnea in nonobese men. *Am J Respir Crit Care Med.* 2009;179:241-246.
2. Redolfi S, Arnulf I, Pottier M, Bradley TD, Similowski T. Effects of venous compression of the legs on overnight rostral fluid shift and obstructive sleep apnea. *Respir Physiol Neurobiol.* 2011;175:390-393.

Pediatric Sleep-Disordered Breathing

SIDS and Other Sleep-Related Infant Deaths: Expansion of Recommendations for a Safe Infant Sleeping Environment
Task Force on Sudden Infant Death Syndrome, Moon RY
Pediatrics 128:e1341-e1367, 2011

Despite a major decrease in the incidence of sudden infant death syndrome (SIDS) since the American Academy of Pediatrics (AAP) released its recommendation in 1992 that infants be placed for sleep in a nonprone position, this decline has plateaued in recent years. Concurrently, other causes of sudden unexpected infant death occurring during sleep (sleep-related deaths), including suffocation, asphyxia, and entrapment, and ill-defined or unspecified causes of death have increased in incidence, particularly since the AAP published its last statement on SIDS in 2005. It has become increasingly important to address these other causes of sleep-related infant death. Many of the modifiable and nonmodifiable risk factors for SIDS and suffocation are strikingly similar. The AAP, therefore, is expanding its recommendations from being only SIDS-focused to focusing on a safe sleep environment that can reduce the risk of all sleep-related infant deaths including SIDS. The recommendations described in this report include supine positioning, use of a firm sleep surface, breastfeeding, room-sharing without bed-sharing, routine immunization, consideration of a pacifier, and avoidance of soft bedding, overheating, and exposure to tobacco smoke, alcohol, and illicit drugs. The rationale for these recommendations is discussed in detail in this technical report. The recommendations are published in the accompanying "Policy Statement—Sudden Infant Death Syndrome and Other Sleep-Related Infant Deaths: Expansion of Recommendations for a Safe Infant Sleeping Environment," which is included in this issue (www.pediatrics.org/cgi/doi/10.1542/peds.2011-2220).

▶ The incidence of sudden infant death syndrome (SIDS) has decreased dramatically with the "Back to Sleep" Campaign. In this article, the Task Force on Sudden Infant Death Syndrome has expanded their recommendations to include not only the data regarding SIDS, but also a safe sleep environment. If your sleep medicine practice includes evaluation and management of infants, this is a great document to read. Sleep medicine professionals are consulted regularly on apnea in infants, and familiarity of risk factors and recommendation for a safe sleep environment that can reduce the risk of sleep-related infant deaths is needed. A summary and strength of recommendations are included as well as a nice reference list. Lastly, one of the recommendations of the Task Force is that that all physicians, nurses, and other health care professionals receive education on safe infant sleep.

S. F. Jones, MD, FCCP, DABSM

Non-Pulmonary Sleep

A Brief Sleep Intervention Improves Outcomes in the School Entry Year: A Randomized Controlled Trial

Quach J, Hiscock H, Ukoumunne OC, et al (Univ of Melbourne, Australia; Univ of Exeter, UK)

Pediatrics 128:692-701, 2011

Objective.—To determine the feasibility of screening for child sleep problems and the efficacy of a behavioral sleep intervention in improving child and parent outcomes in the first year of schooling.

Methods.—A randomized controlled trial was nested in a population survey performed at 22 elementary schools in Melbourne, Australia. Intervention involved 2 to 3 consultations that covered behavioral sleep strategies for children whose screening results were positive for a moderate/severe sleep problem. Outcomes were parent-reported child sleep problem (primary outcome), sleep habits, psychosocial health-related quality of life, behavior, and parent mental health (all at 3, 6, and 12 months) and blinded, face-to-face learning assessment (at 6 months).

Results.—The screening survey was completed by 1512 parents; 161 (10.8%) reported a moderate/severe child sleep problem, and 108 of 136 (79.2% of those eligible) entered the trial. Sleep problems tended to resolve more rapidly in intervention children. Sleep problems affected 33% of 54 intervention children versus 43% of 54 control children at 3 months ($P = .3$), 25.5% vs 46.8% at 6 months ($P = .03$), and 32% vs 33% at 12 months ($P = .8$). Sustained sleep-habit improvements were evident at 3, 6, and 12 months (effect sizes: 0.33 [$P = .03$]; 0.51 [$P = .003$]; and 0.40 [$P = .02$]; respectively), and there were initial marked improvements in psychosocial scores that diminished over time (effect sizes: 0.47 [$P = .02$]; 0.41 [$P = .09$]; and 0.26 [$P = .3$]; respectively). Better prosocial behavior was evident at 12 months (effect size: 0.35; $P = .03$), and learning and parent outcomes were similar between groups.

Conclusions.—School-based screening for sleep problems followed by a targeted, brief behavioral sleep intervention is feasible and has benefits relevant to school transition.

▶ Data from the Longtitudinal Study of Australian Children show that sleep problems are common in children age 4 to 5 years. Poor sleep is associated with negative outcomes, such as health-related quality of life, behavior, language, and learning scores.[1] Quach has taken this one step further in this article by examining the effect of a behavioral intervention that included 1 individual session and 2 follow-up phone calls. In this work, screening surveys were sent to 22 schools in Australia, with completion by 1512 parents. The strengths of the study are notable. Seventy-one percent of surveys were completed, and of those children identified with moderate to severe sleep problems, 79% took part in the study. This study had a high retention rate, even 12 months afterwards. Improvements in sleep were notable at 6 months. The improvement in psychosocial scores shows that a brief intervention could be effective. Although these improvements diminished over time, the true effect of the intervention on the psychosocial scores are likely dampened by the number of subjects (n = 47). This study should be expanded to include a more diverse population. This work is significant and is a true example of population health research.

S. F. Jones, MD, FCCP, DABSM

Reference

1. Quach J, Hiscock H, Canterford L, Wake M. Outcomes of child sleep problems over the school-transition period: Australian population longitudinal study. *Pediatrics.* 2009;123:1287-1292.

Efficacy of Brief Behavioral Treatment for Chronic Insomnia in Older Adults
Buysse DJ, Germain A, Moul DE, et al (Univ of Pittsburgh School of Medicine, PA; Cleveland Clinic Sleep Disorders Ctr, OH)
Arch Intern Med 171:887-895, 2011

Background.—Chronic insomnia is a common health problem with substantial consequences in older adults. Cognitive behavioral treatments are efficacious but not widely available. The aim of this study was to test the efficacy of brief behavioral treatment for insomnia (BBTI) vs an information control (IC) condition.

Methods.—A total of 79 older adults (mean age, 71.7 years; 54 women [70%]) with chronic insomnia and common comorbidities were recruited from the community and 1 primary care clinic. Participants were randomly assigned to either BBTI, consisting of individualized behavioral instructions delivered in 2 intervention sessions and 2 telephone calls, or IC, consisting of printed educational material. Both interventions were delivered by a nurse clinician. The primary outcome was categorically defined treatment response at 4 weeks, based on sleep questionnaires and diaries. Secondary outcomes included self-report symptom and health measures, sleep diaries, actigraphy, and polysomnography.

Results.—Categorically defined response (67% [n=26] vs 25% [n=10]; χ^2=13.8) ($P < .001$) and the proportion of participants without insomnia (55% [n=21] vs 13% [n=5]; χ^2=15.5) ($P < .001$) were significantly higher for BBTI than for IC. The number needed to treat was 2.4 for each outcome. No differential effects were found for subgroups according to hypnotic or antidepressant use, sleep apnea, or recruitment source. The BBTI produced significantly better outcomes in self-reported sleep and health (group×time interaction, $F_{5,73}$=5.99, $P < .001$), sleep diary ($F_{8,70}$=4.32, $P < .001$), and actigraphy ($F_{4,74}$=17.72, $P < .001$), but not polysomnography. Improvements were maintained at 6 months.

Conclusion.—We found that BBTI is a simple, efficacious, and durable intervention for chronic insomnia in older adults that has potential for dissemination across medical settings.

Trial Registration.—clinicaltrials.gov Identifier: NCT00177203.

▶ Insomnia is frequently encountered in the primary care office, and its prevalence is greater than that of obstructive sleep apnea syndrome in the general population. The use of hypnotics for the treatment of insomnia, although effective, is particularly problematic for older patients who may experience side effects and increased risk of falls. Knowledge of the effectiveness of cognitive behavioral therapy is not new. This has been reported again and again.[1-3] The uniqueness of the findings of Buysse lies within the delivery of the intervention.

Cognitive behavioral therapy has for too long been sequestered in specialized sleep centers and offered by behavioral sleep medicine experts. Its application has been limited by the number of qualified personnel and the time limitations/constraints within a health care practice to create effective change in the habits and beliefs of those affected. We need better ways to deliver effective care to those who need it. In this article, cognitive behavioral therapy was delivered for 4 weeks (which is shorter than other studies) by a masters-level mental health nurse practitioner with no prior experience in sleep medicine or behavioral interventions for insomnia. Furthermore, half of the sessions were delivered by telephone. The results were impressive and most importantly sustainable at 6 months. There are some limitations to the study that introduce bias, but the design of the study was in the spirit of a real-world primary care practice. We should look into incorporating the author's strategies within our own health care systems.

S. F. Jones, MD, FCCP, DABSM

References

1. Shochat T, Umphress J, Israel AG, Ancoli-Israel S. Insomnia in primary care patients. *Sleep.* 1999;22:S359-S365.
2. Ohayon MM. Epidemiology of insomnia: what we know and what we still need to learn. *Sleep Med Rev.* 2002;6:97-111.
3. Jennum P, Riha RL. Epidemiology of sleep apnoea/hypopnoea syndrome and sleep-disordered breathing. *Eur Respir J.* 2009;33:907-914.

Increasing Walking and Bright Light Exposure to Improve Sleep in Community-Dwelling Persons with Alzheimer's Disease: Results of a Randomized, Controlled Trial
McCurry SM, Pike KC, Vitiello MV, et al (Univ of Washington, Seattle; et al)
J Am Geriatr Soc 59:1393-1402, 2011

Objectives.—To test the effects of walking, light exposure, and a combination intervention (walking, light, and sleep education) on the sleep of persons with Alzheimer's disease (AD).
Design.—Randomized, controlled trial with blinded assessors.
Setting.—Independent community living.
Participants.—One hundred thirty-two people with AD and their in-home caregivers.

Interventions.—Participants were randomly assigned to one of three active treatments (walking, light, combination treatment) or contact control and received three or six in-home visits.

Measurements.—Primary outcomes were participant total wake time based on wrist actigraphy and caregiver ratings of participant sleep quality on the Sleep Disorders Inventory (SDI). Secondary sleep outcomes included additional actigraphic measurements of sleep percentage, number of awakenings, and total sleep time.

Results.—Participants in walking ($P = .05$), light ($P = .04$), and combination treatment ($P = .01$) had significantly greater improvements in total wake time at posttest (effect size $0.51-0.63$) than controls but no significant improvement on the SDI. Moderate effect size improvements in actigraphic sleep percentage were also observed in active treatment participants. There were no significant differences between the active treatment groups and no group differences for any sleep outcomes at 6 months. Participants with better adherence (4 d/wk) to walking and light exposure recommendations had significantly less total wake time ($P = .006$) and better sleep efficiency ($P = .005$) at posttest than those with poorer adherence.

Conclusion.—Walking, light exposure, and their combination are potentially effective treatments for improving sleep in community-dwelling persons with AD, but consistent adherence to treatment recommendations is required.

▶ Sleep disturbances in patients with dementia are associated with caregiver stress. Care-recipient sleep disturbances are a common reason for institutionalization of a person with dementia.[1,2] Although pharmacologic therapy is used in the management of sleep disturbances in patients with dementia, medications such as benzodiazepines, antihistamines, or tricyclic antidepressants can produce untoward side effects. Nonpharmacologic therapy using light or activity has been successful in improving sleep in institutionalized patients with dementia. This study is unique in that it examines the effect of light versus activity versus combination plus education in community-dwelling patients with Alzheimer dementia. Objective measurements of sleep-wake activity using actigraphy improved at 2 months in all treatment arms but were not sustainable at 6 months. Interestingly, measures of sleep quality using questionnaires of caregivers did not improve at 2 months. The authors discussed several possibilities for this.

This was a challenging study to perform because of the number of factors related to quality of sleep, adherence to the protocol, education of the caregivers, the population, setting, etc. The findings of the study lend hope to the possibility of finding nonpharmacologic interventions for improvements in sleep in a vulnerable population. Examining the factors preventing longer treatment adherence are needed. Effective ways to improve sleep and possibly prolong or eliminate the need for institutionalization in this population are needed.

S. F. Jones, MD, FCCP, DABSM

References

1. McCurry SM, Logsdon RG, Teri L, Vitiello MV. Sleep disturbances in caregivers of persons with dementia: contributing factors and treatment implications. *Sleep Med Rev.* 2007;11:143-153.
2. Hope T, Keene J, Gedling K, Fairburn CG, Jacoby R. Predictors of institutionalization for people with dementia living at home with a carer. *Int J Geriatr Psychiatry.* 1998;13:682-690.

Prospective Evaluation of Consultant Surgeon Sleep Deprivation and Outcomes in More Than 4000 Consecutive Cardiac Surgical Procedures

Chu MWA, Stitt LW, Fox SA, et al (Univ of Western Ontario, London, Canada)
Arch Surg 146:1080-1085, 2011

Objective.—To determine the effect of consultant surgeon sleep hours on patient outcomes in cardiac surgery.

Design.—Prospective observational cohort study.

Subjects.—Between January 2004 and December 2009, we prospectively collected sleep hours of 6 consultant surgeons, ranging in age from 32 to 55 years, working in a tertiary care academic institution. The prospective study cohort included all patients undergoing coronary artery bypass, valve, combined valve—coronary artery bypass, and aortic surgery. The predicted risk of death and/or any of 10 major complications was calculated using our institutional multivariable model, which was then compared with observed values. Additional prespecified analyses examined the interaction between surgeon age, sleep hours, and postoperative outcomes. This study had more than 90% power to detect a 4% (clinically important) difference in overall complication rates among groups.

Main Outcome Measures.—Complication and mortality rates in operations performed by surgeons with 0 to 3, 3 to 6, or more than 6 hours' sleep the evening prior to surgery.

Results.—Of 4047 consecutive surgical procedures, 83 were performed by a consultant with 0 to 3 hours, 1595 with 3 to 6 hours, and 2369 with more than 6 hours of sleep. Rates of mortality (3 [3.6%], 44 [2.8%], and 80 [3.4%], respectively; $P=.53$) were similar in the 3 groups, as were the observed vs expected ratios of major complications (1.20, 0.95, and 1.07, respectively; $P=.25$). There was no significant interaction between surgeon age, hours of sleep, and occurrence of death or any of 10 major complications ($P=.09$).

Conclusion.—This well-powered prospective study showed no evidence that consultant surgeon sleep hours had an effect on postoperative outcomes.

▶ Restrictions on residency duty hours came into effect nearly 7 years ago. Additional restrictions became effective July 1, 2011. Current guidelines state that postgraduate year 1 residents are limited to 16 continuous hours of duty and must have 10 hours free of duty between scheduled duty periods. Intermediate residents are limited to 24 hours of continuous duty and must have at least

14 hours free of duty after 24 hours of in-house duty.[1] This has led to much heated debate about the evidence behind the guidelines and even more debate about the implications and effects on residency education and patient care. Will new surgery residents be able to adapt in a practice setting in which duty hours are not restricted?

Simulation studies of laparoscopy have reported impairment in fine motor skills following sleep deprivation[2,3]; however, these studies may not be generalized to other surgeries. Chu reports the results of a prospective observational cohort study of data from more than 4000 cardiac surgeries performed by 6 consultant surgeons at an academic center in Canada. Surgeons reported the number of hours of continuous sleep acquired the night prior to performing surgery. Complication and mortality rates did not differ between procedures conducted in which surgeons reported 0 to 3 hours, 3 to 6 hours, or more than 6 hours of uninterrupted sleep. The study also included the effect of surgeon age on outcomes, which showed no statistically significant differences between surgeons younger than 45 years and older than 50 years of age. The authors hypothesize that expertise contributes to habit and patient care without compromise. Furthermore, authors suggest that a team-based approach to the care of the cardiac surgery patient is able to compensate for possible fatigue-related errors. Certainly, checklists and protocolized perioperative management may exert positive influence on safety and length-of-stay outcomes. Despite the lack of statistically significant differences between groups in negative patient outcomes, I seriously doubt that this study will alter the proponents of duty hour restriction. There will always be the argument that 1 error is too many, statistical or not.

S. F. Jones, MD, FCCP, DABSM

References

1. ACGME duty hours. Common program requirements. http://www.acgme.org/acWebsite/home/Common_Program_Requirements_07012011.pdf. Published July 1, 2011. Accessed February 21, 2012.
2. Eastridge BJ, Hamilton EC, O'Keefe GE, et al. Effect of sleep deprivation on the performance of simulated laparoscopic surgical skill. *Am J Surg.* 2003;186:169-174.
3. Grantcharov TP, Bardram L, Funch-Jensen P, Rosenberg J. Laparoscopic performance after one night on call in a surgical department: prospective study. *BMJ.* 2001;323:1222-1223.

Quantification of sleep behavior and of its impact on the cross-talk between the brain and peripheral metabolism
Hanlon EC, Van Cauter E (Univ of Chicago, IL)
Proc Natl Acad Sci U S A 108:15609-15616, 2011

Rates of obesity have been steadily increasing, along with disorders commonly associated with obesity, such as cardiovascular disease and type II diabetes. Simultaneously, average sleep times have progressively decreased. Recently, evidence from both laboratory and epidemiologic studies has suggested that insufficient sleep may stimulate overeating and thus play a role in the current epidemic of obesity and diabetes. In the human sleep laboratory it is now possible to carefully control sleep behavior and study the link between sleep duration and alterations in circulating hormones involved in feeding behavior, glucose metabolism, hunger, and appetite. This article focuses on the methodologies used in experimental protocols that have examined modifications produced by sleep restriction (or extension) compared with normal sleep. The findings provide evidence that sleep restriction does indeed impair glucose metabolism and alters the cross-talk between the periphery and the brain, favoring excessive food intake. A better understanding of the adverse effects of sleep restriction on the CNS control of hunger and appetite may have important implications for public health.

▶ Rates of obesity and diabetes are on the rise in the United States. Concomitantly, Americans are getting less sleep. Could sleep deprivation or loss of sleep quality or even certain stages of sleep induce metabolic derangements significant enough to promote hyperphagia, excessive caloric intake, and weight gain? In this nice article, Hanlon reviews the research that we are becoming a society of overweight, sleep-deprived individuals and how sleep deprivation may induce significant metabolic dysfunction through increases in leptin and ghrelin hormones. Both leptin and ghrelin interact with neurons within the hypothalamus suppressing or increasing appetite. In addition, Hanlon reviews the medical literature supporting that sleep deprivation is associated with impaired glucose metabolism and increased risk of diabetes. More research should be devoted to sleep deprivation and its effects on metabolism. Effective strategies to increase sleep time could have a significant impact on health.

S. F. Jones, MD, FCCP, DABSM

Sleep Disorders, Health, and Safety in Police Officers
Rajaratnam SMW, for the Harvard Work Hours, Health and Safety Group (Brigham and Women's Hospital, Boston, MA; et al)
JAMA 306:2567-2578, 2011

Context.—Sleep disorders often remain undiagnosed. Untreated sleep disorders among police officers may adversely affect their health and safety and pose a risk to the public.

Objective.—To quantify associations between sleep disorder risk and self-reported health, safety, and performance outcomes in police officers.

Design, Setting, and Participants.—Cross-sectional and prospective cohort study of North American police officers participating in either an online or an on-site screening (n = 4957) and monthly follow-up surveys (n = 3545 officers representing 15 735 person-months) between July 2005 and December 2007. A total of 3693 officers in the United States and Canada participated in the online screening survey, and 1264 officers from a municipal police department and a state police department participated in the on-site survey.

Main Outcome Measures.—Comorbid health conditions (cross-sectional); performance and safety outcomes (prospective).

Results.—Of the 4957 participants, 40.4% screened positive for at least 1 sleep disorder, most of whom had not been diagnosed previously. Of the total cohort, 1666 (33.6%) screened positive for obstructive sleep apnea, 281 (6.5%) for moderate to severe insomnia, 269 (5.4%) for shift work disorder (14.5% of those who worked the night shift). Of the 4608 participants who completed the sleepiness scale, 1312 (28.5%) reported excessive sleepiness. Of the total cohort, 1294 (26.1%) reported falling asleep while driving at least 1 time a month. Respondents who screened positive for obstructive sleep apnea or any sleep disorder had an increased prevalence of reported physical and mental health conditions, including diabetes, depression, and cardiovascular disease. An analysis of up to 2 years of monthly follow-up surveys showed that those respondents who screened positive for a sleep disorder vs those who did not had a higher rate of reporting that they had made a serious administrative error (17.9% vs 12.7%; adjusted odds ratio [OR], 1.43 [95% CI, 1.23-1.67]); of falling asleep while driving (14.4% vs 9.2%; adjusted OR, 1.51 [95% CI, 1.20-1.90]); of making an error or safety violation attributed to fatigue (23.7% vs 15.5%; adjusted OR, 1.63 [95% CI, 1.43-1.85]); and of exhibiting other adverse work-related outcomes including uncontrolled anger toward suspects (34.1% vs 28.5%; adjusted OR, 1.25 [95% CI, 1.09-1.43]), absenteeism (26.0% vs 20.9%; adjusted OR, 1.23 [95% CI, 1.08-1.40]), and falling asleep during meetings (14.1% vs 7.0%; adjusted OR, 1.95 [95% CI, 1.52-2.52]).

Conclusion.—Among a group of North American police officers, sleep disorders were common and were significantly associated with increased risk of self-reported adverse health, performance, and safety outcomes.

▶ Sleep problems carry significant impact at the population level. Up to 5% of the adult population is estimated to have obstructive sleep apnea syndrome.[1] Chronic insomnia affects approximately 10% of the population,[2] and shift work sleep disorder is estimated to affect 10% of night and rotating shift workers.[3] Sleep disorders account for a significant portion of health care dollars in both direct and indirect costs. Sleep disorders account for many of the complaints of fatigue, sleepiness, and unrestful sleep. Sleep deprivation and fatigue has been found to affect performance and safety.[4] Many, including the Accreditation Council for Graduate Medical Education, are taking a stand in limiting work hours in hopes of reducing fatigue and its negative outcomes. Police officers, like residents, may be vulnerable to the negative outcomes associated with sleep problems.

The investigators in this study performed a cross-sectional and prospective cohort study of nearly 5000 North American police officers to examine associations between sleep disorder risk and self-reported health safety and performance outcomes. The findings are significant in that certain sleep disorders affect a greater number of police officers than the general population. The most frequent was obstructive sleep apnea, which is not a surprise, as over 70% of subjects were overweight or obese. A total of 14.5% of those who worked shift screened positive for shift work sleep disorder. Even more significant is the number of self-reported errors, comorbid disease, and drowsy driving.

While the limitations of this study include recall bias, underreporting of events out of concern for self and his or her job, and the lack of a validated questionnaire for shift work sleep disorder, the findings nevertheless are impressive. I believe that this article will draw great interest and perhaps creation of fatigue and sleep-related education for police departments. Studies examining the effect of fatigue in and performance errors by police officers may soon come. I think this article emphasizes the impact of sleep disorders on population health.

S. F. Jones, MD, FCCP, DABSM

References

1. Young T, Peppard P, Gottlieb DJ. Epidemiology of obstructive sleep apnea: a population health perspective. *Am J Resp Crit Care Med.* 2002;165:1217-1239.
2. National Institutes of Health. National Institutes of Health State of the Science Conference statement on Manifestations and Management of Chronic Insomnia in Adults, June 13-15, 2005. *Sleep.* 2005;28:1049-1057.
3. Drake CL, Roehrs T, Richardson G, Walsh JK, Roth T. Shift work sleep disorder: prevalence and consequences beyond that of symptomatic day workers. *Sleep.* 2004;27:1453-1462.
4. Gaba DM, Howard SK. Patient safety: fatigue among clinician and safety of patients. *N Engl J Med.* 2002;347:1249-1255.

Sleep Duration or Bedtime? Exploring the Relationship between Sleep Habits and Weight Status and Activity Patterns
Olds TS, Maher CA, Matricciani L (Univ of South Australia, Adelaide, Australia)
Sleep 34:1299-1307, 2011

Study Objectives.—To assess the effects of early and late bedtimes and wake up times on use of time and weight status in Australian school-aged children.

Design.—Observational cross-sectional study involving use of time interviews and pedometers.

Setting.—Free-living Australian adolescents.

Participants.—2200 9- to 16-year-olds from all states of Australia.

Interventions.—NA.

Measurements and Results.—Bedtimes and wake times were adjusted for age and sex and classified as early or late using median splits. Adolescents were allocated into 4 sleep-wake pattern groups: Early-bed/Early-rise; Early-bed/Late-rise; Late-bed/Early-rise; Late-bed/Late-rise. The groups were compared for use of time (screen time, physical activity, and study-related time), sociodemographic characteristics, and weight status. Adolescents in the Late-bed/Late-rise category experienced 48 min/d more screen time and 27 min less moderate-to-vigorous physical activity (MVPA) (P < 0.0001) than adolescents in the Early-bed/Early-rise category, in spite of similar sleep durations. Late-bed/Late-rise adolescents had a higher BMI z-score (0.66 vs. 0.45, P = 0.0015). Late-bed/Late-rise adolescents were 1.47 times more likely to be overweight or obese than Early-bed/Early-rise adolescents, 2.16 times more likely to be obese, 1.77 times more likely to have low MVPA, and 2.92 times more likely to have high screen time. Late-bed/Late-rise adolescents were more likely to come from poorer households, to live in major cities, and have fewer siblings.

Conclusions.—Late bedtimes and late wake up times are associated with an unfavorable activity and weight status profile, independent of age, sex, household income, geographical remoteness, and sleep duration.

▶ The number of studies examining the relationship between sleep time and weight status are increasing. Specifically, shorter sleep durations are associated with weight gain. Mechanisms continue to be explored including how caloric intake or diversity of food choices (ie, more carbohydrates) may change with less sleep duration. Olds and colleagues take a different approach. This work examines a less explored relationship between sleep timing and outcomes of weight and physical activity in a large sample of adolescents in Australia. This goes beyond the classification system of morning or evening types, instead classifying sleep timing behavior into 4 groups: early bed/early rise, early bed/late rise, late bed/early rise, and late bed/late rise. The most interesting findings challenge the linkages between sleep duration and weight, instead drawing a new relationship between sleep timing and patterns with weight status and activity patterns. The largest differences were seen between the early bed/early rise and late bed/late rise despite any real significance in sleep duration. Late bed/late rise adolescents had the highest odds ratio for obesity, lower physical activity, and more sedentary activities such as television watching or playing computer games.

This study has important implications. Some propose adjusting school start and end times to later hours to accommodate the natural phase delay associated with this age group. The findings in this article challenge this move to adjust times. I believe that additional research needs to confirm these findings. A longitudinal research study examining these relationships is in order.

S. F. Jones, MD, FCCP, DABSM

The Effect of Melatonin, Magnesium, and Zinc on Primary Insomnia in Long-Term Care Facility Residents in Italy: A Double-Blind, Placebo-Controlled Clinical Trial

Rondanelli M, Opizzi A, Monteferrario F, et al (Univ of Pavia, Italy; et al)
J Am Geriatr Soc 59:82-90, 2011

Objectives.—To determine whether nightly administration of melatonin, magnesium, and zinc improves primary insomnia in long-term care facility residents.

Design.—Double-blind, placebo-controlled clinical trial.

Setting.—One long-term care facility in Pavia, Italy.

Participants.—Forty-three participants with primary insomnia (22 in the supplemented group, 21 in the placebo group) aged 78.3 ± 3.9.

Intervention.—Participants took a food supplement (5 mg melatonin, 225 mg magnesium, and 11.25 mg zinc, mixed with 100 g of pear pulp) or placebo (100 g pear pulp) every day for 8 weeks, 1 hour before bedtime.

Measurements.—The primary goal was to evaluate sleep quality using the Pittsburgh Sleep Quality Index. The Epworth Sleepiness Scale, the Leeds Sleep Evaluation Questionnaire (LSEQ), the Short Insomnia Questionnaire (SDQ), and a validated quality-of-life instrument (Medical Outcomes Study 36-item Short Form Survey (SF-36)) were administered as secondary end points. Total sleep time was evaluated using a wearable armband-shaped sensor. All measures were performed at baseline and after 60 days.

Results.—The food supplement resulted in considerably better overall PSQI scores than placebo (difference between groups in change from baseline PSQI score = 6.8; 95% confidence interval = 5.4−8.3, $P < .001$). Moreover, the significant improvements in all four domains of the LSEQ (ease of getting to sleep, $P < .001$; quality of sleep, $P < .001$; hangover on awakening from sleep, $P = .005$; alertness and behavioral integrity the following morning, $P = .001$), in SDQ score ($P < .001$), in total sleep time ($P < .001$), and in SF-36 physical score ($P = .006$) suggest that treatment had a beneficial effect on the restorative value of sleep.

Conclusion.—The administration of nightly melatonin, magnesium, and zinc appears to improve the quality of sleep and the quality of life in long-term care facility residents with primary insomnia.

▶ Insomnia is a frequently encountered problem, particularly in the elderly. Poor sleep is associated with an increased risk of falls in community-dwelling adults age 64 to 99 years of age.[1] Use of hypnotics such as benzodiazepines and antihistamines can have untoward side effects, including sedation. So therapy with fewer side effects is extremely important. Nursing home residents particularly pose challenges in treatment of insomnia. Furthermore, treatment therapies, such as cognitive behavioral therapy, that are effective for primary insomnia, are usually limited to sleep clinics, and thus, their true effect is not reached in the institutionalized elderly.

Rondanelli conducted a randomized, double-blind, placebo-controlled trial of a food supplement containing melatonin, 5 mg, magnesium, 225 mg, and zinc, 11.25 mg, in pear pulp. There were significant improvements in both the primary and secondary measures. Objective measures of total sleep time also increased in the treatment arm. There were no reported significant side effects of the medication and no dropouts related to the use of the medication. It appears to be safe and well tolerated.

Certainly, the study should be repeated in community-dwelling adults. Specific bedtime and daytime schedules of those residing in nursing home residents may differ quite significantly from those of community-dwelling adults. Also, the population of Italian elders, along with the degree of comorbid disease and disabilities, may differ from American populations. Again, the study should be repeated, but results are promising.

S. F. Jones, MD, FCCP, DABSM

Reference

1. Brassington GS, King AC, Bliwise DL. Sleep problems as a risk factor falls in a sample of community-dwelling adults aged 64-99 years. *J Am Geriatr Soc.* 2000;48: 1234-1240.

8 Critical Care Medicine

Introduction

Wow! I can't believe another whole year has passed. The articles continue to be first rate and fascinating!

Our lead-off article by Drs Schweickert and Kress shows that there is continued innovation in Critical Care. This article about early mobilization goes over the "how to," "why," and "it works"—the interaction of mind, body and just the fact that this (early mobilization) is the cutting edge of what we need to be doing. Of course, there is a lot involved with this. It means that restraint plans have to be changed and that traditional roles have to be changed since physical therapists can't do this alone. There must be a team effort to have patients stand or walk. In addition, it has been proven to be safe. Obviously, medications have to be markedly decreased. We can't just have the patients tied down in bed asleep on high levels of sedation. In fact, medications will need to be turned off. But we are learning as we approach intensive care unit (ICU) delirium more scientifically that our medications are probably making delirium worse instead of better. I hope you enjoy this great article.

Secondly, many of us hear about proportional assist ventilation. The nice article from Italy with Dr Costa and partners outlines how proportional assist looks when set up next to pressure support. I found this really useful in helping me understand the concepts as we move into, again, a more scientific approach to mechanical ventilation.

The third article is likewise very practical yet very helpful. Dr Yeh and partners from Taiwan show us that it is possible to decrease pneumonia in acute strokes. The way to do this is to focus on dysphasia early. Pneumonia has been associated with up to 70% in people with new strokes. Clearly this adds to morbidity and mortality. Thus focusing on what we can do to prevent this is the right thing to do.

I have been a fan of air pressure release ventilation for a long time. Yet the literature has lagged or else I am just an outlier! The fifth article comparing airway pressure release ventilation (APRV) to conventional ventilation in a smoke inhalation acute lung injury (ALI) swine model is definitely worth reading. Unfortunately, for my own hypotheses, the APRV animals did worse than the conventional ventilation. Again, this means that we should follow the acute respiratory distress syndrome (ARDS) net first in all ALI/ARDS patients.

The article about noninvasive ventilation for acute respiratory failure with hematologic malignancies again is very useful. This is quite practical. These patients do have high rates of acute lung injury and ARDS. It's common practice to use noninvasive ventilation. Articles have been written on both sides of this. This study, again, confirms that noninvasive is probably the way to go unless the patient is moribund. Please enjoy reading it.

If you have to read only one article, I would recommend you read the article by Dr Gupta and partners about developing and validating a risk calculator for postoperative respiratory failure. This question comes up all the time. There is a website link provided. I've tried it and it is quite easy and practical to use. This allows us to avoid heuristic thinking and be more scientific in giving advice or planning for very ill patients after operations. The most high risk operations are brain, foregut, hepatopancreatobiliary, and aortic. Likewise, emergency cases, high American Society of Anesthesiologists (ASA) score, patients with low functional status and patients with ongoing systematic inflammatory response syndrome also will do worse. Please see my comments for the direct reference to the website.

The Glide Scope has revolutionized the teaching intubation and observing intubation on very ill patients. It is now also shown that it can be useful in morbidly obese patients. This supplants my previous practice primarily using fiber optic bronchoscope to intubate these patients. Andersen and partners have nicely demonstrated this in a prospective way.

Another must-read article is the one by Drs Nolan and Kelly about airway challenges in critical care. This is thoughtful and comprehensive. ICU intubations are truly high risk. The observation of 10% rate as being very high risk is certainly accurate. The solutions outlined are completely appropriate and reasonable. Please see the nice article here and my comments which go through it.

Many of us don't see anaphylaxis very often. Yet we do treat it a few times a year. The science of anaphylaxis and how to approach the treatment is very well discussed in the 10th article by Estelle Simons.

New technology is very exciting! The Massimo Company has released an oximeter that is able to give excellent trending of hemoglobin levels. This is a nice scientific study from researchers Dr Frasca and partners in France. It shows that the hemoglobin from lab data correlates extremely well with the oximetry of this.

The 13th article is another important one to read. Dr Walkey and collaborators have done an excellent service to us all by demonstrating that new onset atrial fibrillation occurring with severe sepsis increased death and hospital stroke. This is common. These people are very ill, and I think it is an important concept for those of us working in ICU to know. Probably it should change our practice so we anticoagulate all these patients if possible. I know it is not generally practiced on people who have transatrial fibrillation as part of septic shock. The risk factors for atrial fibrillation were really of no surprise and, again, were well discussed in the article and in my comments. Please take time to look at this.

The remaining articles have all packed a lot of punch. I would encourage you to read this entire section. I think it is fantastic. For example, the 14th article by some very experienced authors from the US military covers the current approach to acute nonmassive pulmonary. There is a business case for quality improvement on reducing sepsis. Dr Mavros et al challenges the old concept that atelectasis causes postoperative fever. These are great articles.

Please read and enjoy!

James A. Barker, MD, FACP, FCCP

Ventilator Weaning

Implementing Early Mobilization Interventions in Mechanically Ventilated Patients in the ICU

Schweickert WD, Kress JP (Univ of Pennsylvania, Philadelphia; Univ of Chicago, IL)
Chest 140:1612-1617, 2011

As ICU survival continues to improve, clinicians are faced with short- and long-term consequences of critical illness. Deconditioning and weakness have become common problems in survivors of critical illness requiring mechanical ventilation. Recent literature, mostly from a medical population of patients in the ICU, has challenged the patient care model of prolonged bed rest. Instead, the feasibility, safety, and benefits of early mobilization of mechanically ventilated ICU patients have been reported in recent publications. The benefits of early mobilization include reductions in length of stay in the ICU and hospital as well as improvements in strength and functional status. Such benefits can be accomplished with a remarkably acceptable patient safety profile. The importance of interactions between mind and body are highlighted by these studies, with improvements in patient awareness and reductions in ICU delirium being noted. Future research to address the benefits of early mobilization in other patient populations is needed. In addition, the potential for early mobilization to impact long-term outcomes in ICU survivors requires further study.

▶ There are many potential pitfalls and roadblocks to ambulating ill patients. Certainly, connection to high-tech devices is one of them. Nonetheless, early mobilization of ventilator patients is rapidly becoming state-of-the-art practice. It makes sense. Truncal stability and strengthening has to improve cough and ventilator weaning. Patients must be awake and interactive to walk. And mental outlook will certainly be improved in patients who are awake and alert and can see some new scenery.

This article is a combination how to and state of the art. It is nicely written and informative.

J. A. Barker, MD, FACP, FCCP

A physiologic comparison of proportional assist ventilation with load-adjustable gain factors (PAV+) versus pressure support ventilation (PSV)

Costa R, Spinazzola G, Cipriani F, et al (Catholic Univ of Rome, Italy)
Intensive Care Med 37:1494-1500, 2011

Purpose.—To compare patient—ventilator interaction during PSV and PAV+ in patients that are difficult to wean.

Methods.—This was a physiologic study involving 11 patients. During three consecutive trials (PSV first trial—PSV1, followed by PAV+, followed by a second PSV trial—PSV2, with the same settings as PSV1) we evaluated mechanical and patient respiratory pattern; inspiratory effort from excursion Pdi ($swing_{Pdi}$), and pressure—time products of the transdiaphragmatic (PTPdi) pressures. Inspiratory ($delay_{trinsp}$) and expiratory ($delay_{trexp}$) trigger delays, time of synchrony ($time_{syn}$), and asynchrony index (AI) were assessed.

Results.—Compared to PAV+, during PSV trials, the mechanical inspiratory time (Ti_{flow}) was significantly longer than patient inspiratory time (Ti_{pat}) ($p < 0.05$); Ti_{pat} showed a prolongation between PSV1 and PAV+, significant comparing PAV+ and PSV2 ($p < 0.05$). PAV+ significantly reduced $delay_{trexp}$ ($p < 0.001$). The portion of tidal volume (VT) delivered in phase with Ti_{pat} (VT_{pat}/VT_{mecc}) was significantly higher during PAV+ ($p < 0.01$). The time of synchrony was significantly longer during PAV+

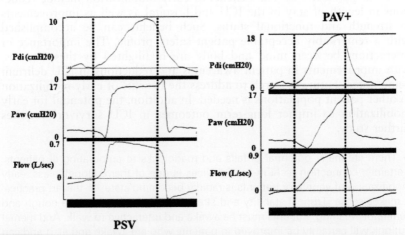

FIGURE 1.—Sample tracings from a patient during PSV and PAV+. Ti_{pat} is represented by the two *dotted lines*. (With kind permission from Springer Science+Business Media: Costa R, Spinazzola G, Cipriani F, et al. A physiologic comparison of proportional assist ventilation with load-adjustable gain factors (PAV+) versus pressure support ventilation (PSV). *Intensive Care Med.* 2011;37:1494-1500.)

than during PSV ($p < 0.001$). During PSV 5 patients out of 11 showed an AI greater than 10%, whereas the AI was nil during PAV+.

Conclusion.—PAV+ improves patient—ventilator interaction, significantly reducing the incidence of end-expiratory asynchrony and increasing the time of synchrony (Fig 1).

▶ Will proportional assist ventilation (PAV) replace pressure support ventilation (PSV) as newer generation ventilators replace older fleets? Is there much difference? Fig 1 demonstrates that airway pressure and flow curves are different in this small pilot study. This was largely an observational study looking at physiologic responses rather than weaning success. And of course, the small patient numbers are not designed to power a large weaning study.

Ventilator synchrony is improved in PAV. Asynchrony at end expiration is also reduced. However, gas exchange and respiratory patterns are not particularly changed. So will PAV be superior to PSV in weaning difficult-to-extubate patients? I would guess it will. But for now, this is only a guess. More data will follow in future years, I hope.

J. A. Barker, MD, FACP, FCCP

Ventilator-Associated Pneumonia

Dysphagia screening decreases pneumonia in acute stroke patients admitted to the stroke intensive care unit
Yeh S-J, Huang K-Y, Wang T-G, et al (Yun-Lin Branch of Natl Taiwan Univ Hosp, Douliu City, Yunlin County, Taiwan; Natl Taiwan Univ Hosp, Taipei City; et al)
J Neurol Sci 306:38-41, 2011

Dysphagia increases the risk of pneumonia in stroke patients. This study aimed to evaluate bedside swallowing screening for prevention of stroke-associated pneumonia (SAP) in acute stroke patients admitted to the intensive care unit (ICU). Consecutive acute stroke patients admitted to the stroke ICU from May 2006 to March 2007 were included. Patients were excluded if they were intubated on the first day of admission or had a transient ischemic attack. A 3-Step Swallowing Screen was introduced since October 2006 and therefore patients were divided into pre-screen and post-screen groups. A binary logistic regression model was used to determine independent risk factors for SAP and in-hospital death. There were 74 and 102 patients included in the pre- and post-screen groups, respectively. Pneumonia was associated with higher National Institutes of Health Stroke Scale (NIHSS) score, older age, nasogastric and endotracheal tube placement. After adjusting for age, gender, NIHSS score and nasogastric and endotracheal tube insertion, dysphagia screening was associated with a borderline decrease in SAP in all stroke patients (odds ratio, 0.42; 95% CI, 0.18—1.00; $p = 0.05$). However, dysphagia screening was not associated with reduction of in-hospital deaths. Systematic bedside swallowing screening is helpful for prevention of SAP in acute stroke patients admitted to the ICU.

▶ Pneumonia occurs in 30% of patients admitted with new stroke. This simple intervention looks promising for reducing this incidence. I doubt that it will eliminate all pneumonia in these patients, however, because probably a significant number aspirate near the time of the stroke. This nicely done study should change our practice for the better.

J. A. Barker, MD, FACP, FCCP

Acute Respiratory Disorder Syndrome

A Description of Intraoperative Ventilator Management in Patients with Acute Lung Injury and the Use of Lung Protective Ventilation Strategies
Blum JM, Maile M, Park PK, et al (Univ of Michigan Health System, Ann Arbor)
Anesthesiology 115:75-82, 2011

Background.—The incidence of acute lung injury (ALI) in hypoxic patients undergoing surgery is currently unknown. Previous studies have identified lung protective ventilation strategies that are beneficial in the treatment of ALI. The authors sought to determine the incidence and examine the use of lung protective ventilation strategies in patients receiving anesthetics with a known history of ALI.

Methods.—The ventilation parameters that were used in all patients were reviewed, with an average preoperative $Paco_2/Fio_2$ ratio of ≤ 300 between January 1, 2005 and July 1, 2009. This dataset was then merged with a dataset of patients screened for ALI. The median tidal volume, positive end-expiratory pressure, peak inspiratory pressures, fraction inhaled oxygen, oxygen saturation, and tidal volumes were compared between groups.

Results.—A total of 1,286 patients met criteria for inclusion; 242 had a diagnosis of ALI preoperatively. Comparison of patients with ALI *versus* those without ALI found statistically yet clinically insignificant differences between the ventilation strategies between the groups in peak inspiratory pressures and positive end-expiratory pressure but no other category. The tidal volumes in cc/kg predicted body weight were approximately 8.7 in both groups. Peak inspiratory pressures were found to be 27.87 cm H_2O on average in the non-ALI group and 29.2 in the ALI group.

Conclusion.—Similar ventilation strategies are used between patients with ALI and those without ALI. These findings suggest that anesthesiologists are not using lung protective ventilation strategies when ventilating patients with low $Paco_2/Fio_2$ ratios and ALI, and instead are treating hypoxia and ALI with higher concentrations of oxygen and peak pressures.

▶ Old habits die hard. Or should we say, when we turn over rocks we find toadstools?

These authors have painstakingly revealed that patients with acute lung injury who require surgery do NOT receive ARDSnet best care with optimal positive end expiratory pressure and low tidal volumes. Anesthesiology as a profession has led the way in best practices. I am confident that these data are the first step in a necessary recalibration. It will require re-education and preoperative checklists. Follow-up studies will be of interest here.

J. A. Barker, MD, FACP, FCCP

Comparison of airway pressure release ventilation to conventional mechanical ventilation in the early management of smoke inhalation injury in swine

Batchinsky AI, Burkett SE, Zanders TB, et al (United States Army Inst of Surgical Res, Fort Sam Houston, TX; Brooke Army Med Ctr, Fort Sam Houston, TX)
Crit Care Med 39:2314-2321, 2011

Objective.—The role of airway pressure release ventilation in the management of early smoke inhalation injury has not been studied. We compared the effects of airway pressure release ventilation and conventional mechanical ventilation on oxygenation in a porcine model of acute respiratory distress syndrome induced by wood smoke inhalation.

Design.—Prospective animal study.

Setting.—Government laboratory animal intensive care unit.

Patients.—Thirty-three Yorkshire pigs.

Interventions.—Smoke inhalation injury.

Measurements and Main Results.—Anesthetized female Yorkshire pigs (n = 33) inhaled room-temperature pine-bark smoke. Before injury, the pigs were randomized to receive conventional mechanical ventilation (n = 15) or airway pressure release ventilation (n = 12) for 48 hrs after smoke inhalation. As acute respiratory distress syndrome developed (PaO_2/FIO_2 ratio <200), plateau pressures were limited to <35 cm H_2O. Six uninjured pigs received conventional mechanical ventilation for 48 hrs and served as time controls. Changes in PaO_2/FIO_2 ratio, tidal volume, respiratory rate, mean airway pressure, plateau pressure, and hemodynamic variables were recorded. Survival was assessed using Kaplan-Meier analysis. PaO_2/FIO_2 ratio was lower in airway pressure release ventilation vs. conventional mechanical ventilation pigs at 12, 18, and 24 hrs ($p < .05$) but not at 48 hrs. Tidal volumes were lower in conventional mechanical ventilation animals between 30 and 48 hrs post injury ($p < .05$). Respiratory rates were lower in airway pressure release ventilation at 24, 42, and 48 hrs ($p < .05$). Mean airway pressures were higher in airway pressure release ventilation animals between 6 and 48 hrs ($p < .05$). There was no difference in plateau pressures, hemodynamic variables, or survival between conventional mechanical ventilation and airway pressure release ventilation pigs.

Conclusions.—In this model of acute respiratory distress syndrome caused by severe smoke inhalation in swine, airway pressure release ventilation-treated animals developed acute respiratory distress syndrome faster than conventional mechanical ventilation-treated animals, showing a lower PaO_2/FIO_2 ratio at 12, 18, and 24 hrs after injury. At other time points, PaO_2/FIO_2 ratio was not different between conventional mechanical ventilation and airway pressure release ventilation.

▶ I am a fan of airway pressure release ventilation (APRV). Many patients are quite comfortable on the mode; spontaneous breathing is allowed, which decreases need for sedation and paralytics; peak and mean airway pressures are inherently controlled; and oxygenation often seems improved compared with conventional ventilation. However, there is a paucity of evidence to support my biases. This article provides evidence, but it is not pro-APRV for us fans of the technique.

Mortality and late findings are not different between the 2 groups. However, the conventional treated swine group has improved findings in the critical first 48 hours. Thus, in acute respiratory distress syndrome (in smoke inhalation injured swine, at least), early APRV has no advantage over conventional mechanical ventilation with optimal positive-end expiratory pressure and is potentially harmful. I stand corrected!

J. A. Barker, MD, FACP, FCCP

Noninvasive versus invasive ventilation for acute respiratory failure in patients with hematologic malignancies: A 5-year multicenter observational survey
Gristina GR, on behalf of the GiViTI (Italian Group for the Evaluation of Interventions in Intensive Care Medicine) (San Camillo-Forlanini Hosp, Rome, Italy; et al)
Crit Care Med 39:2232-2239, 2011

Background.—Mortality is high among patients with hematologic malignancies admitted to intensive care units for acute respiratory failure. Early noninvasive mechanical ventilation seems to improve outcomes.

Objective.—To characterize noninvasive mechanical ventilation use in Italian intensive care units for acute respiratory failure patients with hematologic malignancies and its impact on outcomes vs. invasive mechanical ventilation.

Design, Setting, Participants.—Retrospective analysis of observational data prospectively collected in 2002–2006 on 1,302 patients with hematologic malignancies admitted with acute respiratory failure to 158 Italian intensive care units.

Measurements.—Mortality (intensive care unit and hospital) was assessed in patients treated initially with noninvasive mechanical ventilation vs. invasive mechanical ventilation and in those treated with invasive mechanical ventilation *ab initio* vs. after noninvasive mechanical ventilation failure. Findings were adjusted for propensity scores reflecting the probability of initial treatment with noninvasive mechanical ventilation.

Results.—Few patients (21%) initially received noninvasive mechanical ventilation; 46% of these later required invasive mechanical ventilation. Better outcomes were associated with successful noninvasive mechanical ventilation (vs. invasive mechanical ventilation *ab initio* and vs. invasive mechanical ventilation after noninvasive mechanical ventilation failure), particularly in patients with acute lung injury/adult respiratory distress syndrome (mortality: 42% vs. 69% and 77%, respectively). Delayed vs. immediate invasive mechanical ventilation was associated with slightly but not significantly higher hospital mortality (65% vs. 58%, $p = .12$). After propensity-score adjustment, noninvasive mechanical ventilation was associated with significantly lower mortality than invasive mechanical ventilation.

Limitations.—The population could not be stratified according to specific hematologic diagnoses. Furthermore, the study was observational, and treatment groups may have included unaccounted for differences in covariates although the risk of this bias was minimized with propensity score regression adjustment.

Conclusions.—In patients with hematologic malignancies, acute respiratory failure should probably be managed initially with noninvasive mechanical ventilation. Further study is needed to determine whether immediate invasive mechanical ventilation might offer some benefits for those with acute lung injury/adult respiratory distress syndrome.

▶ This is clearly a controversial area because there are previous studies with results falling on both sides of the question. Once again, it appears that noninvasive ventilation not only yields better outcomes but is preferred. Probably those patients who meet acute respiratory distress syndrome criteria (low peak flow ratios) should be the only ones intubated first.

J. A. Barker, MD, FACP, FCCP

Acute Respiratory Failure

Development and Validation of a Risk Calculator Predicting Postoperative Respiratory Failure

Gupta H, Gupta PK, Fang X, et al (Creighton Univ, Omaha, NE; et al)
Chest 140:1207-1215, 2011

Background.—Postoperative respiratory failure (PRF) (requiring mechanical ventilation >48 h after surgery or unplanned intubation within 30 days of surgery) is associated with significant morbidity and mortality. The objective of this study was to identify preoperative factors associated with an increased risk of PRF and subsequently develop and validate a risk calculator.

Methods.—The American College of Surgeons National Surgical Quality Improvement Program (NSQIP), a multicenter, prospective data set (2007-2008), was used. The 2007 data set (n = 211,410) served as the training set and the 2008 data set (n = 257,385) as the validation set.

Results.—In the training set, 6,531 patients (3.1%) developed PRF. Patients who developed PRF had a significantly higher 30-day mortality

(25.62% vs 0.98%, P < .0001). On multivariate logistic regression analysis, five preoperative predictors of PRF were identified: type of surgery, emergency case, dependent functional status, preoperative sepsis, and higher American Society of Anesthesiologists (ASA) class. The risk model based on the training data set was subsequently validated on the validation data set. The model performance was very similar between the training and the validation data sets (c-statistic, 0.894 and 0.897, respectively). The high c-statistics (area under the receiver operating characteristic curve) indicate excellent predictive performance. The risk model was used to develop an interactive risk calculator.

Conclusions.—Preoperative variables associated with increased risk of PRF include type of surgery, emergency case, dependent functional status, sepsis, and higher ASA class. The validated risk calculator provides a risk estimate of PRF and is anticipated to aid in surgical decision making and informed patient consent.

▶ This is a terrific and useful article. These questions come up all the time. Now instead of guessing or heuristic thinking—"Gee, my last case of a septic 90-year-old with aortic dissection and bowel infarct died; I bet this 40-year-old otherwise healthy person will too"—we can actually use real data. I downloaded the calculator, and it works handily.

The website is http://www.surgicalriskcalculator.com/prf-risk-calculator. Download is free.

The types of operation that were the highest risk were the following: brain, foregut, hepatopancreatobiliary, and aortic. Emergency cases, high American Society of Anesthesiologists score, patients with low functional status, and cases with systemic inflammatory response syndrome or sepsis were also much more likely to be accompanied by respiratory failure.

Why is all this so important when only 3% of cases lead to postoperative respiratory failure? Because 25% of these patients will die, and the other 75% will have increased length of stay as well.

J. A. Barker, MD, FACP, FCCP

Airway Management

GlideScope videolaryngoscope vs. Macintosh direct laryngoscope for intubation of morbidly obese patients: a randomized trial

Andersen LH, Rovsing L, Olsen KS (Copenhagen Univ Hosp, Glostrup, Denmark)
Acta Anaesthesiol Scand 55:1090-1097, 2011

Background.—Morbidly obese patients are at increased risk of hypoxemia during tracheal intubation because of increased frequency of difficult and impossible intubation and a decreased apnea tolerance. In this study, intubation with the GlideScope videolaryngoscope (GS) was compared with the Macintosh direct laryngoscope (DL) in a group of morbidly obese patients.

Methods.—One hundred consecutive patients (body mass index ≥ 35 kg/m^2) scheduled for bariatric surgery were randomized 1 : 1 to intubation with GS (group GS) or DL (group DL). The primary outcome was intubation time. Secondary outcomes were number of attempts, Cormack-Lehane grade, intubation difficulty scale score (IDS), subjective difficulty of intubation, desaturation, airway bleeding, postoperative sore throat, and hoarseness. Group assignment was not blinded.

Results.—Intubation in group GS and group DL lasted 48 (22−148) and 32 s (17−209), respectively (median (range); $P = 0.0001$); median difference 11 s (95% confidence interval 6−17). Laryngoscopic views were better in group GS with Cormack-Lehane grades 1/2/3/4 distributed as 35/13/2/0 vs. 23/13/10/4 in group DL ($P = 0.003$). IDS scores were significantly lower with GS than with DL. No other statistically significant differences were found. Two cases of failed intubation occurred in group DL vs. none in group GS (non-significant). Both patients were intubated with the GlideScope without problems.

Conclusion.—Intubation of morbidly obese patients with GS was slightly slower than with DL. The increased intubation time was of no clinical consequence as no patients became hypoxemic. Both devices generally performed well in the studied population, but the GS provided better laryngoscopic views and decreased IDS scores.

▶ The GlideScope (GS) is revolutionizing critical care intubations. These authors have nicely performed a systematic research project on potentially difficult airway patients and shown a slight advantage of the GS to a MacIntosh curved blade approach.

Personally, I will continue to use fiberoptic intubations for this particular group of patients.

J. A. Barker, MD, FACP, FCCP

Airway challenges in critical care
Nolan JP, Kelly FE (Royal United Hosp, Bath, UK)
Anaesthesia 66:81-92, 2011

Airway management in the intensive care unit is more problematic than during anaesthesia. In general, critically ill patients have less physiological reserve and complications are more common, both during the initial airway intervention (which includes risks associated with induction of anaesthesia), and later once the airway has been secured. Despite these known risks, those managing the airway of a critically ill patient, particularly out of hours, may be relatively inexperienced. Solutions to these challenging airway problems include: recognition of those patients with a potential airway problem; implementation of a plan to deal with their airway; immediate availability of a difficult airway trolley; use of capnography for every airway intervention and continuously in all ventilator-dependent patients; and appropriate training of all intensive care unit staff including use of simulation.

▶ This is a thoughtful, comprehensive discussion of an important everyday problem in the intensive care unit (ICU). The estimation of 10% ICU intubations as being difficult airways is accurate. The off-hours timing, inexperience of operators, and human factors are all important. The risks, of course, are tremendous: death or significant morbidity.

The solutions suggested again are appropriate and reasonable:

1. Plan for difficult airways. Have equipment available and access to experienced operators.
2. Have equipment at the ready.
3. Plan, plan, plan. This includes standardized anesthetics such as ketamine and etomidate.
4. Given the poor results of cricothyrotomy, standardized training in this technique should be included in all advanced airway courses.
5. Have protocols for displaced trach tubes. I totally agree with this. This seems to be an area that is frequently overlooked in airway management planning.
6. Use simulators and repetition to control for human factors.

I think all trainees and program directors should read this article.

J. A. Barker, MD, FACP, FCCP

Anaphylaxis pathogenesis and treatment
Simons FER (Univ of Manitoba, Winnipeg, Canada)
Allergy 66:31-34, 2011

Anaphylaxis is a serious allergic reaction that is rapid in onset and sometimes leads to death. Understanding mechanisms, triggers, and patient-specific risk factors for severe or fatal anaphylaxis is critically important. Diagnosis of anaphylaxis is currently based on established clinical criteria. Epinephrine (adrenaline) is the first-line medication for anaphylaxis treatment and delay in injecting it contributes to biphasic reactions, hypoxic-ischemic encephalopathy, and fatality. Here, we focus on four important areas of translational research in anaphylaxis: studies of potential new biomarkers to support the clinical diagnosis of anaphylaxis, laboratory tests to distinguish allergen sensitization from clinical risk of anaphylaxis, the primary role of epinephrine (adrenaline) in anaphylaxis treatment, and strengthening the overall evidence base for anaphylaxis treatment (Fig 1).

▶ Anaphylaxis is fortunately a rather uncommon critical care problem. However, there is much room for more evidence-based information. Therapy with epinephrine remains state of the art. However, the author points out the lack of information

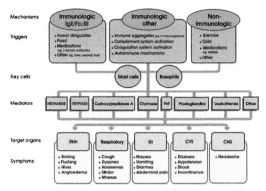

FIGURE 1.—Anaphylaxis pathogenesis. Reprinted from The Journal of Allergy and Clinical Immunology, 121/2, Simons FER, Anaphylaxis. 2008 Mini-primer on allergic and immunologic diseases, S402-S407, Copyright (2008), with permission from Elsevier. (Reprinted from Simons FER, Anaphylaxis pathogenesis and treatment. *Allergy*. 2011;66:31-34, with permission from John Wiley and Sons (www.interscience.wiley.com).)

as to dosing or even efficacy of antihistamines and steroids, which are routinely given. Fig 1 very nicely outlines the current ideas as to pathophysiology.

J. A. Barker, MD, FACP, FCCP

Imaging and Monitoring in the ICU

Accuracy of a continuous noninvasive hemoglobin monitor in intensive care unit patients

Frasca D, Dahyot-Fizelier C, Catherine K, et al (Centre Hospitalier Universitaire de Poitiers, France)
Crit Care Med 39:2277-2282, 2011

Objective.—To determine whether noninvasive hemoglobin measurement by Pulse CO-Oximetry could provide clinically acceptable absolute and trend accuracy in critically ill patients, compared to other invasive methods of hemoglobin assessment available at bedside and the gold standard, the laboratory analyzer.

Design.—Prospective study.

Setting.—Surgical intensive care unit of a university teaching hospital.

Patients.—Sixty-two patients continuously monitored with Pulse CO-Oximetry (Masimo Radical-7).

Interventions.—None.

Measurements and Results.—Four hundred seventy-one blood samples were analyzed by a point-of-care device (HemoCue 301), a satellite lab CO-Oximeter (Siemens RapidPoint 405), and a laboratory hematology analyzer (Sysmex XT-2000i), which was considered the reference device. Hemoglobin values reported from the invasive methods were compared to the values reported by the Pulse CO-Oximeter at the time of blood draw. When the case-to-case variation was assessed, the bias and limits of agreement were 0.0 ± 1.0 g/dL for the Pulse CO-Oximeter, 0.3 ± 1.3 g/dL for the point-of-care device, and 0.9 ± 0.6 g/dL for the satellite lab CO-Oximeter compared to the reference method. Pulse CO-Oximetry showed similar trend accuracy as satellite lab CO-Oximetry, whereas the point-of-care device did not appear to follow the trend of the laboratory analyzer as well as the other test devices.

Conclusion.—When compared to laboratory reference values, hemoglobin measurement with Pulse CO-Oximetry has absolute accuracy and trending accuracy similar to widely used, invasive methods of hemoglobin measurement at bedside. Hemoglobin measurement with pulse CO-Oximetry has the additional advantages of providing continuous measurements, noninvasively, which may facilitate hemoglobin monitoring in the intensive care unit.

▶ It would seem that this technology has many important advantages. Because this study now independently verifies that it is indeed accurate technology, we will have to assess how our care will change. For example, do we still wait for equilibration effect in gastrointestinal bleeding patients while we give blood and saline, or will we react differently if we know actual hemoglobin trends? I think we will adjust and change practice patterns.

J. A. Barker, MD, FACP, FCCP

Cardiopulmonary Interactions

Prognostic implications of arterial blood gases in acute decompensated heart failure

Miñana G, Núñez J, Bañuls P, et al (Universitat de Valencia, Spain)
Eur J Intern Med 22:489-494, 2011

Background.—The prognostic value of arterial blood gases (ABG) in patients with acute decompensated heart failure (ADHF) is not well-established. We therefore conducted the present study to determine the relationship between ABG on admission and long-term mortality in patients with ADHF.

Methods.—We studied 588 patients consecutively admitted to our department with ADHF. ABG and classical prognostic variables were determined at patients' arrival to the emergency department. The independent association among the main variables of ABG (pO2, pCO2 and pH) and mortality was assessed with Cox regression analysis.

Results.—At a median follow-up of 23 months, 221 deaths (37.6%) were registered. 308 (52.4%), 54 (9.2%) and 50 (8.5%) patients showed hypoxemia (pO2 <60 mm Hg), hypercapnia (pCO2 >50 mm Hg) and acidosis (pH <7.35), respectively. Patients with hypoxemia, hypercapnia and acidosis did not show higher mortality rates (38% vs. 37.1%, 42.6% vs. 37.1%, and 48% vs. 36.6%, respectively; p-value = ns for all comparisons). In multivariate analysis, after adjusting for well-known prognostic covariates, pO2, pCO2 and pH did not show a significant association with mortality. Hazard ratios (HR) for these variables were: pO2, per increase in 10 mm Hg: 0.99 (95% CI: 0.90-1.09), p = 0.861; pCO2, per increase in 10 mm Hg: 1.12 (95% CI: 0.91–1.39), p = 0.262; pH per increase in 0.1: 1.01 (95% CI: 0.99–1.04), p = 0.309. When dichotomizing these variables according to established cut-points, the HR were: hypoxemia (pO2 <60 mm Hg): 1.07 (95% CI: 0.81–1.40), p = 0.637; hypercapnia (pCO2 >50 mm Hg): 0.98 (95% CI: 0.62–1.57), p = 0.952; acidosis (pH <7.35): 1.38 (95% CI: 0.87–2.19), p = 0.173.

Conclusion.—In patients admitted with ADHF, admission arterial pO2, pCO2 and pH were not associated with all-cause long-term mortality.

▶ I am surprised that this study has negative results. This does emphasize the dogma that we in Pulmonary Medicine will teach, "If it clears in 24 hours, think heart failure." There are some positive correlations that we might expect: hypoxemia is common in those with low ejection fractions, and hypercarbia is quite common in those with underlying chronic obstructive pulmonary disease as well.

I agree with these authors. The negative correlations with arterial blood gases findings clearly indicate that a lot of reversibility is possible in acute decompensations of heart failure. Blood gases should not be used for prognostication in these patients.

J. A. Barker, MD, FACP, FCCP

Incident Stroke and Mortality Associated With New-Onset Atrial Fibrillation in Patients Hospitalized With Severe Sepsis

Walkey AJ, Wiener RS, Ghobrial JM, et al (Boston Univ School of Medicine, MA; Univ of Washington School of Medicine, Seattle; et al)
JAMA 306:2248-2255, 2011

Context.—New-onset atrial fibrillation (AF) has been reported in 6% to 20% of patients with severe sepsis. Chronic AF is a known risk factor for stroke and death, but the clinical significance of new-onset AF in the setting of severe sepsis is uncertain.

Objective.—To determine the in-hospital stroke and in-hospital mortality risks associated with new-onset AF in patients with severe sepsis.

Design and Setting.—Retrospective population-based cohort of California State Inpatient Database administrative claims data from nonfederal acute care hospitals for January 1 through December 31, 2007.

Patients.—Data were available for 3 144 787 hospitalized adults. Severe sepsis (n = 49 082 [1.56%]) was defined by validated *International Classification of Diseases, Ninth Revision, Clinical Modification (ICD-9-CM)* code 995.92. New-onset AF was defined as AF that occurred during the hospital stay, after excluding AF cases present at admission.

Main Outcome Measures.—A priori outcome measures were in-hospital ischemic stroke (*ICD-9-CM* codes 433, 434, or 436) and mortality.

Results.—Patients with severe sepsis were a mean age of 69 (SD, 16) years and 48% were women. New-onset AF occurred in 5.9% of patients with severe sepsis vs 0.65% of patients without severe sepsis (multivariable-adjusted odds ratio [OR], 6.82; 95% CI, 6.54-7.11; $P<.001$). Severe sepsis was present in 14% of all new-onset AF in hospitalized adults. Compared with severe sepsis patients without new-onset AF, patients with new-onset AF during severe sepsis had greater risks of in-hospital stroke (75/2896 [2.6%] vs 306/46 186 [0.6%] strokes; adjusted OR, 2.70; 95% CI, 2.05-3.57; $P<.001$) and in-hospital mortality (1629 [56%] vs 18 027 [39%] deaths; adjusted relative risk, 1.07; 95% CI, 1.04-1.11; $P<.001$). Findings were robust across 2 definitions of severe sepsis, multiple methods of addressing confounding, and multiple sensitivity analyses.

Conclusion.—Among patients with severe sepsis, patients with new-onset AF were at increased risk of in-hospital stroke and death compared with patients with no AF and patients with preexisting AF (Table 2).

▶ As intensivists, we are used to the onset of atrial fibrillation and other atrial arrhythmias with our very ill patients. This outcomes article nicely elucidates

TABLE 2.—Factors Associated With New-Onset Atrial Fibrillation Among Patients With Severe Sepsis[a]

Variables	Odds Ratio (95% CI)
Age, per 10 y	1.52 (1.47-1.56)
Female sex	0.83 (0.76-0.90)
Race/ethnicity	
White	1 [Reference]
Black	0.67 (0.58-0.78)
Hispanic	0.58 (0.50-0.63)
Other	0.78 (0.69-0.87)
Comorbidities[b]	
Hypertension	0.88 (0.81-0.95)
Diabetes mellitus	0.82 (0.75-0.90)
Obesity	1.20 (1.03-1.40)
Congestive heart failure	1.61 (1.41-1.83)
Metastatic or hematologic malignancy	1.23 (1.09-1.39)
Prior stroke	1.64 (1.35-2.01)
Acute organ dysfunction[b]	
Per organ failure	1.12 (1.05-1.19)
Respiratory failure	2.81 (2.48-3.19)
Renal failure	1.40 (1.26-1.56)
Hematologic failure	1.50 (1.34-1.68)
Acidosis	0.87 (0.77-0.97)
Right heart catheterization[b]	2.25 (1.87-2.70)
Source of infection[b]	
Respiratory tract	1.27 (1.14-1.40)
Urinary tract	0.89 (0.81-0.99)
Abdominal	1.77 (1.59-1.97)
Primary bacteremia	1.17 (1.02-1.36)
Skin or soft tissue	1.33 (1.14-1.55)
Pathogen type[b]	
Gram-positive bacteria	1.29 (1.18-1.55)
Fungal	1.59 (1.27-2.00)

[a]C statistic=0.760.
[b]The reference group for these variables is none present.

many of the issues we should understand with regard to this situation. Of course, the article is focused on septic shock and atrial fibrillation. The risk factors for atrial fibrillation (high odds ratios) are outlined in Table 2. They are not surprising to me: advanced age, congestive heart failure, metastatic malignancy, prior stroke, organ failure of any type, especially respiratory failure, right heart catheterization, abdominal infection, and fungal infection. The highest risk was right heart catheterization. Maybe this explains the increased mortality seen in prior studies of Swan Ganz usage. Pressor types are not discussed but would be important cofactors in future studies. For example, my own practice is to switch, if possible, to phenylephrine (pure alpha) if arrhythmias occur with norepinephrine or dopamine. Does this really work? I don't know.

In addition, stroke rates and mortality do go up in those patients with atrial fibrillation. Knowing this, we should certainly be considering whether we should be anticoagulating all of these patients. If the atrial fibrillation resolves during the admission, should we anticoagulate them at discharge? I don't know that either. There will clearly be more to follow on this issue.

J. A. Barker, MD, FACP, FCCP

Pulmonary Hypertension in the ICU

Current Approach to the Diagnosis of Acute Nonmassive Pulmonary Embolism

Moores LK, King CS, Holley AB (Uniformed Services Univ of the Health Sciences, Bethesda, MD; Beaumont Army Med Ctr, El Paso, TX; Walter Reed Army Med Ctr, Washington, DC)
Chest 140:509-518, 2011

Pulmonary embolism is a common and potentially lethal disease. Given the variable presentation and associated morbidity of this condition, an accurate and efficient diagnostic algorithm is required. Clinical pretest probability serves as the root of any diagnostic approach. We, thus, review several clinical decision rules that may help standardize this determination. Using a review of the literature, the accuracy, predictive values, and likelihood ratios for several diagnostic tests are described. The combination of these tests, based on the pretest probability of disease, can be used in a Bayesian fashion to make accurate treatment decisions. A completely noninvasive diagnostic algorithm for patients presenting with suspected acute pulmonary embolism is proposed (Table 8).

▶ This is a great and tremendously useful article. This information is very much a moving target, so I particularly like this logical yet pragmatic article.

I find Table 8 invaluable. This is the information we are always asked as consultants. Just how good is...?

Likewise, Fig 1 in the original article appears to be a busy algorithm but actually isn't if one just follows each branch. Risk to patients is kept low by

TABLE 8.—Exclusion or Confirmation of Acute PE Using a Noninvasive Diagnostic Algorithm

Exclusion of PE	NLR	Posttest Probability, %	Confirmation of PE	PLR	Posttest Probability, %
Low PTP (prevalence of PE < 10%)					
Normal D-dimer[a]	0.29	<5	Positive CUS	16.2	>65
Normal $\dot{V}/\dot{Q}$ scan	0.05	<1	High prob $\dot{V}/\dot{Q}$	18.3	~70[b]
Low prob $\dot{V}/\dot{Q}$ scan	0.36	<4	Positive CTPA in main or lobar arteries	24.1	>70
Indeterminate $\dot{V}/\dot{Q}$[c]	ND				
Negative CTPA	0.11	<2			
Intermediate PTP (prevalence of PE approximately 35%)					
Normal quantitative ELISA D-dimer	0.08	<5	Positive CUS	16.2	>85
Normal $\dot{V}/\dot{Q}$ scan	0.05	<5	High prob $\dot{V}/\dot{Q}$	18.3	>88
Low prob $\dot{V}/\dot{Q}$[c]	0.36	~10			
Negative CTPA	0.11	<5	Positive CTPA	24.1	>92
High PTP (prevalence of PE >70%)					
Negative CTPA[d]	0.11	<20	Positive CUS	16.2	> 95
			High prob $\dot{V}/\dot{Q}$	18.3	> 95
			Positive CTPA	24.1	> 95

CTPA = CT pulmonary angiography; CUS = compression ultrasonography; ELISA = enzyme-linked immunosorbent assay; ND = not done; NLR = negative likelihood ratio; PLR = positive likelihood ratio; prob = probability. See Table 1 and 7 legends for expansion of other abbreviations.
[a]Standard or rapid ELISA.
[b]Wide CI on PLR; discordant results may warrant further confirmation.
[c]Study by Salaun et al 35 suggest this is safe. May need further validation.
[d]Outcome studies suggest this is safe.[56] Some may perform CUS or obtain follow-up CUS in 5-7 d.

marching through it using likelihoods and least invasive tests first. All of us need to know this information—or have a copy of this article handy.

J. A. Barker, MD, FACP, FCCP

Trauma Issues

Costs of Postoperative Sepsis: The Business Case for Quality Improvement to Reduce Postoperative Sepsis in Veterans Affairs Hospitals

Vaughan-Sarrazin MS, Bayman L, Cullen JJ (Univ of Iowa College of Medicine)
Arch Surg 146:944-951, 2011

Objective.—To estimate the incremental costs associated with sepsis as a complication of general surgery, controlling for patient risk factors that may affect costs (eg, surgical complexity and comorbidity) and hospital-level variation in costs.

Design.—Database analysis.

Setting.—One hundred eighteen Veterans Health Affairs hospitals.

Patients.—A total of 13 878 patients undergoing general surgery during fiscal year 2006 (October 1, 2005, through September 30, 2006).

Main Outcome Measures.—Incremental costs associated with sepsis as a complication of general surgery (controlling for patient risk factors and hospital-level variation of costs), as well as the increase in costs associated with complications that co-occur with sepsis. Costs were estimated using the Veterans Health Affairs Decision Support System, and patient risk factors and postoperative complications were identified in the Veterans Affairs Surgical Quality Improvement Program database.

Results.—Overall, 564 of 13 878 patients undergoing general surgery developed postoperative sepsis, for a rate of 4.1%. The average unadjusted cost for patients with no sepsis was $24 923, whereas the average cost for patients with sepsis was 3.6 times higher at $88 747. In risk-adjusted analyses, the relative costs were 2.28 times greater for patients with sepsis relative to patients without sepsis (95% confidence interval, 2.19-2.38), with the difference in risk-adjusted costs estimated at $26 972 (ie, $21 045 vs $48 017). Sepsis often co-occurred with other types of complications, most frequently with failure to wean the patient from mechanical ventilation after 48 hours (36%), postoperative pneumonia (31%), and reintubation for respiratory or cardiac failure (29%). Costs were highest when sepsis occurred with pneumonia or failure to wean the patient from mechanical ventilation after 48 hours.

Conclusion.—Given the high cost of treating sepsis, a business case can be made for quality improvement initiatives that reduce the likelihood of postoperative sepsis.

▶ The Veterans Affairs Surgical Quality Improvement Program preceded the National Surgical Quality Improvement Program and continues to contribute both to medical literature and to continuous quality improvement. This very nice article outlines just how expensive complications are—not only in the human cost of morbidity and mortality but also in dollars. Clearly, front-end proactive care is better in all instances.

J. A. Barker, MD, FACP, FCCP

Atelectasis as a Cause of Postoperative Fever: Where Is the Clinical Evidence?

Mavros MN, Velmahos GC, Falagas ME (Alfa Inst of Biomedical Sciences (AIBS), Athens, Greece; Massachusetts General Hosp and Harvard Med School, Boston)
Chest 140:418-424, 2011

Background.—Atelectasis is considered to be the most common cause of early postoperative fever (EPF) but the existing evidence is contradictory. We sought to determine if atelectasis is associated with EPF by analyzing the relevant published evidence.

Methods.—We performed a systematic search in PubMed and Scopus databases to identify studies examining the association between atelectasis and EPF.

Results.—A total of eight studies, including 998 cardiac, abdominal, and maxillofacial surgery patients, were eligible for analysis. Only two studies specifically examined our question, and six additional articles reported sufficient data to be included. Only one study reported a significant association between postoperative atelectasis and fever, whereas the remaining studies indicated no such association. The performance of EPF as a diagnostic test for atelectasis was also assessed, and EPF performed poorly (pooled diagnostic OR, 1.40; 95% CI, 0.92-2.12). The significant heterogeneity among the studies precluded a formal metaanalysis.

Conclusion.—The available evidence regarding the association of atelectasis and fever is scarce. We found no clinical evidence supporting the concept that atelectasis is associated with EPF. More so, there is no clear evidence that atelectasis causes fever at all. Large studies are needed to precisely evaluate the contribution of atelectasis in EPF.

▶ "Wound, wind, water, walk." I remember the mantra from third-year Surgery Clerkship. (I probably don't remember much else, come to think of it.) The "wind" part was supposed to remind one of atelectasis or early pneumonia as cause of postoperative fever. Yet these investigators and others in recent years demonstrate that atelectasis doesn't cause fever. One would think that it should. After all, bronchoscopy with bronchoalveolar lavage (BAL) seems to. Perhaps the difference is that bronchoscopy with BAL is actively altering alveoli and thus inducing pyrogen release, whereas atelectasis is passive. Alveoli are not necessarily disturbed.

The other shoe to drop is this one: Incentive spirometry doesn't really work either. It is a brave new evidence based medicine world out there.

J. A. Barker, MD, FACP, FCCP

A Method to Detect Occult Pneumothorax With Chest Radiography
Matsumoto S, Kishikawa M, Hayakawa K, et al (Saiseikai Yokohamashi Tobu Hosp, Kanagawa, Japan; Saiseikai Fukuoka General Hosp, Japan)
Ann Emerg Med 57:378-381, 2011

Small pneumothoraces are often not visible on supine screening chest radiographs because they develop anteriorly to the lung. These pneumothoraces are termed occult. Occult pneumothoraces account for an astonishingly high 52% to 63% of all traumatic pneumothoraces. A 19-year-old obese woman was involved in a head-on car accident. The admission anteroposterior chest radiographs were unremarkable. Because of the presence of right chest tenderness and an abrasion, we suspected the presence of a pneumothorax. Thus, we decided to take a supine oblique chest radiograph of the right side of the thorax, which clearly revealed a visceral pleural line, consistent with a diagnosis of traumatic pneumothorax. A pneumothorax may be present when a supine chest radiograph reveals either an apparent deepening of the costophrenic angle (the "deep sulcus sign") or the presence of 2 diaphragm-lung interfaces (the "double diaphragm sign"). However, in

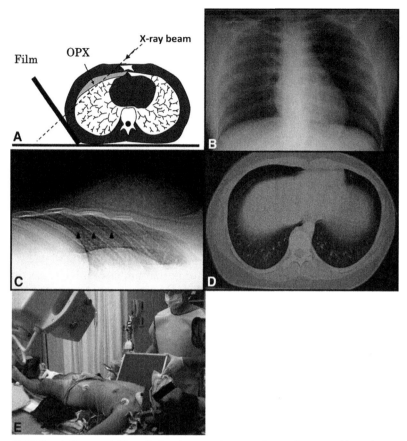

FIGURE.—*A,* We created this method to detect occult pneumothoraces by supine oblique chest radiography without the need for a CT scan. *OPX,* Occult pneumothorax. *B,* Anteroposterior supine radiograph shows no abnormality. Indeed, a left-sided pneumothorax appears unlikely. *C,* Oblique supine chest radiograph on the right side clearly reveals a distinct visceral pleural line (arrowheads). *D,* CT scan proves the existence of an occult pneumothorax on the right side. The pneumothorax size is about 19% of the pleural cavity. *E,* Supine oblique chest radiographs are easily performed in our trauma resuscitation area. (Reprinted from Annals of Emergency Medicine, Matsumoto S, Kishikawa M, Hayakawa K, et al. A method to detect occult pneumothorax with chest radiography. *Ann Emerg Med.* 2011;57:378-381. Copyright 2011, with permission from the American College of Emergency Physicians.)

practice, supine chest radiographs have poor sensitivity for occult pneumothoraces. Oblique chest radiograph is a useful and fast screening tool that should be considered for cases of blunt chest trauma, especially when transport of critically ill patients to the computed tomographic suite is dangerous or when imminent transfer to another hospital is being arranged and early diagnosis of an occult pneumothorax is essential (Fig).

▶ I agree with the inventiveness of these authors. If you think a pneumothorax is present, it is incumbent on us to find it or rule it out. CT scans provide great images in cases such as this, but concern over radiation levels is ever mounting.

In addition, moving patients to scanners increases the risk of complications. So a low-tech approach, such as obtaining an oblique film, is a great way to go.

I am surprised the authors did not use bedside ultrasound scan. It likely would have shown the same thing. Bedside ultrasound scanning is becoming standard of care in emergency department trauma bays. However, this nice example shows one more alternative imaging approach.

J. A. Barker, MD, FACP, FCCP

A comparative study of two- *versus* one-lung ventilation for needlescopic bleb resection

Kim H, Kim HK, Kang D-Y, et al (Korea Univ Guro Hosp, Seoul)
Eur Respir J 37:1183-1188, 2011

This prospective study was conducted to evaluate the feasibility of two-lung (TL) ventilation with low tidal volume anaesthesia compared with one-lung (OL) ventilation for needlescopic bleb resection.

Patients with spontaneous pneumothorax that underwent bleb resection with a 2-mm thoracoscope were enrolled. During the operation, the tidal volume was set at 4.0 mL·kg^{-1} in the TL group and 8.0 mL·kg^{-1} in the OL group; the respiration rate was set at 23 and 12 breaths·min^{-1}, respectively, at the same inspiratory oxygen fraction (50%).

A total of 108 patients (55 patients in the TL group and 53 in the OL group) were included in this study. Airway pressure was significantly lower in the TL group (mean ± SD 8.0 ± 3.3 *versus* 24.0 ± 3.9 mmHg in the OL group; p<0.001). The time from endotracheal intubation to the incision was 17.1 ± 4.0 min in the TL group and 35.3 ± 7.6 min in the OL group, which was significantly different (p<0.001). However, the operation time was not different in comparisons between the two groups. Therefore, the total anaesthesia time was significantly longer in the OL group (77.9 ± 21.6 *versus* 64.9 ± 14.7 min in the TL group; p=0.002).

Needlescopic bleb resection using TL ventilation anaesthesia with low tidal volume was technically feasible, cost-effective and time-saving compared with OL ventilation anaesthesia.

▶ This study reminds us all how important it is to continuously look at our current techniques and decide whether we are using the right ones. Large chest thoracotomy has been replaced by muscle-sparing thoracotomy, and this has since been replaced by video-assisted thoracoscopic surgery (VATS). VATS is now being performed with needle-sized instruments. These investigators challenge (successfully, I might add!) the dogma of deflating 1 lung during thoracoscopy. Dual lumen tubes and single lung ventilation are not always simple to use and do have side effects. I applaud this innovation.

J. A. Barker, MD, FACP, FCCP

Miscellaneous

"CAN WE FEED?" A Mnemonic to Merge Nutrition and Intensive Care Assessment of the Critically Ill Patient

Miller KR, Kiraly LN, Lowen CC, et al (Univ of Louisville, KY; Oregon Health Sciences Univ, Portland)
JPEN J Parenter Enteral Nutr 35:643-659, 2011

As care of the critically ill patient grows more complex, so does the breadth of knowledge required of the intensivist to deliver quality service. Nutrition is one area of many where the complexity of care has grown and the opportunity for improving patient outcomes has become evident. The use of mnemonics has proven successful in compartmentalizing information that must be considered in complex decision-making processes. The authors propose one such mnemonic, "CAN WE FEED?" to assist in the development and initiation of early enteral nutrition therapy in the intensive care unit (ICU). Critical illness severity (C), age (A), and nutrition risk screening (N) are considered when performing a baseline evaluation of the critically ill patient upon presentation to the ICU. Wait for resuscitation (W) is a key component in the care of most critically ill patients and is an important consideration prior to the initiation of feeding. Energy requirements (E) are determined using conventional weight-based equations, indirect calorimetry, or combinations of both techniques. The more practical aspects of support that follow include formula selection (F), enteral access (E), efficacy (E), and the determination of tolerance (D). With careful consideration of these components through the use of the mnemonic "CAN WE FEED?" the intensivist can successfully implement a nutrition plan, and the clinical nutritionist can appreciate where nutrition therapy appropriately intervenes in the initial resuscitation and management of the critically ill patient (Fig).

▶ I love mnemonics. This one is one of the best ever. Not only do the authors have this great mnemonic acronym as a way to remember the assessment and implementation of intensive care unit nutrition, they also cover the rationale and evidence for each point. Appendix B looks very much like it could be modified to a useful scorecard or checklist. Nutritional support of the critically ill patient has come a long way baby! Intensivists should read this article for a quick update.

J. A. Barker, MD, FACP, FCCP

C Comorbidities
Severity of Illness: Calculate score, as indicated by patient ICU admitting diagnosis
APACHE II ____
Ranson criteria ____
SOFA ____
ISS ____

Preexisting conditions:
Diabetes mellitus?	□ Yes	□ No	*If yes, carefully target glucose control*
Liver dysfunction?	□ Yes	□ No	*If yes, carefully monitor protein tolerance*
Renal dysfunction?	□ Yes	□ No	*If yes, carefully monitor protein tolerance*
Alcohol abuse and related malnutrition?	□ Yes	□ No	*If yes, carefully monitor for malnutrition and refeeding syndrome*
Drug abuse and related malnutrition?	□ Yes	□ No	*If yes, carefully monitor for malnutrition and refeeding syndrome*

A AGE _____

N Nutrition Risk Screening (NRS 2002 System)[18]
Initial Screening
BMI <20.5?	□ Yes	□ No
Weight loss in last three months?	□ Yes	□ No
Reduced dietary intake in past week?	□ Yes	□ No
Severe illness?	□ Yes	□ No

Final Screening (Complete if "yes" to any of above questions)

Part I Impaired Nutrition Status
Absent	Score 0:	Normal nutrition status
Mild	Score 1:	Wt loss >5% in three months or food Intake <50–75% normal in last week
Moderate	Score 2:	Wt loss >5% in last two months or BMI 18.5–20.5 Or food intake <25–50% normal in last week
Severe	Score 3:	Wt loss >5% in last month (>15% in last 3 mos) Or BMI < 18.5 + impaired general condition Or food intake 0–25% normal in last week

Part II Severity of Disease
Absent	Score 0:	Normal nutrition requirements
Mild	Score 1:	Hip fracture, chronic patients (hemodialysis, diabetes, cancer, cirrhosis, COPD) with acute complication
Moderate	Score 2:	Major abdominal surgery, stroke, severe pneumonia, hematologic malignancy
Severe	Score 3:	Head injury, bone marrow transplantation, APACHE II score >10

Total Nutrition Risk Score
Part 1 Impaired NS score ____ + Part II Severity of Disease Score ____ + 1 (if age > 70) ____ = ____Total
[If total of 3 or more, nutrition support is indicated.]

W Wait for Resuscitation
Proceed with caution if answer is Yes. Hold feeding if answer is No.
Fluid resuscitation complete?	□ Yes	□ No	CVP 8–12 mm Hg	□ Yes	□ No
Mean arterial pressure ≥65 mm Hg?	□ Yes	□ No	Serum lactate <2 mg/dL	□ Yes	□ No
Stable pressor agents for 24 hours?	□ Yes	□ No	Base excess < 5 mEq	□ Yes	□ No
CVO_2 ≥70% or MVO_2 ≥65%	□ Yes	□ No			

E Estimated Energy Requirements
Calories:
BMI <30: Use 25–30 kcal/ kg ABW/day _____ kcal ABW = Actual Body Weight
BMI ≥30: Use 11–14 kcal/ kg ABW/day _____ kcal IBW = Ideal Body Weight
Protein:
BMI <30 Use 1.2–2.0 gm protein/kg ABW/day _____ gms protein
BMI 30–40: Use ≥2.0 gm protein/kg IBW/day _____ gms protein
BMI >40: Use 2.5 gm protein/ kg IBW/day _____ gms protein

F Formula Selection
Candidate for arginine-containing pharmaconutrition formula:	□ Yes	□ No

Criteria: Major surgery, trauma (ATI score >20), burns (TBSA >30%), head/neck cancer, critically ill on MV
Candidate for Anti-inflammatory Pharmaconutrition:	□ Yes	□ No

Criteria: ARDS or ALI
Candidate for Malassimilation formula: Small peptide/ MCT oil	□ Yes	□ No
Fiber-containing	□ Yes	□ No

If no to all above, then candidate for standard enteral formula.

FIGURE.—ICU "CAN WE FEED?" Nutrition Screening Tool. Adapted from Kondrup J, Allison SP, Elia M, Vellas B, Plauth M. ESPEN guidelines for nutrition support screening 2001. *Clin Nutr.* 2003;22(4):415-421. (Reprinted from Miller KR, Kiraly LN, Lowen CC, et al. "CAN WE FEED?" A mnemonic to merge nutrition and intensive care assessment of the critically ill patient. *JPEN J Parenter Enteral Nutr.* 2011;35:643-659, © 2011 by American Society for Parenteral and Enteral Nutrition. Reprinted by Permission of SAGE Publications.)

E Enteral Access

Access site	Nasoenteric	□ Yes	□ No
	Oroenteric (concern for sinusitis)	□ Yes	□ No
	Percutaneous (anticipate feeds >4 wks)	□ Yes	□ No
Level of infusion	Stomach	□ Yes	□ No
	Postpyloric	□ Yes	□ No
	Below ligament of Treitz	□ Yes	□ No
Need for simultaneous gastric decompression (aspirate/feed tube)		□ Yes	□ No

E Efficacy

Days NPO _____ Cumulative Caloric Balance _____
Initial Rate _____ Rapid ramp-up rate _____
Goal Rate _____ Goal volume/day _____
Initiate volume-based feeds □ Yes □ No [□ gastric (max 280 mL/ hour) □ postpyloric (max 150 mL/hour)]

D Determine Tolerance

First Gastric Residual Volume >500 mL:
    □ Continue current infusion, recheck in four hours   □ Initiate narcan 8 mg in saline per tube q 6 hours
    □ Normalize serum electrolytes   □ Elevate HOB
    □ Initiate metaclopramide 10 mg IV q 6 hours   □ Turn patient to right lateral decubitus position
Second Gastric Residual Volume >500 mL:
    □ Hold enteral infusion   □ Recheck GRV in 2 hours
    □ Restart infusion once GRV <500 mL
Serum Glucose 80–150 mg/dL   □ Yes   □ No   Passage of stool/gas   □ Yes   □ No
Diarrhea (>250 mL/day stool output per rectum **Or** >1000 mL/day output per ileostomy)
    □ Remove sorbitol from oral/enteric medications
    □ Obtain stool cultures/oxin assays to rule out infectious diarrhea
    □ Initiate opiates once infectious etiology ruled out (lomotil, immodium, paregoric)
    □ Consider fiber-containing formula and/or small peptide/MCT formula
    □ Provide fiber additive

FIGURE.—*(continued).*

A Model for Increasing Palliative Care in the Intensive Care Unit: Enhancing Interprofessional Consultation Rates and Communication

Villarreal D, Restrepo MI, Healy J, et al (The Univ of Texas Health Science Ctr, San Antonio; et al)
J Pain Symptom Manage 42:676-679, 2011

Background.—Only a minority of patients who die in the medical intensive care unit (MICU) receive palliative care services. At the South Texas Veterans Health Care System Audie L. Murphy Hospital, only 5% of patients who died in the MICU from May to August 2010 received a palliative care consultation.

Measures.—We measured the percentage of MICU patients for which there was a palliative care consultation during the intervention period.

Intervention.—Starting October 1, 2010 and ending April 30, 2011, the palliative care and MICU teams participated in daily "pre-rounds" to identify patients at risk for poor outcomes, who may benefit from a palliative care consultation.

Outcomes.—Palliative care consultation increased significantly from 5% to 59% for patients who died in the MICU during the intervention period. Additionally, palliative care consultation increased from 5% to 21% for all patients admitted to the MICU during the intervention period.

Conclusions/Lessons Learned.—Daily pre-rounds between the palliative care and MICU teams increased palliative care services for MICU patients at risk for poor outcomes, who may benefit from a palliative care consultation.

▶ I include this article in this year's reading because, quite frankly, one of the largest effects on critical care practice these past few years has been the growth of palliative care services. These authors nicely show that there are multiple ways to "skin a cat." As they point out, full integration of palliative care practice and intensive care is highly desirable. There is a high percentage of patients who are likely to die or are outright terminal in modern critical care units. Palliative care practitioners have much to offer them. In addition, the bedside caregivers (nurses, techs, respiratory therapists, and even physicians) likely benefit by having another perspective shared with patients and families. Several studies have clearly linked increased burnout rates with high rates of futile cases. The prerounds approach used here is a relatively simple, yet effective, approach to the roll-out of a new process, especially when resources are limited.

J. A. Barker, MD, FACP, FCCP

Impact of Nonphysician Staffing on Outcomes in a Medical ICU
Gershengorn HB, Wunsch H, Wahab R, et al (Beth Israel Med Ctr, NY; New York Presbyterian Hosp-Columbia)
Chest 139:1347-1353, 2011

Background.—As the number of ICU beds and demand for intensivists increase, alternative solutions are needed to provide coverage for critically ill patients. The impact of different staffing models on the outcomes of patients in the medical ICU (MICU) remains unknown. In our study, we compare outcomes of nonphysician provider-based teams to those of medical house staff-based teams in the MICU.

Methods.—We conducted a retrospective review of 590 daytime (7:00 AM-7:00 PM) admissions to two MICUs at one hospital. In one MICU staffed by nurse practitioners and physician assistants (MICU-NP/PA) there were nonphysicians (nurse practitioners and physicians assistants) during the day (7:00 AM-7:00 PM) with attending physician coverage overnight. In the other MICU, there were medicine residents (MICU-RES) (24 h/d). The outcomes investigated were hospital mortality, length of stay (LOS) (ICU, hospital), and posthospital discharge destination.

Results.—Three hundred two patients were admitted to the MICU-NP/PA and 288 to the MICU-RES. Mortality probability model III (MPM$_0$-III) predicted mortality was similar ($P=.14$). There was no significant difference in hospital mortality (32.1% for MICU-NP/PA vs 32.3% for MICU-RES, $P=.96$), MICU LOS (4.22 ± 2.51 days for MICU-NP/PA vs 4.44 ± 3.10 days for MICU-RES, $P=.59$), or hospital LOS (14.01 ± 2.92 days for MICU-NP/PA vs 13.74 ± 2.94 days for MICU-RES, $P=.86$). Discharge to a skilled care facility (vs home) was similar (37.1% for MICU-NP/PA vs 32.5% for MICU-RES, $P=.34$). After multivariate adjustment, MICU staffing type was not associated with hospital mortality ($P=.26$), MICU LOS ($P=.29$), hospital LOS ($P=.19$), or posthospital discharge destination ($P=.90$).

Conclusions.—Staffing models including daytime use of nonphysician providers appear to be a safe and effective alternative to the traditional house staff-based team in a high-acuity, adult ICU.

▶ Staffing with advanced practice professionals (nurse practitioners and physician assistants) in critical care is increasingly frequent. Critical care continues to be more specialized. There is an inadequate supply of intensivist physicians to staff all intensive care units. Simultaneously, we are seeing continuous reduction in residency work hours. Thus, the trend for specialized APPs to work in critical care is no surprise.

The results are quite reassuring. Quality measures show no difference in comparing supervised physician trainee teams versus physician/APP teams. This phenomenon will continue to become more prevalent.

J. A. Barker, MD, FACP, FCCP

A Prospective Observational Study of Physician Handoff for Intensive-Care-Unit-to-Ward Patient Transfers
Li P, Stelfox HT, Ghali WA (Univ of Calgary, Alberta, Canada)
Am J Med 124:860-867, 2011

Background.—Poor physician handoff can be a major contributor to suboptimal care and medical errors occurring in the hospital. Physician handoffs for intensive care unit (ICU)-to-ward patient transfer may face more communication hurdles. However, few studies have focused on physician handoffs in patient transfers from the ICU to the inpatient ward.

Methods.—We performed a hospitalized patient-based observational study in an urban, university-affiliated tertiary care center to assess physician handoff practices for ICU-to-ward patient transfer. One hundred twelve adult patients were enrolled. The stakeholders (sending physicians, receiving physicians, and patients/families) were interviewed to evaluate the quality of communication during these transfers. Data collected included the presence and effectiveness of communication, continuity of care, and overall satisfaction.

Results.—During the initial stage of patient transfers, 15.6% of the consulted receiving physicians verbally communicated with sending physicians; 26% of receiving physicians received verbal communication from sending physicians when patient transfers occurred. Poor communication during patient transfer resulted in 13 medical errors and 2 patients being transiently "lost" to medical care. Overall, the levels of satisfaction with communication (scored on a 10-point scale) for sending physicians, receiving physicians, and patients were 7.9 ± 1.1, 8.1 ± 1.0, and 7.9 ± 1.7, respectively.

Conclusion.—The overall levels of satisfaction with communication during ICU-to-ward patient transfer were reasonably high among the stakeholders. However, clear opportunities to improve the quality of physician

TABLE 4.—Recommendations to Improve Physician Communication in ICU-to-Ward Patient Transfer

	Number*
Recommendations made by physicians	
Concise, accurate, and up-to-date ICU discharge summaries focused on key issues of patients	15
ICU discharge summaries completed before patient transfer	12
Face-to-face communication between ICU physicians and receiving physicians	8
Receiving physicians notified about patient's arrival on the ward	8
The patient's medications and orders updated by ICU physicians and confirmed by receiving physicians before patient transfer	5
Clear documentation of acceptance of patient transfer of care by receiving physicians	4
Using rapid response teams as a redundant system during transfer from the ICU	4
Recommendations made by patients or families	
Inform patient and family about current medical conditions and future plans before the transfer	10
Provide earlier notification to patients and family members about the upcoming ICU discharge	6
Allow family members to accompany patients during the transfer	3
ICU staff follow-up on the ward following transfer to ensure continuity of care	2

ICU = intensive care unit.
*Number indicates the number of times that a recommendation was made by interviewees.

communication exist in several areas, with potential benefits to quality of care and patient safety (Table 4).

▶ I would guess that all of us have either run relays in track during school years or at least watched it on television. Surely everyone watches the ubiquitous Summer Olympics every 4 years! It was incredibly easy to drop the baton. Yet when done right, the passing is a thing of beauty. The receiver speeds up rapidly during the transition box. The first runner slows down only minimally, communicates clearly, and makes a firm clear handoff. Number 2 takes the baton in stride and powers on toward the finish.

It is no different with our patients. Unfortunately, as medicine has become more humane to the caregivers in terms of work hours, handoffs have become mandatory. Yet all too often, we adopt the old cowboy approach, where we push the patients out of the intensive care unit (ICU) as fast as possible without always talking to the receiving team. And, it is a 2-way street of dysfunction. Often, the receiving physicians don't want a face-to-face encounter or to come to the ICU. They are busy, and if the transfer is delayed, another team may receive the patient. Communication is real work. And there isn't pay for it either!

These investigators have quantified how often handoffs occur and nicely showed that errors go up when handoffs don't happen or are ineffective. Table 4 lists nicely desired suggestions from all sides: intensivists, hospitalists, and probably most importantly, patients and families. All agree that there can never be too much communication, and the earlier, the better.

J. A. Barker, MD, FACP, FCCP

Association of ICU or Hospital Admission With Unintentional Discontinuation of Medications for Chronic Diseases

Bell CM, Brener SS, Gunraj N, et al (Keenan Res Centre in Li Ka Shing Knowledge Inst at St Michael's Hosp, Toronto, Ontario, Canada; Inst for Clinical Evaluative Sciences, Toronto, Ontario, Canada)
JAMA 306:840-847, 2011

Context.—Patients discharged from acute care hospitals may be at risk for unintentional discontinuation of medications prescribed for chronic diseases. The intensive care unit (ICU) may pose an even greater risk because of the focus on acute events and the presence of multiple transitions in care.

Objective.—To evaluate rates of potentially unintentional discontinuation of medications following hospital or ICU admission.

Design, Setting, and Patients.—A population-based cohort study using administrative records from 1997 to 2009 of all hospitalizations and outpatient prescriptions in Ontario, Canada; it included 396 380 patients aged 66 years or older with continuous use of at least 1 of 5 evidence-based medication groups prescribed for long-term use: (1) statins, (2) antiplatelet/anticoagulant agents, (3) levothyroxine, (4) respiratory inhalers, and (5) gastric acid–suppressing drugs. Rates of medication discontinuation were compared across 3 groups: patients admitted to the ICU, patients hospitalized without ICU admission, and nonhospitalized patients (controls). Odds ratios (ORs) were calculated and adjusted for patient demographics, clinical factors, and health services use.

Main Outcome Measures.—The primary outcome was failure to renew the prescription within 90 days after hospital discharge.

Results.—Patients admitted to the hospital (n=187 912) were more likely to experience potentially unintentional discontinuation of medications than controls (n=208 468) across all medication groups examined. The adjusted ORs (AORs) ranged from 1.18 (95% CI, 1.14-1.23) for discontinuing levothyroxine in 12.3% of hospitalized patients (n=6831) vs 11.0% of controls (n=7114) to an AOR of 1.86 (95% CI, 1.77-1.97) for discontinuing antiplatelet/anticoagulant agents in 19.4% of hospitalized patients (n=5564) vs 11.8% of controls (n=2535). With ICU exposure, the AORs ranged from 1.48 (95% CI, 1.39-1.57) for discontinuing statins in 14.6% of ICU patients (n=1484) to an AOR of 2.31 (95% CI, 2.07-2.57) for discontinuing antiplatelet/anticoagulant agents in 22.8% of ICU patients (n=522) vs the control group. Admission to an ICU was associated with an additional risk of medication discontinuation in 4 of 5 medication groups vs hospitalizations without an ICU admission. One-year follow-up of patients who discontinued medications showed an elevated AOR for the secondary composite outcome of death, emergency department visit, or emergent hospitalization of 1.07 (95% CI, 1.03-1.11) in the statins group and of 1.10 (95% CI, 1.03-1.16) in the antiplatelet/anticoagulant agents group.

Conclusions.—Patients prescribed medications for chronic diseases were at risk for potentially unintentional discontinuation after hospital admission. Admission to the ICU was generally associated with an even higher risk of medication discontinuation.

▶ It is true. We don't continue chronic medications when people are admitted to the intensive care unit. We worry about drug interactions, poor renal or liver clearance, and toxicity. In addition, frequently the patients are too ill to go over the outpatient medications face to face. These investigators have outlined the significant risks of this approach. Patients are on chronic medications for good reasons. In addition, there is considerable confusion when going home if hospital and home medications don't reconcile.

Efforts to reconcile home medications must be redoubled.

J. A. Barker, MD, FACP, FCCP

Diabetes Is Not Associated With Increased Mortality in Emergency Department Patients With Sepsis

Schuetz P, Jones AE, Howell MD, et al (Beth Israel Deaconess Med Ctr, Boston, MA; Carolinas Med Ctr, Charlotte, NC; et al)
Ann Emerg Med 58:438-444, 2011

Study Objective.—Despite its high prevalence, the influence of diabetes on outcomes of emergency department (ED) patients with sepsis remains undefined. Our aim is to investigate the association of diabetes and initial glucose level with mortality in patients with suspected infection from the ED.

Methods.—Three independent, observational, prospective cohorts from 2 large US tertiary care centers were studied. We included patients admitted to the hospital from the ED with suspected infection. We investigated the association of diabetes and inhospital mortality within each cohort separately and then overall with logistic regression and generalized estimating equations adjusted for age, sex, disease severity, and sepsis syndrome. We also tested for an interaction between diabetes and hyperglycemia/hypoglycemia.

Results.—A total of 7,754 patients were included. The mortality rate was 4.3% (95% confidence interval [CI] 3.9% to 4.8%) and similar in diabetic and nondiabetic patients (4.1% versus 4.4%; absolute risk difference 0.4%; 95% CI −0.7% to 1.4%). There was no significant association between diabetes and mortality in adjusted analysis (odds ratio [OR] overall 0.85; 95% CI 0.71 to 1.01). Diabetes significantly modified the effect of hyperglycemia and hypoglycemia with mortality; initial glucose levels greater than 200 mg/dL were associated with higher mortality in nondiabetic patients (OR 2.1; 95% CI 1.4 to 3.0) but not in diabetic patients (OR 1.0; 95% CI 0.2 to 4.7), whereas glucose levels less than 100 mg/dL were associated with higher mortality mainly in the diabetic population (OR 2.3; 95% CI 1.6 to 3.3) and to a lesser extent in nondiabetic patients (OR 1.1; 95% CI 1.03 to 1.14).

Conclusion.—We found no evidence for a harmful association of diabetes and mortality in patients across different sepsis severities. High initial glucose levels were associated with adverse outcomes in the nondiabetic population only. Further investigation is warranted to determine the mechanism for these effects.

▶ This is an important article for 2 reasons: First, I am completely surprised that preexisting diabetes does not increase mortality in sepsis. We know that uncontrolled diabetes does cause immune suppression and is associated with increased incidence of invasive fungal infections. However, apparently either the incidence of community-acquired fungal infections is very low (probably) or the immunosuppression from diabetes is rather minimal.

The second very interesting finding was the increased mortality of patients with hyperglycemia who were not known diabetics. So does this mean that undiagnosed, untreated diabetics have increased mortality? Or does it mean that hyperglycemia is an independent marker for severity of disease? I surmise that both are true. Time will tell.

J. A. Barker, MD, FACP, FCCP

How do I investigate septic transfusion reactions and blood donors with culture-positive platelet donations?
Eder AF, Goldman M (American Red Cross, Rockville, MD; Canadian Blood Services, Ottawa, Ontario, Canada)
Transfusion 51:1662-1668, 2011

Background.—Methods are in place to prevent and to detect bacterial contamination of platelets (PLTs), thereby avoiding transfusion-transmitted infections. These methods have not, however, eliminated the risk of septic transfusion reactions, so the appropriate steps to investigate suspected cases were outlined.

Methods.—Hospitals should have a written protocol outlining the clinical triggers for investigating suspected contamination and the actions to be taken at bedside and in the laboratory. Most septic transfusion reactions are manifest at the time of the transfusion or within 4 hours. Symptoms include fever, chills, tachycardia, dyspnea, and nausea and vomiting. Clinical judgment must consider the patient's pre-transfusion condition as well.

Bedside, the transfusion should be halted immediately and the blood component bag sealed. All bags of transfusions given within the previous 4 hours should be sent to the laboratory for testing. At least one set of blood cultures should be obtained from the patient before beginning antibiotic treatment.

The laboratory should immediately notify the blood supplier. All sampling of blood components is done with aseptic technique. If no blood remains in the bag, 10 to 20 mL of trypticase soy broth, other culture broth, or sterile saline solution is injected into the bag, mixed, and reaspirated for inoculation into culture bottles. If there are blood components

TABLE 1.—Asymptomatic Donor Bacteremia Implicated as Source of Contaminated PLTs

Bacterial Isolate	Donor Investigation	Reference(s)
S. bovis	Adenocarcinoma of the colon	Haimowitz et al.[18]
S. agalactiae (Group B streptococcus)		Stevens et al.[19]
S. aureus	Bacterial endocarditis	Blajchman et al.[20]
Viridans streptococci	Tooth extraction; dental procedures	Goldman and Blajchman[17]
S. aureus		Braine et al.[21]
Salmonella cholerae-suis	Subclinical osteomyelitis	Rhame et al.[22]
Salmonella heidelberg	Salmonella enteritis	Heal et al.[23]
Salmonella enterica	Pet snake owner	Jafari et al.[8]
Pasteurella multocida	Feral cat bites/exposure	Bryant et al.[24]

Editor's Note: Please refer to original journal article for full references.

remaining, samples are inoculated into aerobic and anaerobic blood culture bottles and incubated for 5 to 7 days at 36° to 36°C. All bags should also have a direct slide taken for Gram or acridine orange staining and microscopic examination, especially if the reaction was severe. The laboratory should perform cultures on any visible bacteria or positive blood cultures to determine if the patient and blood component contain the same bacterium and the same strain. The blood supplier is informed of the results of these investigations.

Donor Issues.—Positive bacterial cultures after routine PTL donation should be evaluated on a case-by-case basis to determine the possible significance to the donor's health. Blood donors with culture-positive donations should be counseled and referred for appropriate health screening, with significant associations with specific bacterial isolates considered. Bacterial screening of apheresis PLT donors provides a secondary public health benefit, allowing the early detection of serious medical conditions. However, in most cases finding a contaminated donation has no clear impact on the donor's health status. Donors who have apheresis PLT donations with likely skin contaminants can still donate, even after two similar incidents. Donors with a previous confirmed positive bacterial culture for the same or a similar organism should be deferred for donations as a precautionary measure.

Conclusions.—A written protocol should be followed by all institutions dealing with transfusions and blood donations. Timely actions in cases of transfusion-related infection are essential to provide appropriate care for the affected patient and avoid transfusing other bacterially contaminated components from the same donation (Table 1).

▶ Fever is common with transfusion of blood or blood products. Sometimes, however, patients may become quite ill after transfusion. We are usually thinking about transfusion mismatch and severe reaction. Fortunately, this is very rare. Probably much more common is transfusion-related acute lung injury.

The authors herein point out the unique features of bacteremia related to infected platelet packs. See Table 1 for an outline of this. In addition, they point out how skin contamination may occur. I did not realize that platelets are kept at room temperature, and of course, the risk of culture media brewing organisms is very real.

We are usually at the mercy of our blood banks for investigation of transfusion reactions. Yet that seems an inherent conflict of interest. They don't really want to find anything or put any real resources into an investigation. The authors give a step by step approach to this problem, which I find useful and pragmatic.

J. A. Barker, MD, FACP, FCCP

Article Index

Chapter 1: Asthma, Allergy, and Cystic Fibrosis

Two Days of Dexamethasone Versus 5 Days of Prednisone in the Treatment of Acute Asthma: A Randomized Controlled Trial — 2

Nebulized Budesonide Added to Standard Pediatric Emergency Department Treatment of Acute Asthma: A Randomized, Double-blind Trial — 4

Tiotropium improves lung function in patients with severe uncontrolled asthma: A randomized controlled trial — 6

Point: Efficacy of Bronchial Thermoplasty for Patients With Severe Asthma. Is There Sufficient Evidence? Yes — 8

Internet-based tapering of oral corticosteroids in severe asthma: a pragmatic randomised controlled trial — 9

Management of asthma in pregnancy guided by measurement of fraction of exhaled nitric oxide: a double-blind, randomised controlled trial — 10

Daily exhaled nitric oxide measurements and asthma exacerbations in children — 13

An Official ATS Clinical Practice Guideline: Interpretation of Exhaled Nitric Oxide Levels ($F_{E_{NO}}$) for Clinical Applications — 16

Age and Risks of FDA-Approved Long-Acting β_2-Adrenergic Receptor Agonists — 17

Efficacy of budesonide/formoterol pressurized metered-dose inhaler versus budesonide pressurized metered-dose inhaler alone in Hispanic adults and adolescents with asthma: a randomized, controlled trial — 18

Fluticasone furoate demonstrates efficacy in patients with asthma symptomatic on medium doses of inhaled corticosteroid therapy: an 8-week, randomised, placebo-controlled trial — 19

Reslizumab for Poorly Controlled, Eosinophilic Asthma: A Randomized, Placebo-Controlled Study — 21

Association between childhood asthma and ADHD symptoms in adolescence − a prospective population-based twin study — 22

Results of a phase IIa study of VX-809, an investigational CFTR corrector compound, in subjects with cystic fibrosis homozygous for the *F508del-CFTR* mutation — 23

A CFTR Potentiator in Patients with Cystic Fibrosis and the *G551D* Mutation — 25

Comparative Efficacy and Safety of 4 Randomized Regimens to Treat Early *Pseudomonas aeruginosa* Infection in Children With Cystic Fibrosis — 27

Improved treatment response to dornase alfa in cystic fibrosis patients using controlled inhalation — 28

Chapter 2: Chronic Obstructive Pulmonary Disease

Lifetime risk of developing chronic obstructive pulmonary disease: a longitudinal population study — 30

Geographic Isolation and the Risk for Chronic Obstructive Pulmonary Disease—Related Mortality: A Cohort Study — 32

Lung Cancer in Patients with Chronic Obstructive Pulmonary Disease: Incidence
and Predicting Factors   33

Racial Differences in Quality of Life in Patients With COPD   35

Early-Onset Chronic Obstructive Pulmonary Disease Is Associated with Female
Sex, Maternal Factors, and African American Race in the COPDGene Study   36

The Progression of Chronic Obstructive Pulmonary Disease Is Heterogeneous: The
Experience of the BODE Cohort   38

The Chronic Bronchitic Phenotype of COPD: An Analysis of the COPDGene Study 40

Acute Exacerbations of Chronic Obstructive Pulmonary Disease: Identification of
Biologic Clusters and Their Biomarkers   42

Validation of a Novel Risk Score for Severity of Illness in Acute Exacerbations of
COPD   43

Effect of an action plan with ongoing support by a case manager on exacerbation-
related outcome in patients with COPD: a multicentre randomised controlled trial 45

Azithromycin for Prevention of Exacerbations of COPD   47

Mortality associated with tiotropium mist inhaler in patients with chronic
obstructive pulmonary disease: systematic review and meta-analysis of randomised
controlled trials   49

Risk of fractures with inhaled corticosteroids in COPD: systematic review and
meta-analysis of randomised controlled trials and observational studies   50

The Impact of Anxiety and Depression on Outcomes of Pulmonary Rehabilitation
in Patients With COPD   53

Effect of β blockers in treatment of chronic obstructive pulmonary disease:
a retrospective cohort study   54

Factors Associated With Bronchiectasis in Patients With COPD   56

Chapter 3: Lung Cancer

Cancer Statistics, 2011: The Impact of Eliminating Socioeconomic and Racial
Disparities on Premature Cancer Deaths   62

Lung Cancer Risk Prediction: Prostate, Lung, Colorectal and Ovarian Cancer
Screening Trial Models and Validation   64

Incorporation of a Genetic Factor into an Epidemiologic Model for Prediction of
Individual Risk of Lung Cancer: The Liverpool Lung Project   67

Human Immunodeficiency Virus–Associated Primary Lung Cancer in the Era of
Highly Active Antiretroviral Therapy: A Multi-Institutional Collaboration   69

Serum B Vitamin Levels and Risk of Lung Cancer   70

Quitting Smoking Among Adults — United States, 2001–2010   72

Treating Smokers in the Health Care Setting   74

Reduced Lung-Cancer Mortality with Low-Dose Computed Tomographic
Screening   78

Screening by Chest Radiograph and Lung Cancer Mortality: The Prostate, Lung,
Colorectal, and Ovarian (PLCO) Randomized Trial   80

Baseline Characteristics of Participants in the Randomized National Lung
Screening Trial 82

Identification of Chronic Obstructive Pulmonary Disease in Lung Cancer Screening
Computed Tomographic Scans 83

Seventh Edition of the Cancer Staging Manual and Stage Grouping of Lung
Cancer: Quick Reference Chart and Diagrams 85

Mediastinoscopy vs Endosonography for Mediastinal Nodal Staging of Lung
Cancer: A Randomized Trial 87

Population-Based Risk for Complications After Transthoracic Needle Lung Biopsy
of a Pulmonary Nodule: An Analysis of Discharge Records 89

Cumulative Radiation Dose From Medical Imaging Procedures in Patients
Undergoing Resection for Lung Cancer 91

International Association for the Study of Lung Cancer/American Thoracic
Society/European Respiratory Society International Multidisciplinary
Classification of Lung Adenocarcinoma 94

Trends in Stage Distribution for Patients with Non-small Cell Lung Cancer:
A National Cancer Database Survey 96

Variability of Lung Tumor Measurements on Repeat Computed Tomography Scans
Taken Within 15 Minutes 97

Anaplastic Lymphoma Kinase Inhibition in Non—Small-Cell Lung Cancer 99

Targeting Anaplastic Lymphoma Kinase in Lung Cancer 101

Treatment of Non—Small-Cell Lung Cancer with Erlotinib or Gefitinib 102

Survival Following Lobectomy and Limited Resection for the Treatment of Stage I
Non-small Cell Lung Cancer ≤1 cm in Size: A Review of SEER Data 103

Lung Cancer in Chronic Obstructive Pulmonary Disease: Enhancing Surgical
Options and Outcomes 105

Surgeon Specialty and Long-Term Survival After Pulmonary Resection for Lung
Cancer 106

New driver mutations in non-small-cell lung cancer 108

Frequency of *EGFR* and *KRAS* Mutations in Lung Adenocarcinomas in African
Americans 110

Prognostic and Predictive Gene Signature for Adjuvant Chemotherapy in Resected
Non—Small-Cell Lung Cancer 111

Chapter 4: Pleural, Interstitial Lung, and Pulmonary Vascular Disease

A noninvasive algorithm to exclude pre-capillary pulmonary hypertension 116

Usefulness of Serial N-Terminal Pro—B-Type Natriuretic Peptide Measurements for
Determining Prognosis in Patients With Pulmonary Arterial Hypertension 117

Tricuspid Annular Plane Systolic Excursion Is a Robust Outcome Measure in
Systemic Sclerosis-associated Pulmonary Arterial Hypertension 118

Race and Sex Differences in Response to Endothelin Receptor Antagonists for
Pulmonary Arterial Hypertension 120

Long-term efficacy of bosentan in treatment of pulmonary arterial hypertension in children   121

Long-term effects of inhaled treprostinil in patients with pulmonary arterial hypertension: The TReprostinil sodium Inhalation Used in the Management of Pulmonary arterial Hypertension (TRIUMPH) study open-label extension   122

Long-term Treatment With Sildenafil Citrate in Pulmonary Arterial Hypertension: The SUPER-2 Study   124

Pulmonary Hypertension in Heart Failure With Preserved Ejection Fraction: A Target of Phosphodiesterase-5 Inhibition in a 1-Year Study   125

Intensive Care Unit Management of Patients with Severe Pulmonary Hypertension and Right Heart Failure   127

Proinflammatory and Antiinflammatory Cytokine Levels in Complicated and Noncomplicated Parapneumonic Pleural Effusions   129

Automated Quantification of High-Resolution CT Scan Findings in Individuals at Risk for Pulmonary Fibrosis   130

Ascertainment of Individual Risk of Mortality for Patients with Idiopathic Pulmonary Fibrosis   131

Delayed Access and Survival in Idiopathic Pulmonary Fibrosis: A Cohort Study   133

Gastroesophageal Reflux Therapy Is Associated with Longer Survival in Patients with Idiopathic Pulmonary Fibrosis   134

Short-term safety of thoracoscopic talc pleurodesis for recurrent primary spontaneous pneumothorax: a prospective European multicentre study   135

Chapter 5: Community-Acquired Pneumonia

Validation of the Infectious Diseases Society of America/American Thoratic Society Minor Criteria for Intensive Care Unit Admission in Community-Acquired Pneumonia Patients Without Major Criteria or Contraindications to Intensive Care Unit Care   138

Severity assessment tools to guide ICU admission in community-acquired pneumonia: systematic review and meta-analysis   140

Low CURB-65 is of limited value in deciding discharge of patients with community-acquired pneumonia   142

Procalcitonin Algorithms for Antibiotic Therapy Decisions: A Systematic Review of Randomized Controlled Trials and Recommendations for Clinical Algorithms   144

Inflammatory responses predict long-term mortality risk in community-acquired pneumonia   145

Dexamethasone and length of hospital stay in patients with community-acquired pneumonia: a randomised, double-blind, placebo-controlled trial   146

Hospital-reported Data on the Pneumonia Quality Measure "Time to First Antibiotic Dose" Are Not Associated With Inpatient Mortality: Results of a Nationwide Cross-sectional Analysis   148

Epidemiology, Antibiotic Therapy, and Clinical Outcomes in Health Care—Associated Pneumonia: A UK Cohort Study   150

Patterns of Antimicrobial Use for Respiratory Tract Infections in Older Residents of Long-Term Care Facilities   153

How deadly is seasonal influenza-associated pneumonia? The German Competence
Network for Community-Acquired Pneumonia 154

British Thoracic Society adult community acquired pneumonia audit 2009/10 156

Long-term use of thiazolidinediones and the associated risk of pneumonia or lower
respiratory tract infection: systematic review and meta-analysis 157

The Spectrum of Pneumococcal Empyema in Adults in the Early 21st Century 158

Chapter 6: Lung Transplantation

Predictors of Acute Rejection After Lung Transplantation 161

Timing of basiliximab induction and development of acute rejection in lung
transplant patients 162

The protective role of laparoscopic antireflux surgery against aspiration of pepsin
after lung transplantation 164

High Levels of Mannose-Binding Lectin Are Associated With Poor Outcomes After
Lung Transplantation 166

Circulating Fibrocytes Correlate With Bronchiolitis Obliterans Syndrome
Development After Lung Transplantation: A Novel Clinical Biomarker 167

Cytomegalovirus Replication Within the Lung Allograft Is Associated With
Bronchiolitis Obliterans Syndrome 168

Survival Determinants in Lung Transplant Patients With Chronic Allograft
Dysfunction 169

Comparison of Hospitalized Solid Organ Transplant Recipients and
Nonimmunocompromised Patients With Pandemic H1N1 Infection:
A Retrospective Cohort Study 171

Pneumonia Complicating Pandemic (H1N1) 2009: Risk Factors, Clinical Features,
and Outcomes 172

Invasive Fungal Infections in Lung Transplant Recipients Not Receiving Routine
Systemic Antifungal Prophylaxis: 12-Year Experience at a University Lung
Transplant Center 173

Increased Serum Vitamin A and E Levels After Lung Transplantation 175

Ocular complications in patients with lung transplants 176

Outcomes After Lung Transplantation and Practices of Lung Transplant Programs
in the United States Regarding Hepatitis C Seropositive Recipients 177

Impact of Anastomotic Techniques on Airway Complications After Lung
Transplant 178

Lung transplantation in children with idiopathic pulmonary arterial hypertension:
An 18-year experience 179

Chapter 7: Sleep Disorders

An Integrated Health-Economic Analysis of Diagnostic and Therapeutic Strategies
in the Treatment of Moderate-to-Severe Obstructive Sleep Apnea 182

Therapeutic Decision-making for Sleep Apnea and Hypopnea Syndrome Using
Home Respiratory Polygraphy: A Large Multicentric Study 184

A prospective polysomnographic study on the evolution of complex sleep apnoea   185

Cheyne–Stokes respiration and obstructive sleep apnoea are independent risk factors for malignant ventricular arrhythmias requiring appropriate cardioverter-defibrillator therapies in patients with congestive heart failure   186

Obstructive sleep apnoea: a stand-alone risk factor for chronic kidney disease   188

Obstructive Sleep Apnea: Brain Structural Changes and Neurocognitive Function before and after Treatment   189

Sleep-Disordered Breathing, Hypoxia, and Risk of Mild Cognitive Impairment and Dementia in Older Women   190

Continuous Positive Airway Pressure in Severe Obstructive Sleep Apnea Reduces Pain Sensitivity   191

Early treatment of obstructive apnoea and stroke outcome: a randomised controlled trial   193

Effects of Continuous Positive Airway Pressure Therapy Withdrawal in Patients with Obstructive Sleep Apnea: A Randomized Controlled Trial   194

Attenuation of Obstructive Sleep Apnea by Compression Stockings in Subjects with Venous Insufficiency   195

SIDS and Other Sleep-Related Infant Deaths: Expansion of Recommendations for a Safe Infant Sleeping Environment   197

A Brief Sleep Intervention Improves Outcomes in the School Entry Year: A Randomized Controlled Trial   198

Efficacy of Brief Behavioral Treatment for Chronic Insomnia in Older Adults   199

Increasing Walking and Bright Light Exposure to Improve Sleep in Community-Dwelling Persons with Alzheimer's Disease: Results of a Randomized, Controlled Trial   200

Prospective Evaluation of Consultant Surgeon Sleep Deprivation and Outcomes in More Than 4000 Consecutive Cardiac Surgical Procedures   202

Quantification of sleep behavior and of its impact on the cross-talk between the brain and peripheral metabolism   203

Sleep Disorders, Health, and Safety in Police Officers   204

Sleep Duration or Bedtime? Exploring the Relationship between Sleep Habits and Weight Status and Activity Patterns   206

The Effect of Melatonin, Magnesium, and Zinc on Primary Insomnia in Long-Term Care Facility Residents in Italy: A Double-Blind, Placebo-Controlled Clinical Trial   207

Chapter 8: Critical Care Medicine

Implementing Early Mobilization Interventions in Mechanically Ventilated Patients in the ICU   213

A physiologic comparison of proportional assist ventilation with load-adjustable gain factors (PAV+) versus pressure support ventilation (PSV)   214

Dysphagia screening decreases pneumonia in acute stroke patients admitted to the stroke intensive care unit   215

A Description of Intraoperative Ventilator Management in Patients with Acute Lung Injury and the Use of Lung Protective Ventilation Strategies — 216

Comparison of airway pressure release ventilation to conventional mechanical ventilation in the early management of smoke inhalation injury in swine — 217

Noninvasive versus invasive ventilation for acute respiratory failure in patients with hematologic malignancies: A 5-year multicenter observational survey — 218

Development and Validation of a Risk Calculator Predicting Postoperative Respiratory Failure — 219

GlideScope videolaryngoscope vs. Macintosh direct laryngoscope for intubation of morbidly obese patients: a randomized trial — 220

Airway challenges in critical care — 221

Anaphylaxis pathogenesis and treatment — 222

Accuracy of a continuous noninvasive hemoglobin monitor in intensive care unit patients — 223

Prognostic implications of arterial blood gases in acute decompensated heart failure — 224

Incident Stroke and Mortality Associated With New-Onset Atrial Fibrillation in Patients Hospitalized With Severe Sepsis — 225

Current Approach to the Diagnosis of Acute Nonmassive Pulmonary Embolism — 227

Costs of Postoperative Sepsis: The Business Case for Quality Improvement to Reduce Postoperative Sepsis in Veterans Affairs Hospitals — 228

Atelectasis as a Cause of Postoperative Fever: Where Is the Clinical Evidence? — 229

A Method to Detect Occult Pneumothorax With Chest Radiography — 230

A comparative study of two- *versus* one-lung ventilation for needlescopic bleb resection — 232

"CAN WE FEED?" A Mnemonic to Merge Nutrition and Intensive Care Assessment of the Critically Ill Patient — 233

A Model for Increasing Palliative Care in the Intensive Care Unit: Enhancing Interprofessional Consultation Rates and Communication — 235

Impact of Nonphysician Staffing on Outcomes in a Medical ICU — 236

A Prospective Observational Study of Physician Handoff for Intensive-Care-Unit-to-Ward Patient Transfers — 237

Association of ICU or Hospital Admission With Unintentional Discontinuation of Medications for Chronic Diseases — 239

Diabetes Is Not Associated With Increased Mortality in Emergency Department Patients With Sepsis — 240

How do I investigate septic transfusion reactions and blood donors with culture-positive platelet donations? — 241

Author Index

A

Abrams TE, 32
Accurso FJ, 23
Acencio MM, 129
Agbaje OF, 67
Aguirre-Jaíme A, 38
Albera C, 131
Albert RK, 47
Aliberti S, 142
Allenspach LL, 162
Andersen LH, 220
Annema JT, 87
Arena R, 125
Arnulf I, 195
Avila NA, 130
Ayers L, 194

B

Bafadhel M, 42
Bagiella E, 133
Bailey M, 168
Baker TB, 74
Bakker EM, 28
Bang Y-J, 99
Bañuls P, 224
Baraldi E, 13
Batchinsky AI, 217
Bateman ED, 19
Bayman L, 228
Becker HF, 185
Bell CM, 239
Benza RL, 122
Bitter T, 186
Bleecker ER, 19
Blum JM, 216
Boggs PB, 16
Bonderman D, 116
Bonnin M, 193
Bourbeau J, 45
Bower M, 69
Brambilla E, 94
Brawley O, 62
Brener SS, 239
Bridevaux P-O, 135
Briel M, 144
Brotherwood M, 175
Buckens CFM, 83
Burdick MD, 167
Burgos J, 158
Burkett SE, 217
Busse WW, 19
Buysse DJ, 199

C

Camidge DR, 99
Canessa N, 189
Canisius S, 185
Caporaso NE, 64
Cappa SF, 189
Cardillo G, 135
Carroll KE, 166
Casanova C, 33, 38
Cascagnette P, 30
Cassel W, 185
Castro M, 8, 21
Castronovo V, 189
Cataldo VD, 102
Catherine K, 223
Cavallazzi R, 50
Chalmers JD, 138, 140, 150
Chen A, 8
Chiappa V, 144
Cho YW, 177
Chou Y-T, 188
Christ-Crain M, 145
Chu MWA, 202
Cipriani F, 214
Cipriano LE, 182
Clancy JP, 23
Cosentini R, 142
Costa R, 214
Cullen JJ, 228

D

Dahyot-Fizelier C, 223
Davis CS, 164
Dean MM, 166
DeCamp MM Jr, 105
de Torres JP, 33, 38
Ding K, 111
Disse B, 6
D'Jaen GA, 69
Dominici P, 2
Donat Sanz Y, 56
du Bois RM, 131
Duffy SW, 67
Dweik RA, 16

E

Eder AF, 241
Elder DHJ, 54
Elicker BM, 134

Emaminia A, 167
Enright PL, 49
Erzurum SC, 16

F

Falagas ME, 229
Falcó V, 158
Fan VS, 32
Fang X, 219
Farjah F, 106
Fiore MC, 74
Fisichella PM, 164
Flum DR, 106
Fong T-L, 177
Foreman MG, 36
Forfia PR, 118
Foster H, 121
Fox SA, 202
Frasca D, 223
French B, 120
Furberg CD, 157

G

Gabler NB, 120
Gao F, 96
Garner A, 182
Germain A, 199
Gershengorn HB, 236
Gershon AS, 30
Ghali WA, 237
Ghobrial JM, 225
Gibbons DL, 102
Girard N, 108
Goldman M, 241
Goldstein BS, 179
Granton J, 127
Gristina GR, 218
Groepenhoff H, 117
Guazzi M, 125
Guertler C, 145
Gunraj N, 239
Gupta H, 219
Gupta PK, 219
Gupta S, 175
Guthrie TJ, 178

H

Hamer DH, 153
Hampp C, 173

Han MK, 35
Hanlon EC, 203
Hardeman H, 146
Harrison SL, 190
Hashimoto S, 9
Hawkins KA, 105
Hayakawa K, 230
Healy J, 235
Heatley SL, 166
Hiscock H, 198
Hislop AA, 121
Ho T, 175
Hoeper MM, 127
Holley AB, 227
Hou L, 177
Howell MD, 240
Huang K-Y, 215
Hudgel DW, 191

J

Johannes RS, 43
Johansson M, 70
Johnson ML, 110
Jones AE, 240

K

Kang D-Y, 232
Kates M, 103
Kawut SM, 133
Kelly FE, 221
Kerstjens HAM, 6
Khalid I, 191
Khare RK, 148
Khatib OF, 176
Kim H, 232
Kim HK, 232
Kim V, 40
King CS, 227
Kiraly LN, 233
Kishikawa M, 230
Kohler M, 194
Kravitz J, 2
Kress JP, 213
Kwak EL, 99

L

Lababede O, 85
Laffan AM, 190
Lamas DJ, 133

LaPar DJ, 167
Larsson H, 22
Lee JS, 134
Lee P-H, 188
Lehmann K, 53
Levenson MS, 17
Levvey BJ, 168
Li P, 237
Lim WS, 156
Lipworth SIW, 54
Loke YK, 49, 50, 157
Lowen CC, 233
Lujan M, 158
Lundberg PW, 164
Lundholm C, 22

M

Maher CA, 206
Maile M, 216
Mandal P, 138, 140
Mangi AA, 161
Mansfield LE, 18
Mao J, 179
Marchi E, 129
Marín JM, 33
Martínez-García MÁ, 56
Martischnig AM, 116
Masa JF, 184
Mason DP, 161
Mathai SC, 118
Matricciani L, 206
Matsumoto S, 230
Mauritz G-J, 117
Mavros MN, 229
McCurry SM, 200
McEvoy BW, 17
McKenna S, 42
McLaughlin VV, 122
McMahon AW, 17
Meijvis SCA, 146
Mets OM, 83
Meydani SN, 153
Meziane M, 85
Miller KR, 233
Miñana G, 224
Minnema BJ, 171
Mirza F, 91
Mogensen N, 22
Moledina S, 121
Mollen CJ, 4
Monninkhof EM, 45
Monteferrario F, 207
Moores LK, 227
Morgensztern D, 96

Moul DE, 199
Murphy VE, 10

N

Nemeh HW, 162
Ng SH, 96
Nocero JR, 176
Noguchi M, 94
Nolan JP, 221
Nowicki ER, 161
Núñez J, 224

O

Oken MM, 80
Olds TS, 206
Olsen KS, 220
Opizzi A, 207
Oxnard GR, 97

P

Pantanowitz L, 69
Pao W, 108
Paraskeva M, 168
Park PK, 216
Parra O, 193
Patel M, 171
Pérez-Soler R, 102
Pietzsch JB, 182
Pike KC, 200
Pinney MF, 173
Pinsky PF, 64
Pottier M, 195
Powell ES, 148
Powell H, 10
Prinz C, 186
Puri V, 178

Q

Quach J, 198
Quattromani E, 148

R

Rajaratnam SMW, 204
Raji OY, 67

Ramirez J, 142
Ramsey BW, 25
Raviv S, 105
Redolfi S, 195
Reinersman JM, 110
Relton C, 70
Remmelts HHF, 146
Restrepo MI, 235
Rice T, 85
Riely GJ, 110
Rintoul RC, 87
Rizopoulos D, 117
Roehrs TA, 191
Roldaan AC, 9
Rondanelli M, 207
Rosas IO, 130
Rosenberg AF, 173
Rotstein C, 171
Rovsing L, 220
Rowe SM, 23
Rubin LJ, 124
Ryu JH, 134

S

Salonini E, 28
Sánchez-Armengol Á, 193
Scarfone RJ, 4
Schröder-Babo W, 6
Schuetz P, 144, 240
Schwartz LM, 89
Schweickert WD, 213
Seeger W, 122
Shaw AT, 101
Shifren A, 8
Shorr AF, 43
Short PM, 54
Sibley CT, 118
Siegel R, 62
Sima CS, 97
Simons FER, 222
Singanayagam A, 140, 150
Singh S, 49, 50, 157
Soler-Cataluña JJ, 56
Solomon B, 101
Spinazzola G, 214
Stelfox HT, 237

Stern G, 13
Stiles BM, 91
Stitt LW, 202
Stoewhas A-C, 194
Strom BL, 120
Strumpf D, 111
Sun X, 43
Swanson S, 103
Swarup R, 162
Sweet SC, 179

T

Tammemagi CM, 64
Tarabishy AB, 176
Taube K, 53
Taylor DR, 10
Taylor JK, 138, 150
Ten Brinke A, 9
Terry S, 42
Towe CW, 91
Trappenburg JCA, 45
Travis WD, 94
Treggiari MM, 27
Tschopp J-M, 135

U

Ueland PM, 70
Ufberg J, 2
Ukoumunne OC, 198
Upham BD, 4
Uryniak T, 18

V

van Berkel V, 178
Van Cauter E, 203
van der Valk RJP, 13
van Meerbeeck JP, 87
Vargas FS, 129
Varghese TK Jr, 106
Vaughan-Sarrazin M, 32
Vaughan-Sarrazin MS, 228

Velmahos GC, 229
Vergidis P, 153
Verleden GM, 169
Verleden SE, 169
Viasus D, 172
Vicenzi M, 125
Villarreal D, 235
Vitiello MV, 200
Volpi S, 28
von Baum H, 154
von Leupoldt A, 53
Vos R, 169

W

Wahab R, 236
Walkey AJ, 225
Wang T-G, 215
Ward E, 62
Warner L, 30
Westerheide N, 186
Wexberg P, 116
Weycker D, 131
Wiener RS, 89, 225
Wirz B, 145
Wisnivesky JP, 103
Woloshin S, 89
Wunsch H, 236

Y

Yaffe K, 190
Yang C-T, 188
Yao J, 130
Yeh S-J, 215

Z

Zanders TB, 217
Zanen P, 83
Zangrilli J, 18
Zhao B, 97
Zhu C-Q, 111

Printed and bound by CPI Group (UK) Ltd, Croydon, CR0 4YY

08/05/2025

01864678-0003

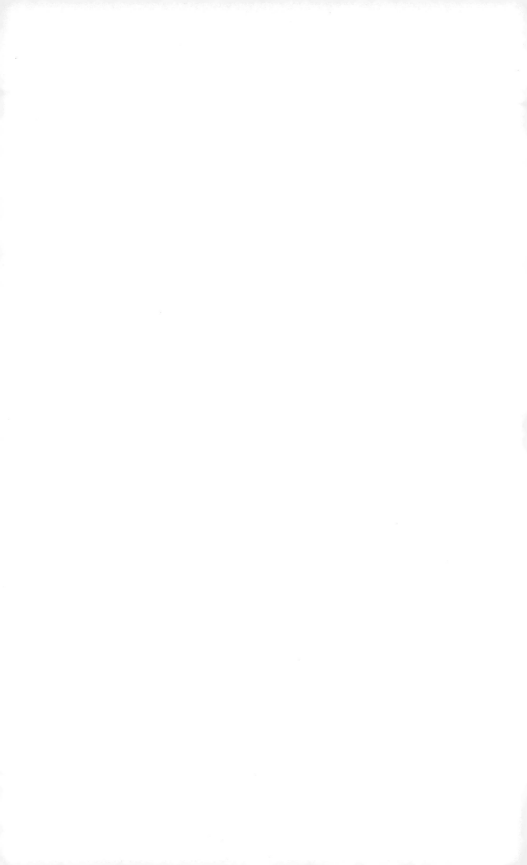